Diabetes in Clinical Practice

Diabetes
dp
in Practice

Diabetes in Clinical Practice

Questions and Answers
from Case Studies

N. Katsilambros

E. Diakoumopoulou
I. Ioannidis
S. Liatis
K. Makrilakis
N. Tentolouris
P. Tsapogas

Translated by K. Makrilakis

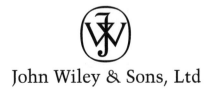

John Wiley & Sons, Ltd

First published in Greek as

Ο Σακχαρώδης Διαβήτης στην Κλινική Πράξη
Ο Διαβήτης από το Α ως το Ω
με Ερωτήσεις και Απαντήσεις

Translated into English by Konstantinos Makrilakis

English language translation copyright   © 2006 John Wiley & Sons Ltd
The Atrium, Southern Gate, Chichester,
West Sussex PO19 8SQ, England
Telephone (+44) 1243 779777

Email (for orders and customer service enquiries): cs-books@wiley.co.uk
Visit our Home page on www.wileyeurope.com or www.wiley.com

Other Wiley Editorial Offices

John Wiley & Sons Inc., 111 River Street, Hoboken, NJ 07030, USA

Jossey-Bass, 989 Market Street, San Francisco, CA 94103-1741, USA

Wiley-VCH Verlag GmbH, Boschstr. 12, D-69469 Weinheim, Germany

John Wiley & Sons Australia Ltd, 42 McDougall Street, Milton, Queensland 4064, Australia

John Wiley & Sons (Asia) Pte Ltd, 2 Clementi Loop #02-01, Jin Xing Distripark, Singapore 129809

John Wiley & Sons Canada Ltd, 6045 Freemont Blvd, Mississauga, ONT, L5R 4J3, Canada

Wiley also publishes its books in a variety of electronic formats. Some content that appears in print may not be available in electronic books.

Library of Congress Cataloging-in-Publication Data

Diabetes in clinical practice : questions and answers from case studies
/ N. Katsilambros ... [et al.] ; translated by K. Makrilakis.
p. ; cm.
Includes bibliographical references and index.
ISBN-13: 978-0-470-03522-1 (alk. paper)
ISBN-10: 0-470-03522-6 (alk. paper)
1. Diabetes–Case studies. 2. Diabetes–Examinations, questions, etc. I. Katsilambros, Nicholas.
[DNLM: 1. Diabetes Mellitus–Case Reports. WK 810 D5375238 2006a]
RC660.D4482 2006
616.4'62–dc22   2006028048

British Library Cataloguing in Publication Data

A catalogue record for this book is available from the British Library

ISBN-13: 978-0-470-03522-1
ISBN-10: 0-470-03522-6

Typeset in 11/13 pt Optima by Thomson Digital
Printed and bound in Great Britain by Antony Rowe Ltd, Chippenham, Wiltshire
This book is printed on acid-free paper responsibly manufactured from sustainable forestry in which at least two trees are planted for each one used for paper production.

CONTENTS

LIST OF AUTHORS

Nicholas Katsilambros
Professor of Internal Medicine
1st Department of Propaedeutic Medicine of the Athens University
Medical School
The Diabetes Center, 'Laiko' General Hospital
Athens, Greece

Evanthia Diakoumopoulou
1st Department of Propaedeutic Medicine of the Athens University
Medical School
The Diabetes Center, 'Laiko' General Hospital
Athens, Greece

Stavros Liatis
1st Department of Propaedeutic Medicine of the Athens University
Medical School
The Diabetes Center, 'Laiko' General Hospital
Athens, Greece

Ioannis Ioannidis
2nd Department of Internal Medicine
Diabetes Clinic, Agia Olga General Hospital
Athens, Greece

Konstantinos Makrilakis
1st Department of Propaedeutic Medicine of the Athens University Medical School
The Diabetes Center, 'Laiko' General Hospital
Athens, Greece

Nicholas Tentolouris
1st Department of Propaedeutic Medicine of the Athens University Medical School
The Diabetes Center, 'Laiko' General Hospital
Athens, Greece

Panagiotis Tsapogas
1st Department of Propaedeutic Medicine of the Athens University Medical School
The Diabetes Center, 'Laiko' General Hospital
Athens, Greece

Preface to Greek Edition

As the title of this book indicates, it deals with diabetes mellitus. The field of this disease is very broad, since diabetes, together with its complications, covers many aspects of general internal medicine. In addition, it is widely accepted that progress in the field of diabetes, especially as concerns its therapy, is fast-moving and sometimes booming. This was the reason for writing this up-to-date and in-depth book. The 30 chapters cover the whole spectrum of diabetes. Special effort was made to ensure that the reader is able to approach the various subjects both theoretically and from the point of daily clinical practice. I believe that constructing and presenting information in the form of questions and answers, as well as analysing many cases, makes the text particularly interesting and clear. In addition, the questions raised in the book are based on queries that have arisen in daily clinical practice. It should be noted that the book is aimed at not only physicians of every specialty, but also diabetic individuals. The diabetic person today is, and needs to be, knowledgeable of many details regarding the disease.

I would like to thank my six colleagues, whose names appear on the cover of the book, for their significant efforts. All specialists in the field of diabetes, I had the honour to closely guide and collaborate with them on a daily basis. I would like especially to thank Dr Konstantinos Makrilakis for his constructive cooperation in the general organization of the book. Similarly, I would like to thank Dr Nicholas Tentolouris for editing the extensive index. Of course, each author has his or her own writing style, however, the undersigned expended much effort to ensure that a level of homogeneity exists between the various chapters, without sacrificing the individual style of each author.

Finally, I would like to thank 'Litsas Publications' for their significant effort in publishing the book.

Professor N. Katsilambros
Director, 1st Department of Propaedeutic Medicine of the Athens
University Medical School and the Diabetes Center, 'Laiko'
General Hospital

Preface to English Edition

Although this book is a translation of the Greek one – first published in April 2005 – it is actually a new book in many ways, since it contains updated information regarding new aspects of diabetes mellitus management that have been introduced into clinical practice since the original publication. New information regarding insulin pumps, continuous glucose monitoring, inhaled insulin, GLP-1 analogues and islet transplantation has been incorporated into this edition, giving the reader the opportunity to obtain up-to-date understanding and anticipate further forthcoming innovations.

It should be emphasized that the book continues to present information concerning diabetes mellitus in a very clear and interesting way. It uses a helpful format of questions and answers and clinical case analysis, mixed with explanatory text, that focuses on practical issues of diabetes management in daily clinical practice.

I would like to thank John Wiley & Sons, Ltd for the great honour in giving us the opportunity to show our work worldwide, and to contribute to the educational efforts addressed by the various medical professionals dealing with diabetes mellitus (diabetologists, endocrinologists, internists, nurses, diabetes educators and diabetic patients).

Professor N. Katsilambros, MD, PhD (Athens University), FACP
Director, 1st Department of Propaedeutic Medicine of the
Athens University Medical School and the Diabetes Center,
'Laiko' General Hospital

Overview of diabetes

Nicholas Tentolouris

What is the definition of diabetes mellitus?

Diabetes mellitus (DM) is a group of metabolic disturbances, characterized mainly by hyperglycaemia, and finally resulting in the appearance
of various complications (macro- and micro-angiopathy, etc.). These
complications relate basically to the heart, the vessels, the eyes, the
kidneys and the nervous system. Hyperglycaemia is a result of defects in
the secretion or action of insulin, or both.

How many types of DM exist?

According to the latest classification, there are four main types of DM
(Table 1.1).

Type 1 diabetes mellitus is characterized by an absolute lack of insulin,
and survival of persons affected by this type of DM is dependent on the
exogenous administration of insulin. This form of the disease is divided
into autoimmune and idiopathic DM (Type 1A and 1B, respectively; see
also Chapter 2). In Type 1A, there is an autoimmune destruction of the
β-cells and auto-antibodies are detected in the serum. In Type 1B, the
exact mechanism of β-cell destruction is unknown and auto-antibodies
are not detected in the serum; this is why this type of DM is called
idiopathic. Type 1B is a relatively rare disturbance, mainly encountered
in persons of African and Asian descent. Patients with idiopathic Type 1
DM have severe insulinopenia and so frequently develop diabetic

Diabetes in Clinical Practice: Questions and Answers from Case Studies. Nicholas Katsilambros *et al.*
© 2006 John Wiley & Sons, Ltd.

Table 1.1. Classification of diabetes mellitus

I. Type 1. Destruction of β-cells, which means total lack of insulin
- A. Autoimmune
- B. Idiopathic

II. Type 2. Includes the whole spectrum of combinations from mainly insulin resistance with relative lack of insulin to mainly impaired secretion of insulin accompanied by a lesser degree of insulin resistance

III. Other specific Types of diabetes mellitus (see Table 1.2)

IV. Gestational diabetes mellitus

---

ketoacidosis. Also, this type of DM is not associated with the major histocompatibility complex antigens.

Type 2 diabetes mellitus comprises a heterogeneous group of metabolic disorders, characterized by either a defect in the secretion or a defect in the action of insulin, in proportions that vary from person to person (or even within the same person) during the course of the disease, depending on its duration. It is accepted today that, in the majority of cases, Type 2 DM is manifested when both secretion and insulin disturbances are present.

With the expected future recognition of specific disturbances in the secretion or action of insulin, it is expected that the category of Type 2 DM is going to shrink, and cases that are now characterized as Type 2 are going to be shifted to the group of *other specific types of diabetes* (a list of which appears in Table 1.2).

Gestational diabetes comprises those cases in which the disease appears for the first time during pregnancy (usually after the 28th week of pregnancy).

What is the frequency of DM?

Diabetes mellitus frequency, both Type 1 and Type 2, varies from country to country. In western countries, it is estimated that DM affects, on average, 6–8 percent of the adult population. Type 2 DM is, however, very frequent in persons over 60 years old (frequency around 20 percent) of both sexes. Type 2 comprises 85–90 percent of cases of Caucasians and 95 percent of other races. Type 2 DM frequency is increasing worldwide, but the biggest increase is seen in the developing countries.

Table 1.2. Other specific Types of diabetes mellitus

A. Genetic defects of beta-cell function
1. Chromosome 12, Hepatocyte Nuclear Factor (HNF)-1-alpha (MODY 3)
2. Chromosome 7, glucokinase (MODY 2)
3. Chromosome 20, HNF-4-alpha (MODY 1)
4. Chromosome 13, insulin promoter factor (IPF)-1 (MODY 4)
5. Chromosome 17, HNF-1β (MODY 5)
6. Chromosome 2, NeuroD1 (MODY 6)
7. Mitochondrial DNA
8. Others

B. Genetic defects in insulin action
1. Type A insulin resistance
2. Leprechaunism
3. Rabson-Mendenhall syndrome
4. Lipoatrophic diabetes
5. Others

C. Diseases of the exocrine pancreas
1. Pancreatitis
2. Trauma (pancreatectomy)
3. Neoplasia
4. Cystic fibrosis
5. Haemochromatosis
6. Fibrocalculous pancreatopathy
7. Others

D. Endocrinopathies
1. Acromegaly
2. Cushing's syndrome
3. Glucagonoma
4. Pheochromocytoma
5. Hyperthyroidism
6. Somatostatinoma
7. Aldosteronoma
8. Others

E. Drug- or chemical-induced
1. Vacor
2. Pentamidine
3. Nicotinic acid
4. Glucocorticoids
5. Thyroid hormone
6. Diazoxide
7. Beta adrenergic agonists
8. Thiazides
9. Phenytoin
10. Interferon alpha
11. Others

F. Infections
1 Congenital rubella
2 Cytomegalovirus
3 Others

G. Uncommon forms of immune-mediated diabetes
1. 'Stiff-man' syndrome
2. Anti-insulin receptor antibodies
3. Others

H. Other genetic syndromes sometimes associated with diabetes
1. Down's syndrome
2. Klinefelter's syndrome
3. Turner's syndrome
4. Wolfram's syndrome
5. Friedreich's ataxia
6. Huntington's chorea
7. Lawrence-Moon-Biedl syndrome
8. Myotonic dystrophy
9. Porphyria
10. Prader-Willi syndrome
11. Others

For example, in India, prevalence of Type 2 DM in 1972 was 2.3 percent whereas in the year 2000, it was 12.1 percent (a five-fold increase). It is estimated that the number of people suffering from DM by the year 2025 will have doubled worldwide. Therefore, DM is correctly referred to as a disease with epidemic proportions.

Type 1 DM incidence is also showing an incremental tendency, with an increase of 3 percent between 1960 and 1996 in many countries. For example, the incidence of Type 1 DM in Greece during the last decade was ten cases of the disease for every 100000 people. This frequency is around five times higher in northern European countries and in the island of Sardinia. A preponderance of males are affected, especially when disease onset happens during puberty.

CASE STUDY 1

A 52 year old man was diagnosed with DM 15 days ago. The patient reports a history of high dose corticosteroid ingestion (methylprednisolone) ten years ago, for a period of six months, due to glomerulonephritis (minimal change disease). During that time he had developed DM, which was treated with a combination of insulin and pills, but the diabetes subsequently disappeared after discontinuation of corticosteroid therapy. Plasma glucose levels during the last few years had been normal (fasting plasma glucose < 100 mg/dl [5.5 mmol/L]), but were found to be elevated recently. One year ago the patient was diagnosed with hypertension, for which he was prescribed a small dose of diuretics (hydrochlorthiazide 12.5 mg/day). What type of DM does this patient have?

According to the history, this patient had steroid-induced DM ten years ago, which subsided after discontinuation of steroids. This happens in about 50 percent of patients developing steroid-induced DM; in the rest, DM persists after termination of steroids. Chronic administration of thiazide diuretics is known to cause a small increase in blood glucose levels; a significant increase, however, is extremely rare. In the majority of cases, these patients already have Type 2 DM, and diuretic administration simply exacerbates the already existent hyperglycaemia.

This case shows that DM can be the final result of the effect of various factors. For example, a woman with DM diagnosed for the first time during pregnancy has Type 2 DM, unless she has pre-existent Type 1.

Reference to the above cases is made in order to emphasize the fact that, regardless of the pathogenetic mechanism, for the patient and his treating physician it is more important to treat the metabolic disturbance than strictly classify the disease into Type 2 or one of the 'other specific types of diabetes'. Of course, the attempt to categorize the type of DM will help in the correct, rational use of therapy (pills, insulin or combination of the two).

CASE STUDY 2

A patient who has had Type 2 DM for seven years receives full dose combination oral antidiabetic therapy (sulfonylurea and metformin) and has had poor glycaemic control for the previous five months (mean fasting blood glucose 170 mg/dl [9.4 mmol/L], HbA$_{1c}$ = 8 percent), despite adequate dietetic advice. The patient had had good glycaemic control with this therapeutic regimen for the previous six years. He also reports a weight loss of around 5 kg (11 lb) during the last five months. What will you recommend to the patient?

Since the patient has been in poor glycaemic control for a relatively long time, it is most likely a secondary failure of antidiabetic treatment. The United Kingdom Prospective Diabetes Study (UKPDS, 1998) showed that up to 70 percent of Type 2 DM patients with a known duration of DM of 7–8 year will require insulin to achieve good glycaemic control. Also, the unexplained weight loss is an indication of lack of insulin.

In the present case, it is obvious that the patient needs insulin for good diabetic control. If we want to be more accurate, we can do a glucagon stimulation test to evaluate more objectively the insulin secretory ability of the pancreas.

What are the indications for performing a glucagon test?

The glucagon test evaluates the ability of the pancreatic β-cells to secrete insulin. During the test, the fasting serum C-peptide concentration is measured at baseline and six minutes after the intravenous administration of 1 mg glucagon. Measurement of the C-peptide concentration is preferred to measurement of the insulin levels. It should be noted that C-peptide and insulin are secreted in equimolar quantities from the pancreas. Although, a proportion of around 40–60 percent of insulin is metabolized during the first pass from the liver, C-peptide is not metabolized and is slowly excreted. Thus, C-peptide level is, in comparison to insulin level, a more reliable index of insulin secretion.

The indications for performing a glucagon test are as follows:

1. the differential diagnosis of Type 1 from other types of DM in some clinically indiscernible cases;
2. the evaluation of residual insulin secretion from the pancreas in some pancreatic diseases due to various causes (pancreatectomy, trauma, chronic pancreatitis);
3. as a criterion for initiation of insulin therapy in people with long-standing Type 2 DM when they do not respond to oral antidiabetic therapy.

The test is performed in the morning, in a fasting state of at least eight hours, without previous administration of insulin or oral antidiabetic medicines. It should also be noted that glucagon should be stored in the refrigerator (maintenance temperature of 4°C) until it is used.

How are the results interpreted?

When serum C-peptide concentrations are very low (< 0.06 ng/ml), this is compatible with lack of insulin and an indication of Type 1 DM presence. C-peptide concentrations at the 6th minute after glucagon administration are better able to discern people with adequate residual ability for insulin secretion (positive for C-peptide) than those with inadequate secretion (negative for C-peptide). The normal values for serum C-peptide levels six minutes after 1 mg of glucagon injection are 3.03–12.12 ng/ml in non-diabetic and in Type 2 diabetic persons, but < 1.81 ng/ml in C-peptide negative (insulin-dependent) persons (patients with Type 1 DM). A C-peptide increment of less than 1.06 ng/ml from the baseline value after injection of glucagon predicts with great accuracy a failure of oral antidiabetic medicines and need for insulin initiation.

What are the contraindications and the side effects of a glucagon test?

Glucagon can produce 'a crisis' in people with pheochromocytoma and can even be used as a diagnostic tool for the presence of the disease. Thus, the test is contraindicated in people with pheochromocytoma.

Side effects of glucagon administration include allergic reactions (rarely anaphylactic reactions), nausea, vomiting, dizziness, headache and increase of blood glucose levels (due to glycogenolysis and gluco-neogenesis in the liver).

CASE STUDY 3

A 42 year old man comes to the office with the probable diagnosis of 'diabetes mellitus'. Recent biochemistry results show a fasting plasma glucose level of 120 mg/dl (6.7 mmol/L). He denies polyuria, polydipsia or weight loss. His family history is positive for Type 2 DM in his mother, diagnosed at the age of 54 years. The patient's height is 1.74 m (5 ft, 8.5 in) and his weight 95 kg (209.5 lb). Does this patient have DM?

According to the diagnostic criteria for diabetes mellitus of the American Diabetes Association (ADA) in 1997 and the World Health Organization (WHO) in 1999, this patient does not fulfil the criteria for the diagnosis of DM. There are three criteria for diagnosing DM:

1. Fasting plasma glucose level > 126 mg/dl (7.0 mmol/L). Fasting means abstinence from calorie intake for at least eight hours.
2. Random plasma glucose level > 200 mg/dl (11.1 mmol/L) with simul-taneous presence of symptoms compatible with DM (i.e., polyuria, polydipsia and unexplained weight loss). Random plasma glucose level means that measurement of plasma level is done at any time during the day, irrespective of food intake.
3. Plasma glucose level > 200 mg/dl (11.1 mmol/L) two hours after oral administration of 75 g glucose.

When one of the above criteria is positive, it should be verified with one of the others on a different day.

According to the above results, does this patient have a disturbance of glucose metabolism?

According to the latest classification of disturbances of glucose metabo-lism, the above patient has impaired fasting glucose (IFG). The previous classification of glucose metabolism disturbances (made by WHO in 1985) did not include this entity. Normal fasting plasma glucose values are 70–109 mg/dl (3.9–6.0 mmol/L). This upper limit of normal values is basically arbitrary, but is a level above which a loss of the first phase of insulin secretion, during the intravenous administration of glucose, is observed. Furthermore, values above 109 mg/dl (6.0 mmol/L) are associated with an increase in the risk of micro- and mainly macro-vascular complications. The category of impaired fasting glucose (fasting glucose 110–125 mg/dl [6.1–6.9 mmol/L]) was established in order to include those glucose values that, although not fulfilling the criteria for diabetes diagnosis (fasting glucose >126 mg/dl [>7.0 mmol/L]), are not entirely normal.

In 2003, the American Diabetes Association proposed a level of 100 mg/dl (5.6 mmol/L) as an upper limit of normal for fasting plasma glucose. The reason for this decrease was that the level of 100 mg/dl is better associated with the future appearance of DM than the level of 110 mg/dl (6.1 mmol/L).

Impaired fasting glucose and impaired glucose tolerance are poten-tially reversible conditions that are associated with the risk of developing Type 2 DM in the future and, as mentioned above, with the risk for cardiovascular events. Impaired fasting glucose and impaired glucose tolerance are collectively called 'pre-diabetes'.

The disturbances of glucose metabolism are shown in Table 1.3.

Table 1.3. Criteria for diagnosis of diabetes mellitus and impaired glucose control

Fasting plasma glucose	<100 mg/dl (5.6 mmol/L)	Normal
Fasting plasma glucose	100–125 mg/dl (5.6–6.9 mmol/L)	Impaired Fasting Glucose (IFG)
Fasting plasma glucose	≥ 126 mg/dl (7.0 mmol/L)	Diabetes mellitus
Plasma glucose 2 hrs after 75 g glucose	<140 mg/dl (7.8 mmol/L)	Normal glucose tolerance
Plasma glucose 2 hrs after 75 g glucose	140–199 mg/dl (7.8–11.0 mmol/L)	Impaired Glucose Tolerance (IGT)
Plasma glucose 2 hrs after 75 g glucose	≥ 200 mg/dl (11.1 mmol/L)	Diabetes mellitus

The above values are valid for USA. In Europe normal fasting plasma glucose is considered to be a value <110 mg/dl (6.1 mmol/L) and impaired fasting glucose 110–125 mg/dl (6.1–6.9 mmol/L).

What will you recommend to the patient?

This is a slightly obese person (body mass index: $31.38\,kg/m^2$). Additionally, he has a positive family history of diabetes (first degree relative with Type 2 DM). Therefore, he has two risk factors for development of Type 2 DM. Several studies have shown that, in obese persons, fasting plasma glucose values are often normal, even though the two hour glucose value during an oral glucose tolerance test is abnormal (above the level for diagnosis of DM: $> 200\,mg/dl$). Therefore, the repeat of fasting glucose measurement in this patient (even though it is an easier, quicker, cheaper, and more widely accepted test by the examinees, with a higher reproducibility than the oral glucose tolerance test) is probably not the most appropriate test in this case. Measurement of a random glucose level is also not indicated, since there are no symptoms compatible with DM. Thus, in order to exclude DM or coexistence of impaired glucose tolerance in this patient, an oral glucose tolerance test (OGTT) is indicated.

CASE STUDY 4

A 48 year old woman comes to the office because she is worried she might be suffering from DM. The reason for her worries is that her father was diagnosed with Type 2 DM at the age of 55 years and died from an acute myocardial infarction at 74. Her cousin has also suffers from Type 2 DM (for ten years) and recently started treatment with insulin injections. A chemistry profile a year ago showed a fasting plasma glucose level of 96 mg/dl (5.3 mmol/L). She has two children: the first child was born 3.6 kg (7.9 lb) and the second 4.5 kg (9.9 lb). She does not report any diabetic symptoms. Her weight is 77.8 kg (171.5 lb) and her height 1.67 m (5 ft, 5.7 in). What will you recommend to the patient?

The patient has three risk factors for developing Type 2 DM: i) she is overweight (body mass index: $27.9\,kg/m^2$); ii) she has a positive family history of Type 2 DM (one first degree relative with Type 2 DM); and iii) she most likely had gestational DM in one of her pregnancies (a neonate's birth weight of $> 4\,kg$ is considered to be evidence of macrosomia, most likely due to gestational DM).

According to the recommendations of international scientific organizations, pre-symptomatic screening for Type 2 DM is indicated in all persons over 45 years of age, especially if they have a high body mass index ($> 25\,kg/m^2$). If the results do not show presence of DM, the

Table 1.4. Risk factors for development of Type 2 diabetes mellitus

---

- Age $\geq$ 45 years
- Increased body weight (body mass index $\geq$ 25 Kg/m^2)
- Family history of Type 2 diabetes
- Sedentary lifestyle
- History of gestational diabetes or child birth weighing > 4 kg
- Hypertension ($\geq$ 140/90 mmHg)
- Dyslipidaemia (HDL-cholesterol $\leq$ 35 mg/dl [0.9 mmol/L] or/and fasting triglycerides $\geq$ 250 mg/dl [2.8 mmol/L])
- Polycystic ovary syndrome
- History of impaired fasting glucose or impaired glucose tolerance
- History of atherosclerotic disease
- People of certain ethnic groups (African Americans, Hispanics, Asians, Pima Indians, inhabitants of certain Pacific islands)

---

screening test should be repeated every three years. The three year interval is set because even if DM is to manifest in the meantime, it is not expected to cause any complications. It is advised, however, that people above 45 years of age who have at least one of the risk factors mentioned in Table 1.4, are screened more frequently. Also, overweight persons (BMI> 25 kg/m^2), of lower age (<45 years) with one additional risk factor from those mentioned in Table 1.4, should be screened for Type 2 DM as for persons aged > 45 years. For all these reasons, therefore, the woman in question should be screened for DM.

The bigger the number of risk factors present, the higher the risk of developing Type 2 DM.

Which method will you choose for diagnosis?

The patient does not have symptoms of DM, so it is not indicated to measure plasma glucose in a random sample of blood. The easiest way, for reasons analysed in the previous case, is to measure fasting plasma glucose level. A different approach would be to perform an oral glucose tolerance test. This is preferred to the measurement of fasting plasma glucose level as a screening test for DM, according to the recommendations of the World Health Organization. A drawback of the method is its poor reproducibility, whereas an advantage is its slightly higher sensitivity compared to fasting plasma glucose in diagnosing DM.

How do you perform an oral glucose tolerance test (OGTT)?

In order to get correct results from an oral glucose tolerance test it is essential that the patient has a proper preparation. The test is performed early in the morning after an overnight fast of 8–14 hours, although drinking water is permitted. In addition, it is essential that for the three days prior to the test the patient does not abstain from carbohydrates (he or she should consume at least 150 g of carbohydrates daily). The evening before the test the patient should eat supper with an overage quantity of carbohydrates (30–50 g).

During the test the patient should remain in the office, seated. Smoking cigarettes, drinking coffee or other beverages (even those that do not contain calories) is not allowed in the morning before or during the test.

After drawing blood for measuring fasting plasma glucose, the adult patient receives, within five minutes, 75 g anhydrous glucose, diluted in 230–250 ml of water. This quantity of anhydrous glucose corresponds to 82.5 g of monohydric glucose. In children, 1.75 g of anhydrous glucose per kg of body weight is given, with a maximum quantity of 75 g. The quantity of anhydrous glucose given for diagnosing gestational diabetes can be different (see Chapter 10). The OGTT starts from the moment the glucose is consumed. A blood sample is drawn two hours after the glucose load.

The blood samples drawn should be quickly centrifuged. If centrifugation is not going to be performed within 60 minutes of the blood being drawn, the blood should be stored in a test tube with an inhibitor of glycolysis (usually sodium fluoride, 2.5 mg per ml of blood). It should be noted that glycolysis is slowed but not completely abolished by the addition of glycolysis inhibitors. The measurement of plasma glucose concentration should also be performed without delay, preferably with an enzymatic method (hexokinase or glucose oxidase method). Measurement of blood glucose concentrations during an OGTT with portable glucose meters (using capillary or venous blood) is not acceptable, since these meters do not have the required accuracy.

The interpretation of the results of the OGTT is shown in Table 1.3.

An oral glucose tolerance test was performed on the patient. The results were as follows: fasting plasma glucose level of 98 mg/dl (5.4 mmol/L); plasma glucose level two hours after glucose load of 130 mg/dl (7.2 mmol/L). What will your instructions to the patient be?

The patient is not suffering from DM nor does she have a disturbance in glucose metabolism (according to the criteria of Table 1.3). Since she is at increased risk of developing DM in the future, however, she should be advised to repeat a screening test for DM in 1–3 years. Since, additionally, there is ample evidence that development of Type 2 DM can be prevented or postponed with the application of lifestyle changes, we would recommend that this woman try and lose some of her excess body weight, and increase her physical activity and proper nutrition. Prevention of Type 2 DM is analysed in Chapter 30.

CASE STUDY 5

A 70 year old man, diagnosed with Type 2 DM two months ago, comes to the office for a follow-up visit. His blood sugar levels are high, both fasting and after meals (250–350 mg/dl [13.9–19.4 mmol/L]). The patient was started initially on treatment with gliclazide (40 mg twice a day), which was gradually increased on a weekly basis. For the last 15 days, he has received the maximum dose of 320 mg/day. His weight is 68 kg (149.9 lb) and his height 1.78 m (5 ft, 10 in). The patient had not had a ketoacedotic coma at diagnosis, although before the diagnosis he had noticed significant weight loss accompanied by symptoms compatible with DM (polyuria, polydipsia), which continue despite nutritional treatment. There is no family history of DM. How will you treat this patient?

The patient in question is not overweight (BMI: 21.46 kg/m^2) and does not have a family history of Type 2 DM (for conditions that usually accompany Type 2 DM, see Table 1.5). Appearance of diabetes at an older age is not a reliable criterion for diagnosing Type 2 DM. In the present case we have to consider the possibility of Type 1 DM, which appears at an older age. One such form of DM is LADA (Latent Autoimmune Diabetes in Adults). This Type of DM accounts for about 10 percent of new cases of DM in northern European countries, although it is rarer in the south. It is generally known that in up to 25 percent of patients with Type 1 DM, diagnosis of the disease is made after the age of 35 years. LADA is characterized by a slower autoimmune destruction of the β-cells compared to younger persons and so its clinical presentation is not very noticeable. It is often mistaken initially for Type 2 DM. There are, however, some differences from Type 2 DM that help in the differential diagnosis: i) in LADA there is no family history of Type 2 DM, although there may be first degree relatives with Type 1 DM;

Table 1.5. Main differences between Type 1 and Type 2 diabetes

	Type 1	Type 2	Comments
Age at presentation	Mainly <40 years (peak = 12th year)	mainly > 40 years (peak = 60–70th year)	10% of older people have Type 1 diabetes (LADA). 20% of diabetic children in some countries have Type 2 diabetes.
Weight	Thin persons, as a rule there is weight loss at presentation	As a rule overweight or obese persons	The number of people with Type 1 diabetes who are obese at the time of diagnosis increases. Weight loss may more rarely happen at the time of diagnosis in Type 2 diabetes as well.
Ketoacidosis	May be present	Is seen rarely and under special conditions	Ketoacidosis may be the presenting symptom in Type 1 diabetes. It is rare in Type 2 diabetes and occurs during a serious infection, trauma, surgery or acute myocardial infarction.
Need for insulin administration	Insulin is necessary for survival	Insulin is not necessary for survival	During the 'honeymoon phase' in a person with Type 1 diabetes, insulin administration may not be necessary or insulin needs may be very small. Insulin may be the only effective treatment for controlling persons with

(continued)

Table 1.5. (*Continued*)

	Type 1	Type 2	Comments
Ability of insulin secretion from β-cells	Absent	Adequate	Type 2 diabetes who have long standing diabetes. Some patients with Type 1 diabetes may have some ability of insulin secretion at the time of diagnosis of the disease. In some patients with Type 2 diabetes and long duration of the disease, the ability of insulin secretion may be seriously decreased.
Auto-antibodies	Positive	Negative	Falsely positive and falsely negative results can occur in both Types of diabetes.

ii) affected persons are lean at diagnosis of DM, whereas persons with Type 2 diabetes are in the majority of cases (80 percent) overweight or obese; iii) these patients do not respond well to oral antidiabetic treatment and quickly require insulin to control their blood sugar; iv) it is more common in northern European countries; v) determination of auto-antibodies against components of the pancreatic islets and β-cells, which characteristically appear in Type 1 DM, is positive in these patients. The major differences between Type 1 and Type 2 DM are shown in Table 1.5.

In the present case, based on the medical history and clinical picture, it seems likely that this is DM of the LADA Type and insulin therapy should be recommended. Diagnosis could be confirmed with determination of specific auto-antibodies in the patient's serum and a glucagon stimulation test (which will show low levels of serum C-peptide and small response of after injection of 1 mg glucagon). If auto-antibodies are negative, it may be the case that it is Type 2 DM with primary failure of oral antidiabetic medicines, or Type 1 DM without auto-antibodies (idiopathic). In either case insulin therapy is indicated.

CASE STUDY 6

A 54 year old woman comes to the clinic for evaluation of possible DM. She was referred by an ophthalmologist, because during fundoscopy for a glaucoma check-up, microaneurysms and haemorrhages were found in the retina. The patient is asymptomatic, without any significant medical history. Her mother had Type 2 DM, diagnosed at the age of 76. Can diabetic complications precede the clinical presentation and diagnosis of the disease?

The United Kingdom Prospective Diabetes Study (UKPDS, 1990) showed that at the time of diagnosis a significant proportion of the patients already had microvascular complications. Retinopathy was especially common (25 percent), although peripheral neuropathy (7 percent) and nephropathy (3 percent) were less common. In some cases, maculopathy, a condition that threatens vision, was also present. Erectile dysfunction was common as well (20 percent). Rarely, there can be neurotrophic ulcers in the soles due to severe diabetic peripheral neuropathy. This happens because the disease can be present for many years without being detected. In population studies it has been shown that for every ten cases of diagnosed diabetes, another five cases are undiagnosed.

Regarding macrovascular complications, UKPDS (1990) showed that up to 40 percent of patients at the time of diagnosis had one such complication (stroke, coronary artery disease or peripheral vascular disease). Hypertension was also especially common (40 percent), in both sexes.

How does Type 2 DM manifest?

In about half of patients there are the classic symptoms of DM (polyuria, polydipsia, rarely weight loss) in a mild form, whereas a proportion of up to 20 percent presents with characteristic infections (especially fungal infections of the genital tract). In 30 percent of the cases, diagnosis of Type 2 DM is made accidentally during examinations for various other reasons (check-up or pre-operative evaluation, examinations for insurance, etc.). Visual disturbances are also common, even when there are no lesions in the retina. These are due to accumulation of glucose and water in the lens owing to the hyperglycaemia. Some patients develop muscular cramps in the lower extremities, burning sensation in the soles and the toes, or hyperalgesia. In a small proportion of patients, especially of older age, the first manifestation of Type 2 DM can be hyperglycaemic hyperosmolar coma, due more frequently to a concomitant infection. As already mentioned, in a non-negligible percentage of patients, diagnosis of DM can happen after the manifestation of one of its complications.

How does Type 1 DM manifest?

In typical cases, Type 1 DM presents with sudden weight loss (in the order of 1–2 kg/week) accompanied by intense polyphagia, polydipsia and polyuria, especially during the night, in persons aged < 30 years old. Usually there is concomitant generalized feelings of fatigue, weakness, sleepiness and significant loss of muscular mass. Visual disturbances as well as skin infections (fungal infections of the genital organs, staphylococcal skin infections, etc.) are also common. Physical examination can reveal evidence of dehydration, muscular atrophy, especially in the thigh area, and acetone breathing, when there is concomitant ketosis.

If diagnosis is delayed, the patient displays deterioration of the symptoms and signs of severe dehydration, while the increase of ketone bodies in the blood causes anorexia, nausea, vomiting, diffuse abdominal pains (which can mimic acute abdomen) and muscle cramps. In a small proportion of patients, especially in very young children, the presenting feature can be a ketoacidotic coma.

Contrary to Type 2 DM, the characteristic microvascular complications of the disease are not present at the time of diagnosis of Type 1 DM.

CASE STUDY 7

A 67 year old patient with Type 2 DM for six years, treated with sulfonylureas and metformin, comes to the clinic for a scheduled follow-up visit. His fasting blood sugar levels in the morning are 130–170 mg/dl (7.2–9.4 mmol/L), before lunch 130–150 mg/dl (7.2–8.3 mmol/L) and before dinner 120–160 mg/dl (6.7–8.9 mmol/L). His post-prandial levels (two hours after a meal) range between 140–200 mg/dl (7.8–11.1 mmol/L). His HbA$_{1c}$ is 7.6 percent. Is his blood sugar control adequate?

This patient's blood sugar control is inadequate. Glycaemic control goals in both types of DM are shown in Table 1.6.

We emphasize that glycaemic control goals should be individualized. In persons living alone, it may be dangerous to attempt very strict control, because a serious hypoglycaemic episode can be fatal. In persons with hypoglycaemia unawareness or frequent hypoglycaemic episodes, as

Table 1.6. Goals of glycaemic control in diabetes

	American Diabetes Association	International Diabetes Federation	American College of Clinical Endocrinologists
HbA$_{1c}$	<7%	<6.5%	<6.5%
Pre-prandial glucose level	90–130 mg/dl (5.0–7.2 mmol/L)	<100 mg/dl (5.6 mmol/L)	<110 mg/dl (6.1 mmol/L)
Post-prandial glucose level	<180 mg/dl (10.0 mmol/L)	<135 mg/dl (7.5 mmol/L)	<140 mg/dl (7.8 mmol/L)

Post-prandial measurements should be performed 1–2 hours after meal. The American Diabetes Association recommends an effort for a further decrease of the proposed post-prandial blood glucose levels when pre-prandial glucose levels are normal but HBA1c values are high.

well as in children, it is preferable to allow higher glucose values. Also, in people with a short life expectancy, the goal is to eliminate hyperglycaemia symptoms. However, in DM during pregnancy we should try to achieve normal HbA$_{1c}$ values individually, whenever possible, since most studies have shown a linear correlation between HbA$_{1c}$ values and frequency of microvascular complications. Of course, the penalty for such a strict control is frequent hypoglycaemias, and especially serious instances in people with Type 1 DM. In the Diabetes Control and Complications Trial (DCCT, 1993), the frequency of all hypoglycaemic episodes was three times higher in the group with intensive insulin treatment, whereas the frequency of serious hypoglycaemias was five times higher when HbA$_{1c}$ values were < 6 percent, compared with persons who had HbA$_{1c}$ values > 8 percent. In the UKPDS (1990) study, people with better glycaemic control had double the frequency of serious hypoglycaemic episodes. There are now newer insulin analogues with pharmacokinetic properties that help in reaching the goals of glycaemic control with a lower risk of hypoglycaemias.

Why must the patient have good glycaemic control?

In both Types of DM, good glycaemic control protects from microvascular complications. In the DCCT (1993) study of Type 1 diabetics, it was shown that during a follow-up period of six and a half years the frequency of appearance and evolution of microvascular complications could be reduced by up to 76 percent in the group with good, compared to those with not so good, glycaemic control. Specifically, better control (HbA$_{1c}$ values 7.1 versus 9.0 percent) resulted in a decreasd risk of:

- microalbuminuria by 39 percent
- proteinuria by 54 percent
- neuropathy by 60 percent
- development of retinopathy by 76 percent
- deterioration of retinopathy by 54 percent
- major cardiovascular events by 42 percent.

Additionally, better glycaemic control was associated with a decrease in the levels of total cholesterol, LDL-cholesterol and triglycerides and an increase in HDL-cholesterol. Also, the intima-media thickness of the carotid arteries, an index of premature atherosclerosis, was significantly lower in persons with better glycaemic control. Cardiovascular events (myocardial infarctions, strokes, peripheral vascular disease) were not significantly lowered in this study ($p = 0.08$), but this was due to the small number of events (40 events in the conventional treatment group versus 23 events in the group with intensive insulin treatment) since participants in the study were young persons without macrovascular complications.

In persons with Type 2 DM, the UKPDS and other smaller studies as well, showed that in a period of ten years better glycaemic control (HbA$_{1c}$ values 7.0 percent versus 7.9 percent) resulted in a decreased risk of:

- all DM-related events by 12 percent
- microvascular complications by 25 percent
- cataract surgeries by 24 percent
- retinopathy by 21 percent
- microalbuminuria by 33 percent
- myocardial infarction by 16 percent.

Decrease in the risk for myocardial infarction in the UKPDS was borderline ($p = 0.052$). Although there is no proof from large studies that improvement in glycaemic control decreases the risk of cardiovascular events (which are very common in people with Type 2 DM), it seems that in order to decrease that risk an optimal control of blood sugar is needed in addition to aggressive treatment of the other concomitant risk factors (hypertension, obesity, dyslipidaemia, smoking).

How feasible is the achievement and attainment of the proposed glycaemic control goals in DM?

All long-term studies in DM (DCCT and UKPDS) have shown that although achievement of glycaemic goals is relatively easy, long-term attainment of the glycaemic control in normal levels is extremely difficult. In the DCCT (1993) study, in which, it should be emphasized, there was provision of full and continuous support of the patients, only about 5 percent of patients managed to retain HbA$_{1c}$ values < 6 percent over the whole length of the study. Variations of HbA$_{1c}$ values in the intensive insulin treated group were between 6.5 and 8 percent during the 10-year follow-up. Also, in the intensively treated group, both fasting glucose levels and post-prandial ones had great deviations from desirable targets.

A steadily continuous deterioration of blood sugar levels and HbA_{1c} values was observed in Type 2 DM, such that a frequent escalation of the therapeutic regimen was necessitated, in order to retain mean HbA_{1c} values at an acceptable level. HbA_{1c} values in the groups that followed an intensive versus conventional therapeutic regimen, per 5-year periods, were as follows: 0–5 years 6.6 versus 7.4 percent; 5–10 years 7.5 versus 8.4 percent; and 10–15 years: 8.1 versus 8.7 percent.

Data from various studies have shown that a small proportion of diabetics achieve values of $HbA_{1c} < 7$ percent, (around 37 percent) while only 7 percent of them had achieved the total of all therapeutic diabetic goals ($HbA_{1c} < 7$ percent, blood pressure $< 130/80$ mmHg and total cholesterol < 200 mg/dl [5.17 mmol/L]).

Further reading

American Diabetes Association (1997) Expert Committee on the Diagnosis and Classification of Diabetes Mellitus. Report of the expert committee on the diagnosis and classification of diabetes mellitus. *Diabetes Care* **20**, 1183–97.

Expert Committee on the Diagnosis of Diabetes Mellitus (2003) Follow-up report on the diagnosis of diabetes mellitus. *Diabetes Care* **26**, 3160–67.

Diabetes Control and Complications Trial Research Group (1993) The effect of intensive treatment of diabetes on the development and progression of long-term complications in insulin-dependent diabetes mellitus. *N Engl J Med*, **329**, 977–86.

Katsilambros, N. and Aliferis, K., Darviri, C., Tsapogas, P., Alexiou, Z., Tritos, N., Arvanitis, M. (1993) Evidence for an increase in the prevalence of known diabetes in a sample of an urban population in Greece. *Diabet Med*, **10**, 87–90.

Katsilambros, N., Hatzakis, A., Perdicaris, G., Pefanis, A., Touloumi, G. (1991) Total and cause-specific mortality in a population based cohort of diabetes in Greece. *Diabete Metab*, **17**, 410–14.

Katsilambros, N. and Tentolouris, N. (2003) Type 2 diabetes: an overview, in *Textbook of Diabetes*, 3rd edn (eds J. Pickup and G. Williams Blackwell Science Ltd, Oxford), **4**, pp. 1–19.

Pinkney, J. (2003) Clinical research methods in diabetes, in *Textbook of Diabetes*, 3rd edn, (eds) J. Pickup and G. Williams Blackwell Science Ltd, Oxford, **35**, pp. 1–20.

Sacks, D.B., Bruns, D.E., Goldstein, D.E., Maclaren, N.K., McDonald, J.M., Parrott, M. (2002) Guidelines and recommendations for laboratory analysis in the diagnosis and management of diabetes mellitus. *Clinical Chemistry*, **48**, 436–72.

UKPDS Study Group. UK Prospective Diabetes Study 6 (1990) Complications in newly diagnosed Type 2 diabetic patients and their association with different clinical and biochemical risk factors. *Diabetes Research*, **13**, 1–11.

UKPDS Study Group (1998) Intensive blood glucose control with sulfonylurea or insulin compared with conventional treatment and risk of complications in patients with Type 2 diabetes (UKPDS 33). *Lancet*, **352**, 837–53.

World Health Organization (1999) Definition, Diagnosis and Classification of Diabetes Mellitus and its Complications: Report of WHO Consultation. Part 1: Diagnosis and Classification of Diabetes Mellitus. Geneva, World Health Orgnization.

2

Pathophysiology of Type 1 diabetes

Ioannis Ioannidis

Why do I have diabetes?

This is a very common question asked after the diagnosis of Type 1 diabetes mellitus (DM). Even when not directly addressed to the doctor, it is still in the minds of the diabetic patients and their families. The question is frequently accompanied by feelings of guilt for possible omissions, mistakes or habits that contributed to the appearance of the disease.

We shall try to answer that question in the following pages, outlining the current opinions regarding pathogenesis of Type 1 DM.

According to the latest classification of the disease, Type 1 DM is divided into Type 1A DM (autoimmune destruction of the pancreatic β-cells, which leads to a shortage of insulin) and Type 1B DM (total lack of insulin without signs of autoimmune destruction of the pancreatic β-cells). The great majority of patients with insulin-dependent DM suffer from Type 1A DM.

Type 1A DM is therefore an autoimmune disease. It usually occurs during childhood and adolescence (which is why in previous classifications it was called *juvenile diabetes* mellitus), but can present during adult life as well. According to current estimates, autoimmune Type 1A DM represents 5–10 percent of the cases of DM that occur in adults. Adults that manifest this type of DM are (arithmetically) equal to the children that manifest Type 1 DM.

In Europe and the USA the great majority (> 90 percent) of Caucasian children who develop DM have Type 1A. However, 50 percent of Hispanic or African-American children in the USA who develop diabetes

Diabetes in Clinical Practice: Questions and Answers from Case Studies. Nicholas Katsilambros *et al.*
© 2006 John Wiley & Sons, Ltd.

lack the auto-antibodies that characterize Type 1A DM. Most of these children suffer from diabetes type MODY (Maturity Onset Diabetes of the Young; an adult-type DM that presents at a young age), the various types of which are characterized by hereditary mutations in the genes of glucokinase or the hepatocyte nuclear factors (HNF, see Chapter 1, Table 1.2). Alternatively, these children suffer from Type 2 DM (a significant proportion today, due to the increased prevalence of obesity in the young age)

When someone suffers from Type 1A DM, both themselves and their relatives are at increased risk of developing other autoimmune diseases as well. Coeliac disease, hypothyroidism, hyperthyroidism, Addison's disease and atrophic gastritis (megaloblastic anaemia) are some of the most common autoimmune diseases that develop in these people.

Type 1 DM is characterized by a lack of insulin (total or nearly total), increase of glucagon (a hormone that is secreted by the α-cells of the pancreatic islets and has the opposite actions of insulin), high blood glucose levels, glucosuria and ketonuria. Treatment with insulin decreases the high blood glucose levels, inhibits ketosis and reverses the general catabolic state. Treatment with insulin is mandatory for the rest of the life for survival (*insulin-dependent diabetes mellitus*, according to the older classification).

The *pathophysiology* of the disease can, for didactic reasons, be categorized into 4 stages: i) genetic sensitivity-susceptibility; ii) effect of a stimulus that triggers onset of the disease; iii) autoimmune reaction; and iv) loss of insulin secretion.

Stage I: Genetic sensitivity-susceptibility

There is definitely a hereditary predisposition for the development of Type 1 DM.

Type 1A DM is genetically heterogeneous. Very few patients have a monogenic defect. Such patients are those with a mutation in the AIRE gene (autoimmune regulator), who manifest the Type 1 autoimmune polyendocrinopathy syndrome, and patients with a mutation in the X-linked gene, which resembles the gene that causes pityriasis in mice (they manifest the XPID syndrome: X-linked polyendocrinopathy with immune defect and diarrhoea).

The vast majority of Type 1A DM cases, however, are due to a polygenic defect. The most significant role in the predisposition for the development of the disease is played by polymorphisms (i.e., variations in the genes' nucleotide sequences) in HLA genes.

HLA antigens. The genes that regulate the white blood cell antigens, known as HLA antigens (Human Leukocyte Antigens), are located on chromosome 6. They belong to the system of major histocompatibility complex (MHC) and their main biological role is the modulation of the immune response. These molecules are expressed on the surface of the cells that present the antigens (antigen-presenting cells, i.e., the macrophages) and are recognized by specific receptors of the T-lymphocytes, which they activate. T-lymphocyte activation requires the binding of HLAs with 'foreign' peptides. The specific amino-acid sequence of HLAs determines which peptides they will be bound with, and thus which peptides the body will 'react' to, by activating the immune mechanism. Every single amino-acid sequence is coded in the literature with a different number, facilitating their recognition.

A significant role in the determination of the sensitivity for development of the disease is played by the regions DQ and DR of the major histocompatibility complex on chromosome 6. In DQ molecules, both chains α and β are polymorphic. Thus, in order to describe a DQ molecule, we need to describe both chains. However, in DR molecules, only chain β is polymorphic (DRB chain). Each number after an asterisk denotes a specific sequence of the HLA allele, while the letters and the first number denote the gene (for example, DRB1*0401: DR B chain, gene number 1, allele 0401).

The observation, nearly 20 years ago, that specific HLA types are associated with the development of Type 1 DM, was a landmark in understanding the pathogenesis of the disease. Extensive studies in many countries showed that some antigens are encountered more frequently in people with Type 1 DM. These antigens are the HLA A1, B8, B15, B40, C3 and especially DR3 and DR4. However, some antigens are found more rarely in these people, such as B7 and DR2. Carriers of these genes seem to have a relative risk of developing DM less than one, which shows that these genes exert some protective role for the development of the disease. An attractive hypothesis, which explains the protection that these alleles exert, reports that the expression of these genes inside the thymus gland contributes to the disappearance of T-lymphocytes that recognize a significant peptide in the pancreatic islets. The disappearance of these cells decreases the risk of diabetes development.

For Caucasians with Type 1A DM, haplotypes that are associated with the greatest risk of developing the disease are the DR3 and DR4. Whereas these haplotypes are found in 40–50 percent of the general population, they are encountered in more than 90 percent of the persons with Type 1A DM.

The relative risk for developing the disease in carriers of the DR3 is five, and for DR3/DR4 is 14. Persons who develop Type 1 DM before the age of five years are in about 50 percent heterozygotes for DR3/DR4. It should be noted that despite the relatively high frequency of these antigens in the general population, the frequency of Type 1 DM is about 0.4 percent. This shows that existence of the antigens alone is not enough for the development of the disease. Its association with these specific HLA genes shows that there is a predilection for an abnormal immune response in some antigens. The high risk HLA alleles present specific pancreatic islet peptides to the T-lymphocytes.

Today there is the ability to sub-analyse DR4 haplotype based on DRB1 and DQB1. Table 2.1 shows an estimation of the risk for developing Type 1 DM based on HLA antigens DR and DQ.

It was recently discovered that if there is aspartate in position 57 (Asp57) of the amino-terminal region of the HLA-DQ β-chain, there is resistance to the development of Type 1 DM. However, there is

Table 2.1. Risk of developing Type 1 DM based on DQ and DR antigens

Risk	DRB1	DQA1	DQB1
High	0401,0405,0402 (**DR4**)	0301	0302
	0301 (**DR3**)	0501	0201
	0801	0401	0402
Moderate	0401	0301	0301
	0401	0301	0303
	0403	0301	0302
	0101	0101	0501
	1601	0102	0502
Low	1101	0501	0301
Protection against Type 1 DM	1501	0102	0602
	0701	0201	0303
	1401	0101	0503

Table 2.2. Gene loci associated with development of Type 1 DM

Gene	Chromosome	Gene locus	Reported relation
IDDM1	6p21	**HLA** (DRBI, DQBI)	7.3
IDDM2	11p15.5	**Insulin** TH/VNTR/INS ClassIII	2.1
IDDM3	15q26	D 15S 107(103)	1.2
IDDM4	11q13	FGF3,DIISI337	3.9
IDDM5	6q25	ESR	1.8
IDDM6	18q21	DI8S487(4)/AI8I,2	4.5
IDDM7	2q31	D25S 152	1.6
IDDM8	6q27	D6S281	1.3
IDDM9	3q21-q25	D3S 1303	3.6
IDDM10	10p11	DIOSI93 (7)	2.1
IDDM11	14q24.3-q31	DI4S67	4.6
IDDM12	2q33	CTLA-4 (G)	3.2
IDDM13	2q34	D2S 164	3.3

increased predisposition if aspartate has been replaced by alanine, valine or serine.

Table 2.2 depicts all the genetic loci that are incriminated as participating in the determination of genetic susceptibility to the disease. Among them, a very significant role is played by the insulin gene.

The insulin gene is located on chromosome 11. It is well established that some polymorphisms of this gene increase the risk of developing Type 1 DM. A repeated nucleotide sequence after the (5′ [prime]) end of the insulin gene is called Variable Nucleotide Tandem Repeat (VNTR). This sequence is comprised of three repeated areas of variable size. The biggest part of this repeated sequence is associated with protection for the development of DM. This aggregate of alleles is associated with a larger production of insulin mRNA in the thymus, leading to the conclusion that large proinsulin production in the thymus decreases the autoimmune response against insulin.

A comparative study of the size of DNA polymorphism of this locus revealed that 88 percent of Caucasian persons with Type 1 DM had about 570 base pairs in this locus, whereas only 12 percent had 2470 base pairs. (Note: Incubation of DNA with restrictive enzymes splits DNA into fragments of different length, depending on the sequence of the DNA bases. Changes in the sequence of the bases in the DNA create new split positions or abolish preexisting ones. Differences in the same positions of homologous chromosomes are called DNA polymorphisms and in most cases concern point mutations, i.e., changes in a single DNA base. DNA polymorphisms have attracted significant interest in medicine today, because they can be 'molecular indices' with which differences in the DNA sequences between people can be discerned). However, in non-diabetics, only 67 percent had the short sequence in this locus and 33 percent the long one.

Around 50 percent of the genetic susceptibility is attributed to the HLA (IDDM1), 10 percent to the insulin gene (IDDM2) and the rest to other gene loci shown in Table 2.2.

In conclusion, therefore, it seems that genetic loci DR3 and DR4 on chromosome 6, including subtypes DQ and DP, and possibly other loci, such as those near the insulin gene or others still unknown, create a predisposition for the development of the disease at some point in the lives of those affected. Given the fact that relatives of Type 1 diabetic persons have a small chance of developing the disease and monozygotic twins have only a 50 percent chance of becoming diabetics, it seems that genetic predisposition for the disease is moderate and other non-genetic factors are required for development of the disease.

Stage II: Effect of a stimulus that triggers onset of the disease

We can produce an autoimmune reaction against the pancreatic islets, insulitis and Type 1 DM, in various animal prototype models, by using various immunologic and genetic manipulations. One such manipulation is to administer the poly-IC (poly inosinic cytodilic) acid to rats with a haplotype of histocompatibility antigens rendering them prone to developing DM. The administration of poly-IC causes insulitis in many of these rats, whereas in others it causes DM with destruction of the β-cells. The poly-IC interacts with the receptors Toll 3 on the surface of the cells of the immune system. This interaction leads to a cataract of intracellular reactions and liberation of cytokines. The poly-IC resembles the RNA of various viruses. It is therefore logical to hypothesize that many infections with RNA viruses could cause DM in genetically predisposed persons. The environmental factors that trigger the auto-immune destruction of the islets in humans are mostly unknown.

However, major aetiologic factors for the development of the disease are thought to be infections by certain viruses, like Coxsackie, mumps and others.

The role of viruses in the development of Type 1 DM was mainly based on two types of observations: i) on the description of sporadic patient cases; and ii) on the development of DM in children whose mothers had contracted rubella during the first trimester of pregnancy. A significant number of chemical substances are also reported in the literature that cause DM in experimental animals. Despite lack of complete proof, viruses and chemical factors are thought to exert a direct harmful effect on the pancreatic β-cells and this harm is the inciting factor that triggers the autoimmune process. The destruction of the pancreatic β-cells is the final result of the cellular and humoral immunity. At this point, the HLA class II antigens (they include HLA-DP, -DQ and -DR molecules) interact with the β-cells that are the target of the viruses, the chemicals and other environmental factors. T-lymphocytes play a crucial role in autoimmunity of DM. Without activated T-lymphocytes, the autoimmune mechanism cannot be stimulated. In fact, in order to have a destruction of the β-cells, it is necessary to have a number of activated T CD8+ cells above a certain crucial number.

Hyperantigens are equally important for the aetiopathogenesis of Type 1 DM. Hyperantigens are microbial or viral proteinic products, which are specific for the β-chain of the T-lymphocyte receptor (TCR = T cell receptor). Many T-lymphocytes that express a specific TCR are activated when the hyperantigens are bound to the major histocompatibility complex. It is therefore considered possible that T-lymphocytes activated by a hyperantigen can lead to autoimmunity when they involve a sensitive person.

Viruses and diabetes. Research into the role of viruses in the aetiopathogenesis of Type 1 DM has a long history. Various viruses, possibly diabetogenic for humans, have been identified and continue to be investigated in many research centres. There is ample evidence for the participation of several viral infections in the aetiopathogenesis of Type 1 DM. The most significant evidence for the most important viruses associated with the development of Type 1 DM are examined in this section.

Mumps. For many years, several cases of Type 1 DM following infection from mumps have been described. This virus probably causes activation of an autoimmunity mechanism against the β-cells. This is supported by the observation that the mumps virus in vitro, in β-cell cultures, stimulates production of interleukin 1 and 6 and abnormal expression of HLA antigens class I and II in the cell surface.

In recent years in Finland, there has been a decrease in the incremental tendency for new Type 1 DM cases, which coincides with the generalization of immunization against mumps, measles and rubella.

Rubella. Congenital rubella causes DM in approximately up to 20 percent of cases of intrauterine infection. DM manifests itself after 5–20 years and is due to autoimmunity, given the fact that anti-islet antibodies are found in more than 50 percent of cases. Patients with congenital rubella carry, in a great proportion, the HLA DR3. Generalization of the rubella vaccine has significantly decreased intrauterine infections by the virus, and so cases of Type 1 DM attributed to congenital rubella are today much fewer.

Coxsackie viruses. Coxsackie viruses were incriminated for participating in the aetiopathogenesis of Type 1 DM in recent years. These viruses cause DM in many animal models. The first evidence for participation of these viruses in the development of Type 1 DM in humans was epidemiologic: a seasonal variation of Coxsackie cases and new diagnoses of Type 1 DM in the spring and autumn was observed. Furthermore, increased titers of IgM antibodies against Coxsackie virus B4 were detected in several children with recent diagnosis of Type 1 DM.

Coxsackie viruses can cause Type 1 DM either through a direct cytolytic effect on β-cells or through an autoimmunity mechanism.

There is evidence that, without the mediation of severe lytic effect, an infection by a Coxsackie virus of small virulence can cause a chronic infection, which leads to autoimmunization through liberation of interferon and hyperexpression of HLA antigens class I on the pancreatic β-cells. It was recently shown that other serotypes of Coxsackie virus, apart from B4, are associated with Type 1 DM.

Intrauterine infection with some enteroviruses is associated with an increased risk for Type 1 DM development as well. Antibodies against such viruses were found at the time of delivery with increased frequency in the serum of women whose children later developed Type 1 DM. The conclusion is that intrauterine infection with certain viruses, and not only from rubella, plays a role in the later development of Type 1 DM in the offspring.

Cytomegalovirus. Infection by the Cytomegalovirus (CMV) can cause damage to the β-cells, since the virus resides in them, as seen from characteristic inclusions that are a well-known feature of the cells attacked by the virus. Many researchers have noted a strong association between the CMV genome and anti-islet antibodies in Type 1 diabetic persons, which makes a case for the fact that persistent infection by CMV may participate in the pathogenesis of Type 1 DM.

Retroviruses. Retroviruses are viruses that cause a slow infection. They can remain in the body in a latent state for a long time. There is scientific evidence that infection with retroviruses in experimental animals can cause DM. Endogenous retroviruses have been incriminated as participants in the aetiology of Type 1 DM in humans as well.

Ebstein-Barr virus. This virus has been implicated in many autoimmune reactions and also studied for its possible contribution to the causation of Type 1 DM. Autoimmunization in the case of Ebstein-Barr virus is based on molecular mimicry.

Therefore, lots of evidence exists for the participation of some viruses in the causation of Type 1 DM. These viruses participate aetiologically in the pathogenesis of the disease, mainly through the induced autoimmunity. Since autoimmunity can be induced even without the participation of viruses, and due to the difficulty of proving a causal relationship between each diabetic case and a viral infection, especially when these infections have happened years before, the proportion of aetiological connection of viruses with Type 1 DM incidence was regarded until recently as small (< 5 percent). In recent reviews, however, this proportion seems to be 10–50 percent.

A cohort study in Finland, the country with the highest frequency of Type 1 DM, that draws blood every three months after birth of children prone to develop Type 1 DM, will probably give definitive answers to this matter within the next few years.

Dietary factors and diabetes. Dietary factors also play a role in the development of Type 1 DM. Contrary to what many people might think, sugar consumption is not associated with the development of Type 1 DM. There are, however, other dietary factors that continue to be under investigation for their contribution in the aetiopathogenesis of the disease. These include cow-milk protein and nitrosamines.

Quite a few years ago, the first evidence appeared in the literature that the contribution of premature addition of cow's milk in the neonatal diet caused Type 1 DM. According to this evidence, neonates who are fed with cow's milk during the first two to three months of their lives have an increased risk of developing Type 1 DM in the following years. It is possible that an autoimmunity mechanism is activated, because there is a cross-reaction between part of the cow's milk albumin and a protein of the β-cell surface, and also parts of cow's milk protein can penetrate the immature neonatal intestinal wall. Increased antibody titers against the cow's milk albumin were detected in a group of diabetic children. A Finnish study found that exclusive feeding of the neonates by breast milk during the first months of life is associated with a lower risk of developing Type 1 DM. In another Finnish study, an association of the incidence of DM with the total consumption of cow's milk was observed. Cow's milk contains increased quantities of casein A1 and B. These varieties of casein have the amino-acid histidine at position 67, which regulates the enzymatic degradation of the molecules and results in β-caseomorphine 7. Casein A2 cannot be split in that position, because it has proline instead of histidine there. β-caseomorphine 7 inhibits *in-vitro* the proliferation of the intestinal lymphocytes.

It is possible, therefore, that casein A1 and B molecules act as immunosuppressants and affect development of immune-resistance for proteins in the intestine. Different kinds of cows produce different proportions of A1 and B casein in their milk and this could explain why some people have a low incidence of Type 1 DM, despite high consumption of cow's milk. Various toxins, such as nitrosurias and the rat poison Vacor, can cause DM by destroying the β-cells. The real contribution of toxic substances in the pathogenesis of Type 1 DM is, however, difficult to elucidate.

Stage III: Autoimmune reaction

It has already become clear that what is inherited in Type 1 DM is the predisposition for the disease and not the disease itself. These genes, therefore, are associated with the disease, but are not specific 'diabeto-genic genes'. The influence of an extrinsic factor stimulates a mechanism of autoimmune pancreatic β-cell destruction. The basic histopathologic lesion in the pancreas is *insulitis*, which consists of lymphocytic infiltration of the islets of the pancreas.

This infiltration is due to the presence of circulating auto-antibodies against components of the β-cells of the islets of Langerhans in the pancreas. Our current ability to detect various auto-antibodies in the blood enables the detection of the preclinical phase of the disease. The most important of these antibodies are antibodies against the cytoplasm of the islet cells (islet cell auto-antibodies, ICA), antibodies against insulin (insulin auto-antibodies, IAA), antibodies against the enzyme GAD (glutamic-acid decarboxylase auto-antibodies, GAA) and antibodies against the enzyme tyrosine phosphatase (IA2). More than 90 percent of diabetic people have at least one antibody positive at the time of diagnosis. At the same time, around 3–5 percent of their relatives have such antibodies as well. These relatives are at increased risk of developing Type 1 DM. There are many studies, worldwide, trying to prevent Type 1 DM in these high risk relatives of diabetic persons, and hope exists that these studies will yield positive results.

The circulating auto-antibodies against the cells of the islets of Langerhans (ICA) recognize antigens of the cytoplasm and/or the surface of these cells. Usually, ICA positive sera, detected by indirect immuno-fluorescence, react with all types of islet cells. The principal islet antigens that were identified as auto-antibody targets, are an antigen with molecular weight of 64 kD, finally proven to be glutamic-acid decarboxylase (GAD), insulin, an antigen of 38 kD, carboxypeptidace H, and others.

The identification of the antigenic targets of ICA and the molecular cloning of genes that code for these antigens, opens the way for both a better understanding of the autoimmune process mechanism leading to the development of the disease and the development of new, handy, sensitive and specific immunodiagnostic methods.

ICA. Islet cell auto-antibodies (ICAs), detected by indirect immuno-fluorescence, react mainly with the cytoplasm of the β, α, δ and PP (pancreatic polypeptide) cells of the islets. The antigenic target of ICAs was considered to be a specific sialoganglioside (or glycolipid), found in all types of islet cells, as was shown from the negation of positive sera during immunofluorescence, after process of the pancreatic substrate with neuraminidase. Apart from that, a fragment of ICA reacts exclusively with the cellular membrane of the β-cells. Selective fluorescence for the β-cells has been attributed mainly to GAD.

ICAs are detected by indirect immunofluorescence in frozen sections of human pancreas of blood type O, based on their ability of binding with the islet cells. Detection rates of ICAs in newly diagnosed patients with DM range from 65–90 percent, whereas in non-diabetic, first-degree relatives, they range from 0.9–9 percent. The reasons why ICAs are detected with such varied frequency in the different laboratories, are mainly differences in sensitivity of pancreatic substrates, usage of non-human substrates, subjectivity of the observer in interpreting the results and methodological modulations done at specific cases. In order to avoid these problems and standardize the method of detecting ICAs, specific rules were finally set: i) preferentially to use human pancreatic tissue blood type O as a substrate and alternatively pancreatic tissue from Wistar-Furth mice (the use of conjugates of hyperoxidase-fluorochrom or alternatively conjugates of protein A-fluorochrom is also proposed); ii) expression (quantification) of the results in Juvenile Diabetes Foundation Units (JDF Units), based on a reference curve taken with the use of internationally standardized prototype sera.

ICAs belong to IgG immunoglobulins, look like they exclusively belong to the IgG-I subtype and frequently fix the complement. The method of complement fixation for their detection is based on this ability of ICAs.

A significant finding was the observation that not only are ICAs detected in newly diagnosed persons with Type 1 DM, but also in healthy subjects, several years before manifestation of the disease. Thus, ICAs are potentially used as predictive indices of the disease in monozygotic twins and in first degree relatives of Type 1 DM patients. ICAs are usually not detected in the circulation a few weeks or months after onset of the disease, perhaps due to the significant destruction of the β-cells. However, when Type 1 DM is also accompanied by other autoimmune endocrinopathies, ICAs are detected in the serum and remain for a long time in high titers.

ICAs that fix the complement are usually found in newly diagnosed Type 1 DM patients, in their relatives with genetic predisposition and in patients with other endocrinopathies. Studies in families of diabetic patients for evaluation of the predictive value of ICAs, detected by the classical method and complement fixation (CF) method, showed that: i) a positive result in CF method is associated with a high predictive value (54 percent); ii) a positive result with the classical ICA method, in conjunction with a negative result with the CF method, is associated with a low predictive value (3 percent); iii) nearly all of the relatives of diabetics with an ICA titer > 80 JDF units progress to develop Type 1 DM.

A screening method of the relatives of Type 1 DM patients, as well as for the general population, would be extremely useful. In order to accomplish this, however, a screening assay that is reliable, reproducible and of low cost is needed. Due to the heterogeneity of humoral autoimmunity in Type 1 DM, it is possible for the assay in pre-diabetic persons to require a series of specific autoantigens. A great deal of effort is expended towards this goal, so that new islet antigens can be detected, which in conjunction with those already existent (GAD, insulin, etc.) would be used in clinical practice.

Antibodies against antigen of 64 kD of glutamic-acid decarboxylase (anti-GAD). Glutamic-acid decarboxylase (GAD) is the enzyme that converts glutamic-acid to the neurotransmitter GABA (γ-aminobutyric acid). Despite the fact that the antigen with molecular weight of 64 kD was known since 1982, only in 1990 was it shown to represent a target for autoantibodies in newly diagnosed Type 1 DM. GAD is mainly encountered in the brain and the β-cells of the pancreatic islets, but also in the peripheral nervous system and other tissues (kidneys, liver, endocrine glands). Two isoforms of GAD have been identified, with molecular weights of 65 kD (GAD65) and 67 kD (GAD67), which are coded by two independent genes. Cloning of both types of genes from human pancreas revealed a 70 percent homology between the isoforms. Although both iso-enzymes are composed in the cytoplasm as hydrophilic and soluble molecules, isoform 65 kD, which is especially ample in the β-cells, is incorporated in the membrane of the cellular synaptic micro-vesicles after a post-translational modulation.

GAD65 is the type that predominates in β-cells. Anti-GAD auto-antibodies are found in 75–85 percent of recently diagnosed Type 1 diabetic cases. Their detection rate is increased with the age at diagnosis and are more frequently encountered in persons positive for the HLA DR3. GAD65, compared to other autoantigens, differs in the fact that it tends to remain positive in the serum of Type 1 DM patients for a longer time after diagnosis of the disease. In newly diagnosed Type 2 DM, anti-islet antibodies are detected in the serum in 10–20 percent of cases, and among them anti-GAD antibodies as well. Frequency of anti-GAD positivity in Type 2 DM patients tends to decrease with increasing age of diagnosis and falls to a rate of 7 percent at ages of 60–65 years. According to relative studies, these patients were not obese, had the highest HbA_{1c} and the lowest insulin secretion. Patients with positive assay for anti-GAD antibodies, to a great extent, need premature initiation of insulin therapy due to secondary failure of oral antidiabetic medicines (usually within the first six years after diagnosis). These patients are obviously slowly progressing Type 1 DM patients, wrongly considered initially as Type 2 (LADA: Latent Autoimmune Diabetes in Adults).

The pathogenetic significance of GAD antibodies is still under investigation. Immune response to GAD can be directly involved in the process of β-cell destruction or can simply present as a surrogate phenomenon produced by the immune stimulation of the partial antigens that are liberated from the destroyed β-cells.

Anti-GAD antibodies are mainly detected in two ways:

1. immunoprecipitation of GAD enzymatic function, found in immuno-precipitating membrane complex of the 64 kD antigen of the islet cells;
2. competitive radioimmunoassay (RIA) by using human recombinant GAD.

With these methods, anti-GAD antibodies (mainly anti-GAD65) are detected in 70–85 percent of newly diagnosed DM patients and in persons who later develop Type 1 DM.

The relatively lower anti-GAD antibody rate of detection (70–85 percent) compared to the rate of anti-64 kD antibody detection (75–96 percent) in patients with newly diagnosed Type 1 DM, implies either a poor sensitivity of the methods that detect anti-GAD antibodies or, most likely, that the 64 kD antigen does not consist solely of GAD. At the same time, experiments of inhibition of ICA fluorescence using GAD from mouse brain showed that the majority of sera from Type 1 DM patients contain ICA identical to anti-GAD, and that some anti-64 kD negative IDDM sera contain ICA directed against other antigens, different to GAD. It should be noted that in Type 1 DM, auto-antibodies against 64 kD/ GAD, contrary to classical ICA, remain in the circulation for a long time after development of the disease.

The production of the recombinant molecule of human GAD constitutes significant progress, and is expected to help towards the development of handy and sensitive assays for population screening, as well as towards a better understanding of the role of the molecule in induction and progression of Type 1 DM.

Antibodies against insulin (IAA).   Insulin has a molecular weight of 5.8 kD, and is produced by the β-cells of the islets of the endocrine pancreas. It is composed of two peptide chains, α and β (21 and 30 amino-acid residues, respectively), produced after the splitting of the connecting part (C-peptide) from the initially formed pre-insulin molecule. After connecting to its receptor on cell surface, insulin promotes glucose entry into the cells, glycogen synthesis, protein synthesis and fat synthesis.

After the discovery that Type 1 DM patients have IAA before the administration of exogenous insulin, lots of studies have been conducted to elucidate the significance of these antibodies in predicting incipient Type 1 DM. Thus, applying RIA and ELISA (enzyme linked immunoassay) methods, it was found that up to 53 percent of newly diagnosed Type 1 DM patients have IAA, whereas they are more widespread in young children, in whom β-cell destruction is faster. Although IAA are generally found in low titers, their appearance, in persons positive for ICA (first degree relatives of Type 1 DM) increases the chance of Type 1 DM development and frequently heralds onset of the disease. Despite the combination of ICA and IAA being exceptionally predictive, IAA on their own have a small predictive value when ICA are negative. As with ICA, IAA titers gradually fall after the clinical diagnosis of Type 1 DM.

The whole evidence, however, supports the view that autoimmune response to insulin is a secondary phenomenon that follows onset of β-cell destruction.

Antibodies against IA-2. The gene for tyrosine phosphatase-2 is located on chromosome 7q36. Its DNA analysis showed that this substance consists of 979 amino-acids that form a transmembrane protein. The function of IA-2 has not been elucidated. Diabetic patients' serum reacts only with the intracellular part of the protein. There are two regions (epitopes) where binding with the antibody takes place: on amino-acids 604-776 (40 percent) and 771-979 (60 percent). Configuration of the molecule in space determines the reaction in a significant degree. It was found that around 65 percent of newly diagnosed Type 1 DM patients have auto-antibodies against IA-2, compared to only 2.5 percent of normal persons. After the first year of diagnosis, the frequency of IA-2 antibody detection starts to decrease. Tyrosine phsosphatase-2 protein could be the target of immune response that destroys the insulin-producing cells. However, IA-2 antibodies could also be a result of β-cell destruction.

In conclusion, one could suggest that autoimmunity in Type 1 DM refers basically to proteins (GAD65, insulin, carboxypeptidase H, IA-2) associated with the secretory vesicles of the β-cells. The first studies in the general population have already shown that, although the individual predictive value of IAA (21 percent), ICA (25 percent) and andtiGAD65 (28 percent) antibodies is relatively low, the combination of all three of them increases the positive predictive value of screening (71 percent). For this reason, the new screening assays for prediction and diagnosis of Type 1 DM will have to comprise an adequate number of antigen-targets of auto-antibodies, so that the classical assay of ICA will finally be able to be substituted. This will enable the massive screening of the population in the future and the application of the proper preventive therapy.

As regards the *mechanism of autoimmune destruction of pancreatic β-cells*, the following mechanisms have been proposed:

- **1st mechanism.** A cell of the organism is attacked by a virus, an amino-acid sequence of which resembles a protein of the β-cell surface, for example GAD (molecular mimicry). The infected cell presents the viral antigen to a cytotoxic T-lymphocyte (CD8+) receptor with the help of HLA class I. The sensitized CD8+ T-lymphocytes are then directed against the antigens and, 'by mistake', due to molecular mimicry, destroy the β-cells.

  At the same time, macrophages that have also phagocytized the virus, present the viral antigen to helper T-lymphocytes (CD4+), with the help of HLA class II. The activated T-lymphocytes stimulate B-lymphocytes to produce antibodies. These antibodies, however, due to molecular similarity as already described, are auto-antibodies and are directed against β-cell proteins. These auto-antibodies help in the destruction of β-cells, but are indices of autoimmunity as well.

- **2nd mechanism.** The pancreatic β-cell is attacked by a virus. The infected cell secretes cytokines and various intermediary substances that contribute to initiation of inflammation. Inflammatory cells are subsequently attracted to the islets and an inflammatory reaction commences. Macrophages phagocytize the virus and then both islet β-cells and macrophages present the viral antigens to the CD8+ and CD4+ lymphocytes respectively. This activates the lymphocytes, and β-cells are destroyed through a cellular and humoral immunologic reaction.

- **3rd mechanism.** It is possible that the pancreatic β-cells are attacked by a slowly-growing virus, causing alterations in cellular proteins. These are then recognized as foreign by the body and finally an immune mechanism is activated that destroys these cells. This is the most likely way that congenital rubella and retroviruses work.

Stage IV: Loss of insulin secretion

The combination of the above mentioned events and stimuli (triggering and accomplishment of the autoimmune destruction of the β-cells in a genetically predisposed individual) leads to a destruction of the β-cells and a final loss of their insulin secretory capacity, with ultimate clinical manifestation of DM.

What is the risk of the offspring of a person who suffers from Type 1 DM developing the disease?

Given the fact that Type 1 DM affects mainly young people, it is understandable that there is a need to prevent development of the disease in the offspring of these people. Evaluation of the risk is based on observations of development of the disease and not on the classical laws of genetics (Table 2.3). The risk of developing Type 1 DM in the offspring of Type 1 diabetic mothers ranges from 0.2–8.0 percent. This

Table 2.3. Relationship of presence of Type 1 DM in the parents with the risk of development of the disease in the offspring, up to the age of 25 years

Possibilities	Disease	Risk (%)
1. Father	**Type 1 DM**	
Mother	Healthy	
1st child	–	6
2. Father	Healthy	
Mother	**Type 1 DM**	
1st child	–	2
3. Father	**Type 1 DM**	
Mother	**Type 1 DM**	
1st child	–	15–20
4. Father	**Type 1 DM**	
Mother	Healthy	
1st child	**Type 1 DM**	
2nd child	–	13
5. Father	Healthy	
Mother	Healthy	
1st child	**Type 1 DM**	
2nd child	–	3–5

rate is corrected on the basis of the predicted age of disease development, since it can present at any age. To begin with, the chance of a Type 1 diabetic mother giving birth to a diabetic child is practically zero. The chance of that child developing Type 1 DM during childhood is around 1 percent, which is higher than the mean of the population, but definitely low. Up to the age of 25 years, the chance is 2–3 percent, and up to the age of 80 years, the chance is 5.6 percent. The literature reports that offspring whose father suffers from Type 1 DM have a greater chance of developing Type 1 DM themselves, compared to those whose mother suffers from Type 1 DM. When the father has Type 1 DM, the chance of the disease in the first child is 2.5 percent and becomes 15–20 percent when the mother also has the disease. The same low risk (3 percent) also applies to the second child of a family whose first child has the disease. However, if both the father and the first child have Type 1 DM, the second child has a 13 percent chance of developing the disease.

When a couple already has a child with Type 1 DM and wishes to know the risk of the second child developing the disease, it can be proposed that they have the HLA system of the children examined. If the genotype of the healthy child is similar to the sick one, then the relative risk of developing the disease is very high (118). If the healthy child has similarity only on one haplotype, the relative risk is 31, whereas if the HLA genotype is different, the risk is insignificant. Unfortunately, there is no preventive therapy for the disease today and, in practice, HLA testing will increase anxiety in the family without being able to offer essential help in most cases (see Chapter 10).

Further reading

Christen, U., Juedes, A., Homann, D., von Herrath, M. (2004) Virally induced inflammation and therapeutic avenues in type 1 diabetes. *Endocrinol Metab Clin N Am*, **33**, 45–58.

Dotta, F. and Eisenbarth, G.S. (1997) Immunopathogenesis of type 1 diabetes in western society, in *International Textbook of Diabetes Mellitus* 2nd edition, (eds K.G.M.M. Alberti, P. Zimmet, R.A. DeFronzo), West Sassex, pp. 97–109.

Eisenbarth, G.S. Immunology of Type 1 Diabetes, in *Type 1 diabetes: molecular, cellular, and clinical immunology* (eds Eisenbarth, G.S., Lafferty, K.J). Barbara Davis Center for Childhood Diabetes, University of Colorado Health Sciences Center [online book]. Available at http://www.uchsc.edu/misc/ diabetes/ eisenbook.html. Accessed January 18, 2004.

Hatziagelaki, E., Jaeger, C., Petzoldt, R., Seissler, J., Scherbaum, W.A., Federlin, K., Bretzel, R.G. (1999) The combination of antibodies to GAD-65 and IA-2ic can replace the islet-cell antibody assay to identify subjects at risk of type 1 diabetes mellitus. *Horm Metab Res*, **31**, 564–9.

Hyoty, H. (2004) Environmental causes: viral causes. *Endocrinol Metab Clin N Am*, **33**, 27–44.

Kawasaki, E., Gill, R., Eisenbarth, G.S. (1999) Type I Diabetes Mellitus in *Endocrine and Organ Specific Autoimmunity*. (ed G. S. Eisenbarth).

Pugliese, A. (2004) Genetics of type 1 diabetes. *Endocrinol Metab Clin N Am*, **33**, 1–16.

Tree, TIM. and Peakman, M. (2004) Autoreactive T cells in human type 1 diabetes. *Endocrinol Metab Clin N Am* **33**, 113–33.

Vaarala, O. (2004) Environmental causes: dietary causes. *Endocrinol Metab Clin N Am*, **33**, 17–26.

3

Pathophysiology of Type 2 diabetes

Konstantinos Makrilakis

What are the main pathophysiologic characteristics of Type 2 diabetes mellitus?

Type 2 diabetes mellitus is a heterogeneous syndrome, with a complex interaction of genetic and environmental factors, which affect multiple phenotypic manifestations in the body, such as insulin secretion and action, pancreatic β-cell mass, distribution of body fat and development of obesity. Type 2 DM is generally characterized by two main pathophysiologic entities: i) resistance to the action of insulin; and ii) insufficient secretion of insulin from the β-cells of the pancreas. Both of these pathophysiologic disturbances (insufficient secretion and peripheral insulin resistance) are thought to be necessary for the development of the disease.

What are the physiologic effects of insulin in the body?

Insulin has multiple and varied metabolic and vascular effects. Traditionally, it has been associated with regulation of glucose metabolism, but in fact it also, equally significantly, affects lipid and protein metabolism and has important effects on the vascular function, on the platelets, the nervous system and the electrolyte equilibrium of the body.

Specifically, insulin regulates glucose metabolism, by promoting glucose intake through insulin-sensitive tissues (muscle cells and cells of the adipose tissue) and by inhibiting hepatic glucose production (it

Diabetes in Clinical Practice: Questions and Answers from Case Studies. Nicholas Katsilambros *et al.*
© 2006 John Wiley & Sons, Ltd.

inhibits glycogenolysis and gluconeogenesis and promotes glycogen-synthesis in the liver). Insulin secretion from pancreatic β-cells is under the direct control of the plasma glucose concentration, which is the main regulator of its secretion: increase in plasma glucose (for example, after a meal) causes an increase in the secretion of insulin and vice versa. The fact that insulin secretion from the pancreas occurs directly into the portal vein and therefore is transferred initially to the liver is very important for the initial decrease/inhibition of glycogenolysis and gluco-neogenesis and promotion of glycogen synthesis in the liver after a meal. It is estimated that about 25–50 percent of an oral glucose load is taken up by the liver (and stored as glycogen), while the rest is distributed mainly in the muscle (80–85 percent) and adipose tissue (10–25 percent). Furthermore, β-cells have various cellular receptors for different pep-tides, hormones and neurotransmitters that can affect insulin secretion, as do various substances inside them (for example, hepatocyte nuclear factors 4-α, 1-α and 1-β, mutations of which are responsible for some of the inherited syndromes of MODY [Maturity Onset Diabetes of the Young]). But even insulin itself, through special insulin receptors on the surface of the β-cells, affects its glucose-dependent secretion (at least in experiments in animals).

The effects of insulin on lipid metabolism are very important: they include stimulation of intravascular lipolysis (through an increase of endothelial lipoprotein lipase activity), promotion of lipogenesis, and inhibition of lipolysis in adipose tissue and inhibition of very-low-density lipoprotein (VLDL) synthesis in the liver.

Insulin also stimulates protein synthesis and transfer of amino-acids into muscle and liver cells. The final effect of all these actions is a decrease in the plasma levels of glucose, triglycerides and free-fatty acids after a meal.

Furthermore, apart from these actions, insulin has significant effects on vascular function and overall body metabolism. It decreases rigidity and stiffness of the large arteries and causes vasodilatation in the smaller peripheral vessels. It inhibits platelet aggregation and their interaction with collagen and regulates autonomic nervous system tone, acting centrally on special receptors in the brain to stimulate sympathetic cardiovascular activity. All of these effects are potentially anti-atherogenic and protective as regards hypertension development. There are, however, also conflicting observations regarding vascular effects of insulin: in experimental studies it was shown that insulin promotes sodium and uric acid re-absorption from the kidneys (contributing to hypertension development), promotes endothelin secretion and secretion of both plasminogen activator as well as plasminogen activator inhibitor-1 (PAI-1). It is believed that the varied degrees of hyperinsulinaemia and insulin resistance in these studies are responsible for these conflicting results.

What is insulin resistance and how is it measured?

Insulin resistance is the inability of insulin to produce its usual biologic effects, at circulating plasma levels that are effective in normal subjects. Insulin resistance is not easy to measure in daily clinical practice. It is estimated clinically only as regards the effects of insulin on carbohydrate metabolism, without taking into consideration its other activities. It is theoretically expressed as the insufficient intake of glucose by the muscles and adipose tissue and by the inability of insulin to suppress hepatic glucose production. Given the fact, as mentioned before, that insulin has multiple and varied effects on whole body metabolism (carbohydrates, lipids, proteins, etc.), and that insulin resistance can develop towards all of these effects (in a degree that varies from person to person, or even occasionally in the same person, it can be seen that it is not correct to focus only on carbohydrate metabolism for the expression of insulin resistance. It is also very possible that many of the phenotypic manifestations of DM can be due both to the presence of insulin resistance to some of its actions (e.g., glucose metabolism) as well as to the increased, unopposed effects of the initial compensatory hyper-insulinaemia on unaffected pathways, where no resistance exists (e.g., protein metabolism, proliferative vascular effects, etc.).

In general, the *euglycaemic hyperinsulinaemic clamp technique* is considered the best for measuring insulin resistance, even though it is technically relatively difficult and demanding. According to its methodology, the rate of intravenous glucose infusion that is necessary to maintain normoglycaemia is measured, while insulin is simultaneously infused intravenously, so that steadily high concentrations of insulin are maintained in the plasma. In this case, the need for a low exogenous glucose infusion rate denotes increased resistance (low sensitivity) to insulin action.

Another method of measuring insulin resistance is the Homeostasis Model Assessment (HOMA) technique, where a specific mathematical formula is used, taking into consideration both fasting insulin and plasma glucose levels:

HOMA-R = [plasma insulin (mU/L) × plasma glucose (mmol/L)]/22.5

This method is much easier, but less reliable, than the first, and is widely used in population studies. Its normal reference values are not precisely established (normal values for HOMA: around 2–3).

There are also some other methods for measuring insulin resistance (intravenous glucose tolerance test, insulin-suppression test, etc.), which are mostly used in research settings.

Which pathophysiologic defect first, but temporally, precedes development of Type 2 DM, insulin resistance or impairment of β-cell secretion?

The natural history of Type 2 DM development is usually characterized by three general stages: i) 'normal glucose tolerance'; ii) 'impaired glucose tolerance'; and iii) 'clinical manifestation of DM'. Plasma insulin levels are generally increased long before clinical development of DM. The fact that this hyperinsulinaemia is observed long before impaired glucose tolerance is manifested, led initially to the belief that impaired insulin secretion develops later, secondary to the existence of resistance to the peripheral action of insulin. It was consequently concluded that insulin resistance always precedes β-cell failure. On the other hand, however, it was observed that many obese, non-diabetic people, with insulin resistance, never develop DM; in addition, many of them never develop impaired glucose tolerance. This clearly shows that the pancreas of these people is able to secrete enough insulin to overcome peripheral resistance. Consequently, insulin resistance is not sufficient in itself to lead to dysfunction, insufficient secretion of the β-cell, and later to DM. The acceptance of this view has been facilitated by experimental studies in animals, where mice with induced disruption of certain genes that caused marked insulin resistance to them, never developed diabetes, in the absence of a simultaneous independent insulin secretory β-cell defect.

It seems, therefore, that both of these pathophysiologic disturbances act simultaneously and separately, both on peripheral tissues and the pancreas and are, in most cases, both necessary for diabetes development.

Type 2 DM can thus be considered a consequence of an inability of the pancreatic β-cells adequately to increase their insulin output in order to compensate for the resistance of the peripheral tissues to its actions. It is deemed certain today that these two pathophysiologic defects are subject to both genetic (mainly) and environmental (obesity – intracellular lipid accumulation) influences, which sometimes renders the exact determination of the aetiology of diabetes in a certain person extremely difficult. About 10 percent of the patients who initially seem to be suffering from Type 2 DM, have in fact a delayed form of autoimmune Type 1 DM (called Type 1.5 diabetes or LADA [Latent Autoimmune Diabetes in Adults]). This type is characterized by the presence of auto-antibodies against the pancreas and a faster failure of its insulin secretory capacity, compared to the classic Type 2 DM. Furthermore, an additional proportion (up to 5 percent) of the phenotypically evident Type 2 DM patients, actually have some kind of the dominantly, autosomally inherited, monogenic syndromes MODY (Maturity Onset Diabetes of the Young). Another approximately 1 percent have some rare genetic mutation of the insulin receptor or of one of the components of the cataract of reactions that insulin binding to its receptor on the cell surface activates. The rest (about 85 percent of the patients) have what we call classical Type 2 DM, with the two pathophysiologic disturbances, already mentioned above. Impaired insulin secretion from the β-cell is considered by many investigators to be the primary genetic disturbance leading to Type 2 DM, and insulin resistance to be the primary acquired defect. In general, the available evidence today favours the view that impaired insulin secretion precedes insulin resistance in those people who finally develop Type 2 DM.

What is the cause of peripheral insulin resistance?

Insulin resistance is strongly related to obesity, especially the central distribution of body fat (abdominal or visceral obesity). The fact that more than 80 percent of diabetics are obese led to the opinion that obesity is most likely the main cause of insulin resistance in DM. Studies, however, both in humans and animals, have shown that insulin resistance is basically associated with intramyocellular triglyceride concentration (as assessed by muscle biopsies or nuclear magnetic spectroscopy) and not that well associated with the degree of obesity, as determined by body mass index. 'Shifting' of lipid deposition from adipose tissue (where it should normally be) to other non-adipose areas (muscle cells, liver, etc), therefore seems to play a very important role in the development of insulin resistance. The role of the central (visceral) distribution of fat is probably related to the increased lipolytic activity of the visceral fat (due to its enhanced adrenergic activity and increased insulin resistance compared to peripheral fat), which leads to increased availability of free fatty acids in the periphery for deposition in non-adipose tissues. The exact molecular mechanism that leads to this result has not been completely elucidated; it seems to be complex and multi-variable, and involves multiple sites in the cataract of intracellular reactions that binding of insulin to its cell-surface receptor causes (decreased activation of insulin receptor substrate-1 [IRS-1], phosphati-dylinositol kinase-3 [PI-3 kinase], translocation of glucose transporters-4 [Glut-4] to the cellular membrane, etc.). Recent studies in insulin resistant offspring of diabetic patients show that this defect of intramyo-cellular fatty acid metabolism is probably due to an inherited mitochon-drial dysfunction of oxidative phosphorylation in these people. Disturbances in the recently discovered adipose tissue hormones (resis-tin, adiponectin, tumour necrosis factor-α [TNF-α]) seem to be involved in the development of insulin resistance as well.

Is insulin resistance genetically predetermined or is it due to environmental influences?

Studies in populations at high risk for the development of Type 2 DM have shown that a strong genetic predisposition exists for the develop-ment of insulin resistance, as is the case for the development of Type 2 DM in general, as well. It seems that heritable differences in insulin sensitivity may be one element of the 'susceptibility genotype' predis-posing members of these high-risk populations to Type 2 DM. Further evidence for genetic influences in the development of insulin resistance is derived from twin studies, demonstrating hereditary effects, estimated to range from 47–66 percent. Whether this heritability depends on obesity, however, is unclear. Type 2 DM is considered to be a polygenic disorder and heritable influences are likely to involve alterations in several genes. To date, no genetic defect has been found in patients with typical Type 2 DM that might cause their diabetes to be due solely to insulin resistance. Cases of monogenic heritable Type 2 DM syndromes involve mutations in genes that cause decreased secretion of the β-cell (MODY syndromes), whereas mutations involving the insulin receptor are exceptionally rare causes of DM. Nevertheless, research in this field of molecular biology-genetics continues intensely in large research centres worldwide, and there are already several studies for some candidate genes (for example, the nuclear receptor PPARγ, insulin receptor substrates, PPARγ coactivator-1 [PGC-1], etc.), which may finally demonstrate existence of a genetic defect in the development of insulin resistance.

Furthermore, the epidemiologic correlation of insulin resistance development with environmental factors, mainly intra-abdominal obesity (a consequence of a modern high-fat, high-energy diet and sedentary lifestyle) is very strong. Central adiposity appears to be a major determinant of insulin resistance, not only in obese individuals, but also in apparently healthy, non-obese persons who have evidence of increased abdominal fat, as assessed by special techniques (NMR spectroscopy, etc.). In obese patients with Type 2 DM, weight loss alone is able, in many cases, to normalize insulin sensitivity and improve glycaemic control. Moreover, it can prevent the progression to DM in high-risk populations (including patients with impaired glucose tolerance), proving the significant contribution of this environmental factor to the development of insulin resistance/diabetes. These observations suggest therefore that insulin resistance is most likely not to be the result of specific gene defects (at least there is no strong genetic influence) but rather is simply due to obesity (with the reservation, of course, of possible hereditary predisposition for obesity development, an issue not yet completely clarified).

What is the role of impaired β-cell insulin secretion in Type 2 DM development?

Although the majority of Type 2 diabetics manifest insulin resistance (around 90–92 percent), Type 2 DM can actually occur even in the absence of insulin resistance. Furthermore, as already mentioned, many people with insulin resistance never develop DM, because their pancreatic β-cells are able to secrete enough insulin to compensate for the peripheral resistance to its action. Consequently, insulin resistance is insufficient, by itself, to cause diabetes. Type 2 DM development necessarily requires the existence of impaired insulin secretion from the β-cell. This impaired insulin secretory ability is present for many years before the clinical manifestation of DM. Even diabetics with insulin resistance who, at the early stages of the course of the disease (before DM develops), manifest compensatory hyperinsulinaemia to overcome increased peripheral resistance, have actually been shown to have decreased insulin secretion relative to the degree of peripheral insulin resistance.

How does insulin secretion from the β-cell occur?

Insulin is a peptide hormone, composed of two chains, α and β (with a total of 51 amino-acid residues – 30 and 21 in each chain, respectively). It is produced in the pancreatic β-cells – specialized cells inside special cellular aggregates in the pancreas, called islets of Langerhans. These islets also contain other types of cells that produce various hormones, such as glucagon (α-cells), somatostatin (δ-cells) and pancreatic poly-peptide (PP cells), which communicate with each other via a neurovas-cular net of arterioles and autonomous nerves. Initially, insulin is composed of pre-pro-insulin (Figure 3.1) in the ribosomes of the rough endoplasmic reticulum, to be quickly converted to pro-insulin (a mixture of insulin and C-peptide), after the splitting of a small part from the molecule. Pro-insulin is transferred to the Golgi apparatus of the cell, where it is stored in special secretory granules and remains in this form inside the cytoplasm of the cell until a stimulus for secretion is applied to the granules. It is then split into equimolar quantities of insulin and C-peptide (connecting peptide) and is excreted from the cell (via exocytosis), with only a small quantity (around 10–15 percent) normally secreted as pro-insulin. The Pancreas produces and secretes insulin constantly, the whole 24 hours (basal, non-stimulated secretion), in a pulsatile way, every about 9–14 minutes. This basal secretion aims at regulating hepatic glucose production (glycogenolysis –gluconeogenesis), which in the case of insulin shortage (total or partial) remains unopposed (it is the main cause of fasting hyperglycaemia in DM). The basic stimulus for insulin secretion, however, is plasma glucose concentration after a meal. The β-cell is able to 'measure' plasma glucose concentration constantly and change insulin secretion accordingly. This coupling of

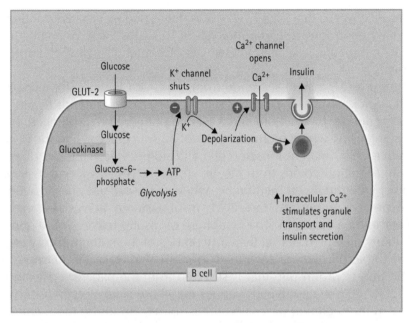

Figure 3.1. Coupling of blood glucose with insulin secretion from the pancreatic β-cell (Reprinted from Textbook of Diabetes, 3rd edn., J. Pickup & G. Williams, Copyright 2003, with permission from Blackwell Science Ltd.)

plasma glucose concentration with insulin secretion is achieved through the ability of glucose to enter the β-cell freely (with the help of special glucose-transporters [GLUT2]), subsequently oxidize itself in the mitochondria and produce energy in the form of ATP. The increased intracellular concentration of ATP causes special potassium channels on the cell-surface to close, which leads to depolarization of the cell-membrane and opening of special calcium channels of the cell-membrane. Intracellular calcium concentration increases (because of the entry of calcium into the cell) and causes exocytosis of the vesicles with the stored insulin (Figure 3.1).

Various substances that are secreted by the intestine after the entry of food in it, the so-called *incretins* (glucagon like peptide-1 [GLP-1] and gastric inhibitory polypeptide or glucose-dependent insulinotropic peptide [GIP]) also seem to play a very significant role in post-prandial production and secretion of insulin. These substances, in a sense, notify the pancreas about the forthcoming entry of glucose into the circulation after a meal and promote both production and secretion of insulin. Since it was discovered that mainly GLP-1 is decreased in Type 2 DM, there is currently enormous research interest for this substance, or analogues of it, for therapeutic use in DM (see also Chapter 29 'New therapies in diabetes').

After a meal, insulin secretion from the β-cell is biphasic: there is an acute, quick (around 5–6 minutes) first phase (which intends to suppress hepatic glucose production) and a second phase, more prolonged, but of lower intensity, which promotes entry of plasma glucose into the insulin-sensitive cells, mainly muscle cells and adipocytes. The first phase of insulin secretion comes from insulin stored in vesicles found near or in contact with the β-cell membrane, whereas the second phase is derived from newly synthesized insulin or insulin stored in vesicles that are deeper in the cytoplasm. The first phase of insulin release is the one that is initially disrupted during the early phases of the natural history of DM (from impaired glucose tolerance to overt diabetes). Furthermore, the proportion of pro-insulin that is secreted from the pancreas rises in DM (up to 30–40 percent), which implies that there is possibly a disturbance either in the secretion or in the process of insulin inside the β-cell.

Apart from glucose, which as mentioned is the most significant stimulus for insulin secretion, an increase in circulating levels of amino-acids, free fatty acids and the gastrointestinal hormones GLP-1 and GIP also promote insulin secretion. In contrast, an increase of other factors, such as catecholamines, cortisol, growth hormone, leptin and tumour necrosis factor-α, decreases insulin secretion.

What is the cause of the impaired secretory ability of the β-cell in Type 2 DM?

The exact aetiology of impaired β-cell secretory ability is not completely elucidated, despite the large number of studies in animals and humans. Specific causes of impaired function can be a decrease in β-cell mass, an increased apoptosis/decreased regeneration of the β-cells, exhaustion of the β-cells secondary to compensatory hyperinsulinaemia (a consequence of long-term peripheral insulin resistance), glucotoxicity and/or lipotoxicity in the pancreas and amyloid deposition in large quantities inside the pancreatic cell. According to findings from the UKPDS (United Kingdom Prospective Diabetes Study), β-cell function was already decreased by 50 percent at the time of diagnosis of Type 2 DM and continued to deteriorate during the following years. Usual defects involve a decrease or absence of the first phase of insulin secretion in response to an intravenous glucose challenge, a decreased response to eating mixed meals, alterations in the pulsatile basal insulin secretion, a decrease in the second phase of insulin secretion, defective responsiveness of the β-cell to insulin-secretory stimuli other than glucose and an increase in the proportion of pro-insulin secretion. Recent studies have proven that β-cell mass is actually decreased in Type 2 DM and this is due to an increase in apoptosis (death) of the β-cells and not to decreased regeneration of the cells. The fact, however, that β-cell mass is decreased by only 20–30 percent in overt DM cannot explain the approximate 80 percent reduction in the functional capacity of the β-cell. This indicates the significance of functional disturbances in the secretory capacity of the β-cell and not simply a decrease in the number of the cells. This decreased mass and functionality of the β-cells precedes the clinical manifestation of DM and is evident even at the stage of pre-diabetes (impaired fasting glucose [IFG] and/or impaired glucose tolerance [IGT]). When β-cell mass decreases below a certain critical level and insulin production cannot compensate for the peripheral needs, hyperglycaemia ensues. A decrease in β-cell function by about 60 percent, in combination with existence of peripheral insulin resistance, is sufficient to cause hyperglycaemia.

This reduced functionality (qualitative and quantitative) of the β-cell is considered to be (as mentioned already) genetically predetermined, although the responsible genes have not yet been determined. Recent studies show that the increased apoptosis of the β-cells at the stage of overt DM is due to amyloid deposition inside the cells and to the effect of environmental factors (hyperglycaemia [glucotoxicity] and dyslipidaemia [lipotoxicity]) on β-cell function. In fact, a series of studies show that prolonged exposure of cultured human islets to high glucose levels and to saturated fatty acids increase β-cell apoptosis in a dose-dependent manner. However, monounsaturated fatty acids seem not to affect adversely islet function and their presence blunts the harmful effects of saturated fatty acids on the β-cell. Nevertheless, although increased apoptotic activity of the β-cells at the stage of overt DM can be explained (by gluco- and lipo-toxicity), it remains unclear what underlies the apoptotic loss of β-cells at the stage of pre-diabetes, before hyperglycaemia and dyslipidaemia ensues. The occurrence of apoptosis in patients with IFG suggests an inherent defect of the β-cell function, presumably of hereditary aetiology, in those people who are predisposed to later develop DM.

Delayed growth during endometrial or first infantile period has also been associated with increased chance of Type 2 DM development later in life, especially in those people who will become obese in their adulthood. It is thought that poor nutrition during endometrial life 'programmes' the β-cell to have reduced responsiveness on extracellular glucose concentrations and leads later to increased apoptosis, especially if insulin resistance develops, as is the case with obesity. However, the fact that DM does not develop in all persons with delayed endometrial growth implies that this element is only one of the events that ultimately lead to disease occurrence.

What is the natural history of Type 2 DM development?

At the early stages of DM development (in the pre-diabetic stage, before occurrence of fasting hyperglycaemia) there is usually hyperinsulinaemia in absolute values (i.e., higher plasma insulin levels compared to non-diabetics), in combination with increased resistance to the action of insulin. These elevated insulin concentrations are considered an augmented reactive response of the pancreas to peripheral insulin resistance and not a real primary hyper-function of the pancreas (in fact, the pancreas of the diabetic person is always functionally deficient, at every stage of DM evolution, compared to a normal pancreas). This relative hyper-function of the pancreas is able to maintain glucose levels (both fasting and post-prandial) in the normal range, for many years. These people's β-cell is genetically predetermined, though, to fail. Thus, gradually, insulin secretory ability deteriorates, which results in an inability of the β-cell to compensate for the increased peripheral needs. Thus, hyperglycaemia ensues, initially only post-prandially (it can be revealed with an oral glucose tolerance test – stage of impaired glucose tolerance [IGT]) and later in the fasting state as well (impaired fasting glucose [IFG] and overt DM), with emergence of the characteristic clinical manifestations of the disease.

Insulin resistance remains generally steady over time (unless the person loses weight and/or increases his or her physical activity, in which case insulin resistance decreases), whereas β-cell functional impairment unfortunately steadily deteriorates over time (regardless of therapy – medicines or diet). Thus, the final result for many patients with

Type 2 DM is that they will need insulin for blood sugar control, a few years after the disease commences (usually 6–15 years).

CASE STUDY 1

A 57 year old obese man (BMI: 32 kg/m², hypertensive for ten years, with positive family history of Type 2 DM in his father, presents with a few months' history of polyuria, polydipsia, polyphagia and easy fatiguability. A random blood sugar measurement reveals a level of 350 mg/dl (19.4 mmol/L) and HbA$_{1c}$ 10.2 percent. What type of diabetes does this man have?

This patient phenotypically has classical Type 2 DM, with positive family history, obesity, hypertension (i.e., components of the metabolic syndrome – see Chapter 16: 'Macroangiopathy in diabetes') and development of the disease at a relatively old age. It is very likely that the patient has insulin resistance (owing to his obesity) and reduced secretory ability of the β-cell relative to his level of peripheral insulin resistance (which explains why hyperglycaemia developed). It is also very likely that the patient already has or will develop in the future dyslipidaemia (see Chapter 23), given the frequent abnormal lipid metabolism that accompanies poor glycaemic control in DM.

CASE STUDY 2

A 14 year old thin man, without any significant past medical history and with no positive family history for DM, is transferred to the Emergency Department of the hospital in a comatose state. His breath is ketotic and his blood sugar level is 850 mg/dl (47.2 mmol/L). Diabetic ketoacidosis is diagnosed. His recent medical history reveals that he had lost about 8 kg (17.6 lb) during the last two months and had experienced polyuria, nocturia and intense thirst during the same time period. What type of DM does this patient have?

This patient manifests the classical picture of Type 1 DM presentation: acute decompensation and manifestation of ketoacidosis in a young, thin person (usual age of Type 1 DM development is 5–6 or 13–15 years of age). Also, a positive family history of DM is usually lacking. This patient needs insulin administration immediately and continuance for the rest of his life in order to survive, because of total lack of insulin secretion from his pancreas.

CASE STUDY 3

A 47 year old man of normal weight (BMI: 22 kg/m²), with no family history of DM, normotensive and with no other medical problems so far in his life,

presents with symptoms compatible with diabetes (polyuria, polydipsia and slight weight loss), during the previous two months. A random blood sugar is 380 mg/dl (21.1 mmol/l), without ketosis. His HbA$_{1c}$ is 9.5 percent. What type of DM does this patient have?

The type of DM in this patient is not easily immediately identifiable. Age at onset is more compatible with Type 2 DM; it is well known, however, that a proportion of up to 25 percent of Type 1 DM can present at an old age (> 35 years old). The fact also that he can tolerate blood sugar levels > 350 mg/dl (19.4 mmol/L) without development of ketoacidosis, implies that he does not have a total lack of insulin. The fact that he is thin (normal BMI) and has no family history of DM, are more compatible with Type 1 DM (it should be noted that hereditary factors are more pronounced in Type 2 rather than in Type 1 DM). Chances are that the patient has either Type 1 DM with delayed onset (type LADA [Latent Autoimmune Diabetes in Adults]) or Type 2 DM (decreased secretion of insulin with or without insulin resistance): despite the fact that he is not obese, insulin resistance can still be present, since it is associated with the presence of increased intramyocellular lipid accumulation – which is difficult to elucidate in daily clinical practice and not well predicted by the BMI).

Management of this patient can in practice be achieved in two ways: first, we can start treatment for possible Type 2 DM with oral antidiabetic medicines (insulin secretagogues [sulfonylurea or meglitinides] and medicines that improve insulin resistance [metformin, glitazones]), and wait to see the response (how quickly he needs insulin treatment). Second, we can measure specific auto-antibodies against components of the pancreas (anti-GAD65, anti-islet cell auto-antibodies [ICA], anti-insulin auto-antibodies [IAA] and anti-IA2 antibodies), which are positive in a great proportion of Type 1 diabetics (including LADA patients) at the time of diagnosis and remain positive for 3–4 years after onset of the disease (see Chapter 2). Positivity for the auto-antibodies will increase the clinical suspicion for LADA and will imply that this patient needs to start insulin much faster that the classic Type 2 diabetic patient (usually within 3–5 years as against 6–15 years, which is typical for classic Type 2 DM).

CASE STUDY 4

A 19 year old woman, of normal weight, with positive family history of DM in her father and grandfather (with onset of the disease at a young age in both)

manifests, at a medical check up, mild hyperglycaemia (blood sugar: 155 mg/dl [8.6 mmol/L]). This is confirmed in repeated measurements. No ketoacidosis is ever present. What type of DM does this patient have?

The positive family history of DM, with a young age at onset in two generations, implies the presence of some hereditary type of DM. The age of disease onset in this patient, the mildness of hyperglycaemia, with no ketoacidosis, are also in favour of the view that this is not a classic Type 1 DM case. It is very likely that this is one of the autosomally inherited syndromes of DM (type MODY [Maturity Onset Diabetes of the Young]), which account for around 1–5 percent of cases of Type 2 DM. Up to date, six different types of MODY have been described, which are due to mutations of specific genes (see Chapter 1, Table 1.2). The clinical characteristics that separate MODY patients from those with classic Type 2 DM, are the positive family history of DM in two, or rather, three generations back (with disease onset at a young age, usually less than 25 years), the young age at disease onset of the affected person and lack of obesity. Diabetes mellitus is caused by a β-cell dysfunction, due to a mutation of a gene that alters β-cell function (insulin levels are frequently normal, but lower for the level of the patient's hyperglycaemia). The most common cause of MODY is a mutation in the transcription factor *hepatocyte nuclear factor-1a* (*HNF-1α, MODY 3*), which accounts for around 69 percent of MODY cases. The second most frequent cause is a mutation in the *glucokinase gene* (MODY 2, frequency 14 percent). The rest of the mutations of the transcription factors (see Chapter 1, Table 1.2) are rarer (up to 3 percent of MODY cases). Treatment of patients with these syndromes is usually with dietary advice or oral antidiabetic medications (due to the usually mild hyperglycaemia), and only very rarely is insulin needed.

The practical approach to the present patient would be either to send a specimen for DNA analysis in a specialized laboratory for possible genetic diagnosis of one of these syndromes or better – which will be necessary anyhow – to place the patient under close monitoring, with self measurements of blood glucose at home and frequent office visits. This is necessary in order to monitor the course of the disease and decide the need for intervention or not (with medicines, insulin or diet alone), given the fact that the various MODY syndromes have a variable severity and course.

Further reading

Creutzfeldt, W. (2001) The entero-insular axis in type 2 diabetes – incretins as therapeutic agents. *Exp Clin Endocrinol Diabetes*, **109**(Suppl 2), S288–S303.

Fajans, S.S., Bell, G.I., Polonsky, K.S. (2001) Molecular mechanisms and clinical pathophysiology of maturity-onset diabetes of the young. *N Engl J Med*, **345**, 971–80.

Yki-Jarvinen, H. (2003) Insulin resistance in type 2 diabetes, in *Textbook of Diabetes*, 3rd edn (eds J. Pickup and G. Williams) Blackwell Science Ltd, Oxford, **22**, pp. 1–19.

Gerich, J.E. and Smith. T.S. (2003) B-cell defects and pancreatic abnormalities in type 2 diabetes, in *Textbook of Diabetes*, 3rd edn, (eds J. Pickup and G. Williams) Blackwell Science Ltd, Oxford, **23**, pp. 1–11.

Matthews, D.R., Cull, C.A., Stratton, I.M., Holman, R.R., Turner, R.C. (1998) UK Prospective Diabetes Study (UKPDS) Group. UKPDS 26: sulphonylurea failure in non-insulin-dependent diabetic patients over six years. *Diabet Med*, **15**, 297–303.

Vionnet, N., Stoffel, M., Takeda, H. *et al.* (1992) Nonsense mutation in the glucokinase gene causes early onset non-insulin-dependent diabetes mellitus. *Nature*, **356**, 721–22.

4

Glycaemic control

Stavros Liatis

What is the role of blood glucose self-monitoring with a glucose meter, in persons with Type 1 DM?

Treatment of choice in most patients with Type 1 DM is intensive insulin therapy, which includes a daily (usually before sleep) injection of basal insulin (slow or medium release), and injections of rapid-acting insulin or rapid-acting insulin analogues before meals. Basal insulin dose is determined by fasting blood sugar level (mainly in the morning) whereas pre-prandial doses are determined by the patients themselves, based on meal carbohydrate content and pre-prandial capillary blood glucose levels.

When intensive insulin therapy is used (see Chapter 28), the patient must necessarily be taught the technique of self-monitoring of blood glucose (SMBG) at home, with a portable glucose meter. Sporadic determination of glucose values is not enough. Glucose values in patients with Type 1 DM vary widely within a 24-hour period. Self-monitoring of blood glucose has been found to improve glycaemic control and constitutes a basic requirement of an intensive insulin regimen. At the same time, the patient is able to monitor disease course and effectiveness of therapy, based on target glucose levels. Blood glucose measurements are useful for prevention and treatment of possible hypoglycaemia, especially in people with reduced hypoglycaemia awareness. Programming and executing physical activities is also facilitated to a great extent by SMBG.

Frequency and timing of SMBG is individualized. Every patient who follows an intensive insulin regimen, either with multiple insulin

Diabetes in Clinical Practice: Questions and Answers from Case Studies. Nicholas Katsilambros *et al.*
© 2006 John Wiley & Sons, Ltd.

injections or with an insulin pump, should measure his or her blood sugar levels at least four times daily. The most important measurements are the pre-prandial and the one before bed-time. Additional measurements are recommended when control is not desirable, in hypoglycaemia, in states of stress (acute disease, trauma, etc.), when hyperglycaemia symptoms emerge, before beginning physical activities, at suspicion of Somogyi or Dawn phenomena and at the discretion of the patient. Sporadic post-prandial measurements (1–2 hours after a meal) are also recommended to evaluate post-prandial glycaemia, although this is reflected, to some degree, in the next pre-prandial blood glucose measurement.

Persons with Type 1 DM who do not follow an intensive insulin regimen should also monitor their blood glucose levels daily. In this case measurements could be less than four. Urine glucose evaluation with special reagent-strips is not preferred in Type 1 DM. In contrast, urine ketone determination can be useful in some cases. Specifically, it is recommended in cases of an acute disease, in pregnancy, and when symptoms of ketoacidosis (nausea, vomiting, abdominal pain) occur. Commercial strips are based on nitroprusside reaction, which gives an intense purple-reddish colour. It should be noted that these strips detect only acetoacetic acid and (when they contain glycine) acetone, but not β-hydroxybutyric acid, which is the most abundant ketone body in the case of ketoacidosis. The test can give falsely positive results when the patient uses medicines with a sulfhydryl group (like captopril), and false negative results when the strips stay in the atmosphere for a long time. In recent years, the ability to measure β-hydroxybutyrate in the blood with certain portable glucose meters and special commercial reagent strips has been developed. More studies are needed to evaluate their usefulness compared to classical methods of self-control.

The patient's measurements are usually recorded in an ad lib or specially constructed diary (Table 4.1). Information from this diary can be used, both by the patient and/or the caring physician, to make appropriate alterations in the medical treatment to achieve the best possible metabolic control.

Most patients rely only on the meter's memory (most modern meters are able to store more than 100 measurements), which they bring to the physician's office. However, this means that the ability to compare older values is lost. Some meters are accompanied by a special software

Table 4.1. Self-monitor blood glucose diary in patient with Type 1 diabetes and indicative measurements marked with X

Date	Breakfast– Preprandial	Breakfast– Postprandial	Lunch– Preprandial	Lunch– Postprandial	Dinner– Preprandial	Before bedtime Notes
Friday	X	X	X		X	X
Saturday	X	X	X	X	X	
Sunday	X		X	X	X	X

program that enables connection to a computer and storage of the data in special programs for recording and statistical analysis.

What is the role of blood glucose self-monitoring with a glucose meter, in persons with Type 2 DM?

The role of SMBG in Type 2 DM has not been precisely determined. All of the recent reviews and meta-analyses have failed to prove that SMBG is associated with an improvement in glycaemic control. Only a few isolated studies have indicated that this relation exists. Newer, better-planned, prospective studies are needed to clarify the role of SMBG in Type 2 DM.

It should also be emphasized that in recent years glycaemic targets have become increasingly stricter, and thus glucose and HbA_{1c} values as close as possible to the normal range are now recommended. It is believed that achievement of these targets requires activation and participation of the patients themselves, so their education is consi- dered indispensable in their treatment regimen. Educated and trained patients can capitalize on the advantages that SMBG offers in a much better way than those who simply passively measure their blood sugar at home.

Today, regular SMBG with a portable meter at home is advised to all patients with Type 2 DM who use insulin, albeit not that frequently as in persons with Type 1 DM. In people using sulfonylureas of meglitinides, SMBG with a portable meter at home is possibly useful, especially at the beginning of therapy, when the dose of a medicine is changed or during periods of acute disease. In persons whose DM is controlled only on diet and remain on a steadily good control, SMBG with a portable meter has not been evaluated and its significance is unknown.

How often should Type 2 diabetics measure their blood glucose levels with a portable meter?

Patients with Type 2 DM do not have the high variability of blood glucose values that Type 1 patients have. Consequently, as already mentioned, much fewer measurements are needed to evaluate blood sugar control. When SMBG is recommended by the treating physician, the precise frequency and timing of the measurements is individualized, depending on the type of therapy, drug doses, achievement or not of glycaemic targets and training of the patients. In those using insulin, SMBG should be daily. In the not so frequent case that the patient uses an intensive insulin regimen, measurements should follow the same pattern as in Type 1 DM. Regardless of the frequency of measurements, determination of some post-prandial values (two hours after a meal) is considered essential, especially in cases where fasting blood sugar values are not compatible with HbA_{1c} values.

Could glycaemic control be based on urine glucose determination?

Glucose is freely filtered by renal glomeruli and completely reabsorbed in the proximal convoluted tubules. When, however, glucose concentration in the plasma exceeds approximately 180 mg/dl (10.0 mmol/L), tubular reabsorption is incomplete. Thus, glucose concentration in the urine is proportional to the increase of glucose in the plasma above 180 mg/dl (10.0 mmol/L).

There are special reagent strips used for detection of glucose in the urine. However, this method of glycaemic control evaluation, although simple, painless and cheap, has some major disadvantages:

- Renal threshold varies among people (even within the same person); as a consequence, when the threshold is high, people with significant hyperglycaemia can exhibit no glucosuria (for example, patients with long-standing diabetes), and when the threshold is low, glucosuria can be present even in persons with normal blood glucose values (for example, children and pregnant women).
- Renal threshold increases with age.
- Renal threshold is affected by the body's hydration status.
- Glucose concentration in the urine does not represent glycaemia at the time of determination.

- Even if renal threshold were to be steady at a level of 180 mg/dl (10.0 mmol/L), glucose determination in the urine would not be able to discern between hypoglycaemia, normoglycaemia and mild hyperglycaemia.

For all these reasons, self monitoring of glucose in the urine is now indicated only for persons who refuse or are unable to use a portable glucose meter for home capillary blood glucose measurements. It could only be accepted for persons with mild and controlled Type 2 DM, who do not receive insulin, and perform regular measurements of plasma glucose and HbA_{1c} at a laboratory.

What is glycosylated haemoglobin and when should it be measured?

Glycosylated (glycated) haemoglobin is formed during the non-enzymatic reaction of glucose with some amino-acid residues of haemoglobin. The fraction of haemoglobin HbA_1, called HbA_{1c}, is predominately measured. This fraction is formed when glucose is bound to amino-acid valine, at the amino-terminal end of one or both β-chains of the haemoglobin molecule.

HbA_{1c} rate of composition is mainly dependent on the glucose concentrations that plasma red blood cells are 'exposed' to. HbA_{1c} is a reliable index of glycaemia for the previous 120 days, which corresponds to the duration of life of red blood cells (Table 4.2). However, it should

Table 4.2. Mean plasma glucose values and respective HbA_{1c} values

MPG–mg/dl (mmol/L)	HbA_{1c} (%)
65 (3.6)	4
100 (5.6)	5
135 (7.5)	6
170 (9.4)	7
205 (11.4)	8
240 (13.3)	9
275 (15.3)	10
310 (17.2)	11
MPG: Mean plasma glucose values	

be noted that glycaemia during the 3–5 weeks preceding the HbA_{1c} measurement contributes much more (around 50 percent) to the formation of HbA_{1c} values, compared to the glucose values 90–120 days before HbA_{1c} determination. That explains the relatively fast change in the HbA_{1c} value when there is a significant change in glycaemia.

According to the large landmark studies in DM, by DCCT (in Type 1 DM) and UKPDS (in Type 2 DM), HbA_{1c} value is a measure of the risk for the development of microvascular complications in diabetes. HbA_{1c} should be determined in all diabetic patients, both at diagnosis of the disease as well as during follow-up, in order to evaluate effectiveness of therapy. Measurement should be repeated every three months. For evaluation of glycaemic control of a patient, both blood glucose values from SMBG (for patients using a portable glucose meter at home) and HbA_{1c} values are appreciated. HbA_{1c} represents the most reliable element of the two and is additionally used to evaluate the precision and reliability of the patient's measurements.

How reliable is the determination of HbA_{1c}?

The biggest problem with HbA_{1c} measurement is the fact that both reference values and a given value of a blood sample may differ significantly among various laboratories. In recent years, principally in the USA but in other countries as well, a serious effort of standardization of the various methods has started, using the method used in the DCCT as a reference. There are, however, technical problems that persist, and it is hoped that development of newer methods of determination will permanently solve them. For these reasons, it should be emphasized that HbA_{1c} determination should not be used for diagnosis of DM.

More than 30 methods for HbA_{1c} determination currently exist, based mainly on two principles. The first principle refers to the reduction of the positive charge of the haemoglobin molecule, brought about by glycosylation. The methods of ion-exchange chromatography – the with most significant representative being High Performance Liquid Chromatography (HPLC) that was used in DCCT and UKPDS – are based on this principle. The second principle refers to the detection of alterations in the structure of haemoglobin, brought about by the presence of glucose. The methods of affinity chromatography and some that use antibody reactions (immunoassays) are based on this principle.

Affinity chromatography methods determine the whole glycosylated haemoglobin and report the result either as total GHb or as corrected equivalent of HbA_{1c}.

Which factors can affect the HbA_{1c} value?

Any condition that reduces the duration of life of the red blood cells or their mean life-span (haemolytic anaemias or an acute haemorrhage), leads to falsely low HbA_{1c} levels, regardless of the method used for its determination. Hypertriglyceridaemia, uraemia, elevated bilirubin and alcoholism have been reported to influence chromatography methods, resulting in falsely elevated HbA_{1c} values. Haemoglobinopathies affect some of the methods regardless of their effect on red blood cells' life span. The results can be false elevations or false decreases, depending on the method used and haemoglobinopathy present. Ion-exchange chromatography methods are affected more, and immunoassays and affinity chromatography methods, less. Nevertheless, most abnormal haemoglobins are recognized during chromatography and their presence should be reported in the result. Fetal haemoglobin (HbF) co-chromatographs with HbA_1 and consequently, when increased (as is the case mainly in homozygous β-thalassaemia and much less so in heterozygous), it falsely elevates HbA_{1c} values in some ion-exchange chromatography methods. Immunoassays are not affected when HbF is < 5 percent, but at higher levels it can give falsely low values. Affinity chromatography methods are not affected by an increase in HbF. Haemoglobins S and C (HbS and HbC, found in sickle cell anaemia) falsely lower HbA_{1c} levels.

When there is suspicion of false results due to a haemoglobinopathy, HbA_{1c} determination should be repeated using an alternative method. If the result is still considered unreliable, it is possible to use the fructosamine method, which also determines glycosylated serum proteins (mainly albumin). Since the mean lifespan of serum proteins is 17 days, fructosamine determines glycaemic control of the previous 2–3 weeks. It should be emphasized though that fructosamine determination is also affected by conditions like hyperuricaemia, hypertriglyceridaemia and haemolysis. It is also affected by albumin concentrations. Fructosamine determination is not a very well standardized method and there are no studies associating it with DM complications. Improvement of HbA_{1c} determination methods has rendered fructosamine determination minimally popular.

CASE STUDY 1

A 72 years old woman with a 15 year history of Type 2 DM, treated with insulin NPH, 24 units in the morning and 14 units in the evening, presented for the first time in the Diabetes Clinic for evaluation. She reported that during the last six months she had been having 'unexpectedly' high blood sugar values in her SMBG measurements. Her weight has been steady (BMI: 29.5 kg/m^2). She reported no symptoms of any disease, neither polyuria nor polydipsia. Her last fundoscopic examination (two years before) had been normal. She also suffers from mild hypertension (and is receiving treatment with an ACE inhibitor).

The patient's SMBG diary indeed showed that during the last six months her blood glucose levels repeatedly exceeded 200 mg/dl (11.1 mmol/L) and very frequently even 300 mg/dl (16.7 mmol/L). In contrast, in the past, values were – mostly – satisfactory. Physical examination was unremarkable; fundoscopy was normal. A complete biochemical profile was ordered (including an HbA$_{1c}$ level) and the NPH dose was increased to 28 units in the morning and 16 units in the evening. A SMBG schedule was advised with pre- and post-prandial measurements and follow-up was arranged in 20 days.

On the follow-up visit, SMBG values (pre- and post-prandial) remained unchanged. HbA$_{1c}$ was 7.2 percent (HPLC method) and the rest of the laboratory results were within normal range.

There is an obvious inconsistency between HbA$_{1c}$ and the SMBG values of the patient. According to SMBG values, HbA$_{1c}$ should be much higher (see Table 4.2). When there is a discrepancy between these two parameters, which anyway are just the basic methods of glycaemic control evaluation, the physician has to discover the cause and clarify which of the two values correctly reflects the patient's glycaemic status. There are, consequently, two alternatives:

- (A) false result of HbA$_{1c}$
- (B) deceptive indications of SMBG.

Possible causes of alternative (A) have been mentioned earlier in this chapter. None of them seems valid for this patient. Despite that, HbA$_{1c}$ measurement was repeated using another method (affinity chromatography) and the result was 7.1 percent.

Possible causes of alternative (B) are shown in Table 4.3.

A frequent and easily detected SMBG problem is the recording of measurements that do not represent the whole 24 hours of the day. In the

Table 4.3. Possible causes of misleading values of SMBG with a portable glucose meter

1. Measurements only in certain selected times
2. Erroneous handling of the meter by the patient
3. Factitious report of results by the patient
4. Exogenous factors that affect measurements
5. Malfunctioning or damaged meter

current patient, after advice to measure her blood sugar level frequently, this problem was ruled out.

When there is suspicion of false measurements, the correct operation of the portable meter by the patient should be ascertained by the physician or trained medical personnel. Despite the fact that modern meters are quite simple as regards their usage, mistakes are not infrequent, especially from elderly people.

Untruthful reports constitute a relatively frequent phenomenon in children and adolescents, although 'beautification' of the results is not rare in adults either. A sincere and truthful relationship between the patient and physician is very important and decreases the chance of such phenomena. Modern glucose meters can store a large number of measurements in their memory, so that retrieval of the past results is possible. Therefore, when doubt exists about the truth of the results, the patient can be asked to bring in the glucose meter to the clinic. Our patient's meter was 10 years old and had no memory storage capabilities.

There are some factors that can affect the precision of measurements. Many of them, like the time of blood drop deposition, the need to remove excess blood and adequacy of the quantity of blood, have been eliminated with the advent of modern, new generation glucose meters. Nevertheless, altitude, temperature, humidity, haematocrit changes, hypotension, hypoxia and hypertriglyceridaemia are factors that can affect the results. It should also be noted that most meters do not have a good precision at very low or very high blood glucose concentrations. Another problem is the variability of the results among different meters, even from the same manufacturer.

All meters use a stripe that contains oxidase or hexokinase and employ a photometric or electrochemical method. The advantages of modern meters, which render them superior to the older ones, are shown in Table 4.4.

Table 4.4. Technical advantages of modern portable glucose meters

- Stripes do not need 'wiping'
- Automatic start of measurement
- Speed of measurement
- Smaller needed of blood volume (0.3–5 μl)
- Indication of 'wrong' when quantity of blood is insufficient
- Automatic reading of barcode
- Storage of many measurements in memory, capability of connection with a computer and analysis of results
- Smaller size and weight

Every meter should be checked regularly (for example, every six months) as regards the precision of its measurements. Evaluation is performed by simultaneous draw of venous blood and measurement of plasma glucose concentration at a reliable biochemical laboratory. For meters that report plasma values, a difference of 10 percent from the laboratory is considered acceptable.

Our patient's meter was compared to the value that the local hospital laboratory was giving and her meter was found to have a significant divergence. She was advised to change the meter and continue with her current regimen. With the new meter, capillary blood glucose values were now compatible with the HbA_{1c} value.

If the discrepancy between HbA_{1c} and SMBG values cannot be resolved from the above mentioned factors, an alternative solution that may help is to place a glucose sensor on the patient that continuously monitors glucose concentration for 24–72 hours. These sensors measure interstitial fluid glucose concentration through a catheter that is placed subcutaneously. The technology used differs according to the manufacturer. The sensor is calibrated using capillary glucose measurements taken with a usual glucose meter, at regular intervals (4–6 times in a day). For the time being, these glucose sensors enable only the recording of the trend of glucose values in order to evaluate the glycaemic status of Type 1 diabetic patients who have great variability in their measurements, unexplained hypo- or hyper- glycaemias or a discrepancy between HbA_{1c} and SMBG values.

Further reading

Bry, L., Chen. P.C., Sacks, D.B. (2001) Effects of hemoglobin variants and chemically modified derivatives on assays for glycohemoglobin. *Clin Chem*, **47**, 153–63.

Christakopoulos, P.D., Karamanos, B.G., Tountas, C.D., Kardatos, C.G. (1975) An unusual haemoglobin fraction found more frequently in non-controlled diabetics. *Diabetes*, **24**(Suppl 2), 392–448.

Diabetes Control and Complications Trial Research Group (1993). The effect of intensive treatment of diabetes on the development and progression of long-term complications in insulin-dependent diabetes mellitus. *N Engl J Med*, **329**, 977–86.

Harris, M.I. (2001) Frequency of blood glucose monitoring in relation to glycemic control in patients with Type 2 diabetes. *Diabetes Care*, **24**, 979–82.

Pickup, J.C. (2003) Diabetic control and its management, in *Textbook of Diabetes*, 3rd edn (eds J. Pickup and G. Williams) Blackwell Science Ltd, Oxford, **34**, pp. 1–17.

American Diabetes Association (2004) Position Statement. Standards of medical care in diabetes. *Diabetes Care*, **27**(Suppl 1):S15–S35.

Rohlfing, C.L., Wiedmeyer, H.M., Little, R.R., England, J.D., Tennill, A., Goldstein, D.E. (2002) Defining the relationship between plasma glucose and HbA$_{1c}$ analysis of glucose profiles and HbA$_{1c}$ in the Diabetes Control and Complications Trial. *Diabetes Care*, **25**, 265–78.

Sacks, D.B., Bruns, D.E., Goldstein, D.E., Maclaren, N.K., McDonald, J.M., Parrott, M. (2002) Guidelines and recommendations for laboratory analysis in the diagnosis and management of diabetes mellitus. *Diabetes Care*, **25**, 750–86.

Weitgasser, R., Gappmayer, B., Pichier, M. (1999) Newer portable glucose meters – analytical improvement compared with previous generation devices? *Clin Chem*, **45**, 1821–25.

Weycamp, C.W., Penders, T.J., Muskiet, F.A.J., Van der Slik, W. (1993) Influence of hemoglobin variants and derivatives of glycohemoglobin determinations, as investigated by 102 laboratories using 16 methods. *Clin Chem*, **39**, 1717–23.

UKPDS Study Group (1998). Intensive blood glucose control with sulfonylurea or insulin compared with conventional treatment and risk of complications in patients with Type 2 diabetes (UKPDS 33). *Lancet*, **352**, 837–53.

5

Hypoglycaemia

Ioannis Ioannidis

CASE STUDY 1

A 19 year old man was brought to the Emergency Department in the early morning hours, in a comatose state. He exhibited tonic-clonic contractions and was extremely agitated. His family members reported that he was suffering from Type 1 DM and that the previous evening he had attended a party; they did not know what he had eaten, but reportedly he had drunk quite a lot of alcohol. His mother got worried when she saw him sleeping very deeply and not responding to her efforts to wake him up. She tried to feed him because she thought he might be having a hypoglycaemic episode, but was unsuccessful (he had 'sealed' his mouth). The treating physician in the Emergency Room, after measuring a blood sugar level with a portable meter and finding it to be 25 mg/dl (1.4 mmol/L), immediately ordered the intravenous administration of dextrose infusion. A 10 percent dextrose in water solution was started and the patient was given an intravenous injection of 5 ampoules 35 percent glucose (10 ml each). What is the diagnosis and cause of this acute situation? How much glucose must be administered?

The patient had a hypoglycaemic coma.

The term hypoglycaemia implies a blood glucose level less than normal (usually below 50 mg/dl [2.8 mmol/L], or according to other authors < 60 mg/dl [3.3 mmol/L]). In daily clinical practice, this term usually implies the clinical consequences of low blood sugar. The classic *triad of Whipple*, i.e., low blood glucose, symptoms compatible with hypoglycaemia and resolution of symptoms after increase of blood sugar level, are accepted by most scientists as necessary for the clinical diagnosis of hypoglycaemia.

Hypoglycaemia is the most common and at the same time the most serious complication of insulin therapy. Its frequency is related to the level

Diabetes in Clinical Practice: Questions and Answers from Case Studies. Nicholas Katsilambros *et al.*
© 2006 John Wiley & Sons, Ltd.

of glycaemic control. Thus, in the DCCT trial, serious hypoglycaemic episodes escalated to 61.2 per 100 person-years in the intensively treated group, versus 18.7 per 100 person-years in the conventional treatment group. It seems, however, that apart from HbA$_{1c}$ levels, hypoglycaemia frequency is also dependent on the quality of the administered services from the health care team and *mainly* on the patient's proper education.

More often than not hypoglycaemia is perceived by the patients themselves and promptly dealt with. Sometimes, however, it is not detected early enough and can lead to a coma (hypoglycaemia is called *serious*, when regardless of the blood glucose level, the intervention of a second person is needed to help treat it).

Severity of hypoglycaemia, therefore, covers a large spectrum, from a practically asymptomatic form (decrease of blood sugar level without overt clinical manifestations), to mild symptomatology (the patient treats it himself or herself), to serious hypoglycaemia and ultimately hypoglycaemic coma.

When the patient is in a coma, treatment of choice is the administration of a glucose solution, intravenously, at a bolus dose of 10–25 g. This is then followed by a continuous infusion of a frequently hypertonic glucose solution 10 percent, under close monitoring, as was the case for the patient under discussion (it should be noted that 1 amp [10 ml] of glucose 35 percent contains 3.5 g glucose, and consequently 3–7 ampoules are needed to reach the 10–25 g that are suggested for the initial treatment of serious hypoglycaemia).

What are the effects of hypoglycaemia?

Decrease in the plasma glucose level is initially accompanied by stimulation of the autonomic nervous system, as well as of various hormones compensatory to insulin (glucagon, catecholamines, growth hormone, cortisol). Afterwards, if blood glucose continues to decrease, neuropsychiatric manifestations occur. Compensatory hormones are secreted from a plasma glucose level of 65 mg/dl (3.6 mmol/L). At the same time, from a level of 70 mg/dl (3.9 mmol/L), insulin secretion from the pancreas, in normal people, has started to decrease significantly (up to the level of complete cessation).

Glucagon and adrenaline (epinephrine) are secreted immediately and act quickly, whereas the actions of cortisol and growth hormone are slow and become evident several hours after onset of hypoglycaemia. Stimulation of α-adrenergic receptors suppresses insulin secretion, and stimulation of β-receptors stimulates glucagon secretion. Glucagon then promotes glycogenolysis and gluconeogenesis in the liver and inhibits glucose disposal from the plasma.

What are the effects of hypoglycaemia in Type 1 DM?

In people with Type 1 DM, the ability of the pancreas to secrete glucagon decreases significantly 2–5 years after onset of the disease. In contrast, epinephrine secretion is preserved and is the main compensatory hormone in the case of hypoglycaemia. After 10–12 years from disease onset, however, epinephrine is secreted at lower glucose levels than in normal people (threshold phenomenon). Therefore, in persons with long-standing disease, both of these abnormalities – lack of glucagon secretion and delayed (at lower glucose levels) epinephrine secretion – raise the risk of severe hypoglycaemia 25-fold. Exogenous insulin administration (that cannot be suppressed any more) exacerbates the problem as well.

Our brain needs a continuous supply of glucose for its proper function. During the intervals between meals, glucose is produced by the liver (mainly), at a rate of 2 mg/kg/min. This process is called gluconeogenesis and uses main substrate amino-acids, derived from proteolysis in the muscles. About 50 percent of this glucose is metabolized in the brain. Glucose can cross the blood-brain barrier, with the help of special receptors. Decreased supply of glucose to the brain causes *neuroglycopenic* symptoms that begin as the inability to concentrate and sluggishness of reflexes, and end up in tonic-clonic convulsions and coma.

What are the causes of hypoglycaemia in diabetic persons?

The causes that frequently lead to hypoglycaemia are:

- administration of an excessive dose of insulin or at a wrong time;
- decreased intake of food;
- delay or omission of a meal, or low carbohydrate content of the food;
- intense muscular activity;

- alcohol consumption without concomitant intake of carbohydrate-containing food;
- presence of gastroparesis due to autonomic neuropathy (delays food absorption from the gastrointestinal tract).

In this particular case is probably due to a combination of factors: the delay or omission of a meal, together with alcohol consumption, most likely led to the hypoglycaemic coma.

What are the symptoms of hypoglycaemia?

Hypoglycaemic symptoms usually start at blood sugar levels around 60–70 mg/dl (3.3–3.9 mmol/L). They are divided into *adrenergic* symptoms (those that are essentially due to the stimulation of the autonomic nervous system – sympathetic and parasympathetic – and to the secretion of compensatory hormones) and *neuroglycopenic* symptoms (those that are due to lack of insulin from the brain).

Adrenergic symptoms come first and the most frequent are:

- hunger
- palpitations
- tremor
- perspiration
- tachycardia
- anxiety

Sometimes these symptoms are lacking or are not prominent. This mainly happens in people with very good glycaemic control and in those with long-standing disease (hypoglycaemia unawareness). The same can also happen when the patient has had multiple hypoglycaemic episodes (usually during the previous few hours). Management of hypoglycaemia unawareness is difficult: usually loosening of strict glycaemic control for a short time can restore awareness of hypoglycaemias.

Neuroglycopenic symptoms are usually the most serious and are due to inadequate supply of glucose to the brain:

- inability to concentrate
- blurring of vision
- diplopia
- alterations in body temperature (often hypothermia)

- sleepiness
- sluggishness in responses
- monotonous talk
- irritable behaviour
- refusal
- aggressiveness

If hypoglycaemia is not managed, then convulsions that even mimic epilepsy and coma may ensue. Central nervous system symptoms are potentially dangerous, especially when the patient performs delicate and responsible acts, drives a car, etc. (resulting in accidents, unexpected and dangerous behaviours, and so on).

After 20–30 minutes the patient resumed conscience. He was sluggish (he had consumed quite a lot of alcohol) and had a soft tremor. Does he need hospitalization?

Hypoglycaemias due to insulin usually do not need hospitalization. Sluggishness and a soft tremor are not worrisome. The patient could go home, after appropriate advice is given. If this episode is considered accidental, no changes in his insulin regimen are necessary. If, however, it has happened before, alterations in his regimen may be considered.

CASE STUDY 2

A 16 year old man suffers from frequent hypoglycaemias. His mother reports that he always consumes chocolates and sweets after such an episode, which later results in extremely high blood sugar levels. His mother wonders about the best way to cope with the problem.

The best treatment regimen for hypoglycaemias is prevention and education of the patient. This means that the diabetic person:

- should not miss a meal or eat less than usual. If this happens, insulin dose should be promptly changed.
- should eat more when he or she plans to exercise.
- should, in case of accidental administration of a higher dose of insulin, immediately consume a carbohydrate-containing food and contact his or her treating physician.
- should prefer a flexible insulin regimen, with pre-prandial administration of rapid-acting insulin together with administration of basal insulin (one injection of insulin glargine or at least two injections of isophane insulin).

If, despite these measures, hypoglycaemia still occurs, the patient should immediately consume 15–20 g glucose or sugar (sucrose). In practice, this means consumption of:

- ½ cup natural fruit juice
- 1–2 teaspoons of sugar or honey
- ½ glass of regular coca-cola
- 1 glass of milk

If after 15 minutes blood sugar is still low, the same is repeated. If blood sugar has risen (to > 70 mg/dl [3.9 mmol/L]) and the next meal is not scheduled for another hour or more, then the following items are suggested:

- crackers or cereal with a glass of milk
- a small sandwich with ham and cheese
- two crackers with some cheese

Administration of a quantity of slowly absorbed carbohydrates (i.e., 2–3 crackers, two pieces of toast, one piece of fruit) together with highly absorbed carbohydrates is recommended, so that repeated decrease of blood sugar is avoided.

Usage of chocolate or other sweets is not advisable. These foods contain quite a lot of fat, which gives additional needless calories, and at the same time slows absorption of contained carbohydrates.

The possibility of intentional hyperinsulinism in order to justify extra sweets should be considered in young children.

If the patient cannot take glucose or sugar by mouth, the subcutaneous or intramuscular administration of glucagon is recommended. This will significantly contribute to an increase in blood sugar levels. The intravenous administration of 1 mg of glucagon, compared to the intravenous administration of 25 g glucose, restores blood sugar levels with the same success rate, but with a small delay (2–3 minutes).

Glucagon injection should and must be administered by a relative or friend of the diabetic patient, as long as the necessary education and training has been provided.

If the patient is in a semi-comatose condition, marmalade, honey or glucose gel can also be given in the mouth followed by massage of the cheeks, which helps with absorption from the buccal mucosa.

CASE STUDY 3

A 78 year old woman was transferred to the Emergency Department with right hemiplegia. The patient has an 8-year history of Type 2 DM. She was taking glibenclamide tablets, 5 mg twice a day. She also suffers from hypertension, treated with slow-release nifedipine tablets, 30 mg twice a day. Urgent laboratory results revealed a blood sugar level of 31 mg/dl (1.7 mmol/L). She was immediately given an intravenous infusion of dextrose in water 10 percent. Computed tomography of the brain was normal. Around an hour later the patient was in complete recovery, without any neurologic sequelae. Is manifestation of hypoglycaemia in this way common?

Elderly persons with DM who are brought to the Emergency Room with atypical, and also even with 'typical', neurologic symptoms must have blood glucose level measured with a portable capillary blood glucose meter. A picture of stroke is one of the possible clinical manifestations of severe neuroglycopenia that accompanies hypoglycaemia in these people.

If, despite restoration of blood glucose levels, the neurologic abnormality persists, a computed tomography of the brain and further examinations for the presence of a stroke or other neurologic abnormality is warranted. Dexamethasone is administered at the same time, which increases blood–brain barrier glucose permeability. A search for a possible suppressive drug effect or alcohol effect should also be initiated.

Is hospitalization of the patient necessary?

YES. Persons with sulfonylurea-induced hypoglycaemias, especially if severe (partial or complete loss of consciousness), should be hospitalized for at least 2–3 days. Hypoglycaemia due to antidiabetic pills usually persists for a few days in these people and thus close monitoring with a continuous glucose supply is needed.

The rest of the biochemical profile of the patient was remarkable for a urea blood level of 98 mg/dl (16.27 mmol/L) and a creatinine level of 1.9 mg/dl (168 μmol/L). Is this renal insufficiency associated with the episode of hypoglycaemia?

Yes. People with renal insufficiency should not generally use sulfonylureas, because they are at risk for more frequent and more severe hypoglycaemias. When, however, renal insufficiency is mild (< 2 mg/dl [176.8 µmol/L]) the administration of very small doses of gliclazide orglimepiride can probably be considered (they are safer in renal insufficiency). Use of metformin is also contraindicated in these people (when creatinine level is > 1.4 mg/dl [123.8 µmol/L] in women or > 1.5 mg/dl [132.6 µmol/L] in men). In elderly persons especially, it is preferable that one determines the creatinine clearance, because plasma creatinine level often underestimates the severity of renal damage. If, therefore, creatinine clearance (as well as from direct measurement in a 24-hour urine specimen, it can be approximately estimated by using the Cockroft formula) is < 60 ml/min, metformin should be avoided.

In these people with renal failure, both the delayed action of dispensed antidiabetic pills and the reduced gluconeogenesis (around 30 percent of gluconeogenesis is derived from the kidneys) contribute to hypoglycaemia occurrence.

What should appropriate therapy be for this patient, after her discharge from the hospital?

The treatment of choice is prescription of insulin. If this is not feasible (refusal of the patient and/or her environment), one of the rapidly acting insulin secretagogues (nateglinide or repaglinide) or one of the newest sulfonylureas in a low dose (gliclazide or glimepiride) could be prescribed. Glitazones are also not contraindicated in cases of renal failure and could be considered as an alternative (either in monotherapy or better in combination with a small dose of an insulin secretagogue).

CASE STUDY 4

A 26 year old man suffers from Type 1 DM and is treated with an intensive insulin regimen. He uses a rapid-acting insulin injection before meals three times a day and one injection of isophane insulin at bedtime every night. His blood sugar in the morning is usually high. He has noticed that whenever he increases his evening insulin dose, things get worse. When asked by the doctor, he admits that he often wakes up 'tired' and during the night he has nightmares. How are these symptoms explained? How can he be helped?

Many factors may contribute to high morning blood glucose levels. Isophane insulins, used before bedtime, exert their peak action early in the night. At the same time, however, the body's insulin sensitivity is at its peak (midnight to 3 a.m.) compared to the morning hours (6 to 8 a.m.). This is due to the secretion of growth hormone in the early morning hours, which has actions contrary to insulin's (dawn phenomenon).

These two factors (peak insulin activity and increased sensitivity) create a high risk for hypoglycaemia at these hours. This night-time hypoglycaemia is often followed by a phenomenon of compensatory hyperglycaemia (rebound phenomenon), contributing in this way to the early morning high glucose levels (Somogyi phenomenon).

It is often necessary to measure a blood sugar level at around 2 to 3 a.m., for a better control of morning blood glucose. Increase of the night-time insulin dose is done by 1–2 units, up to a level so that 2 to 3 a.m. levels range around 110–145 mg/dl (6.1–8.1 mmol/L). Blood sugar should be at least 110 mg/dl (6.1 mmol/L) at this time, so hypoglycaemia can be avoided that morning with certainty. At the same time, the night-time insulin dose should be transferred as late as possible (10 to 11 p.m.), so that its action will last until the morning.

A good alternative is to substitute isophane insulin with a long-lasting insulin analogue (insulin glargine), in this way decreasing significantly the risk of night-time hypoglycaemias.

Night-time hypoglycaemias frequently go unnoticed and are to be suspected by the morning fatigue and nightmares that they cause.

High morning blood glucose levels are often due to such episodes of night-time hypoglycaemia. One should consider other alternatives, though, such as insufficient dose of insulin, large meal the previous night, very high blood sugar level the previous night and poor insulin injection technique.

CASE STUDY 5

A 26 year old woman has suffered from Type 1 DM since the age of five years. Her insulin regimen includes pre-prandial administration of insulin lispro and once a day administration of insulin glargine. Lately, her glucose control has deteriorated significantly and there is great variability in her measurements. She is affected by the occurrence of 'unpredictable' hypoglycaemias, for example, one hour after a meal. When asked by her physician, she reports that her stomach feels full even many hours after a meal. She also reports retching and heartburns. What is the diagnosis and treatment?

Most likely, this patient with long-standing DM, is suffering from gastro-paresis. The significant delay of gastric motility leads to the delayed transfer of food to the intestine and consequently delayed absorption of carbohydrates in the blood. This explains the post-prandial hypoglycae-mia, at the time when insulin lispro exerts its peak activity, whereas there is no respective absorption of glucose from the food.

Delayed and unpredictable propulsion of food in the intestine renders the synchronization of injected insulin with food absorption difficult. A gastric prokinetic agent, like metoclopramide (at a dose of 10 mg before meals), could help with food propulsion. At the same time, changing the type of insulin from a rapid analogue to regular insulin can be effective in ameliorating the problem (regular insulin acts a bit later than the insulin analogue). Another alternative could be the administration of the insulin analogue after the meal or even fragmentation of its dose, with admin-istration of a few units in small intervals after the meal, and monitoring of blood glucose levels.

Administration of insulin via a continuous insulin pump is also indicated in people with this problem.

Note: Hypoglycaemia can occur in non-diabetics when there is hyper-secretion of insulin from tumours, such as insulinomas, some sarcomas, etc. These cases are rare and will not be further analysed in this book.

Also, in non-diabetics, one can frequently find low blood sugar levels 3–5 hours after a meal rich in carbohydrates. This hypoglycaemia is due to hypersecretion of insulin and possibly denotes these people are potential diabetics (decreased initial first phase of insulin secretion, together with delayed hypersecretion at a second phase, comprise a premature detect-able abnormality of carbohydrate metabolism in these people).

Further reading

Diabetes Control and Complications Trial Research Group (1993) The effect of intensive treatment of diabetes on the development and progression of long-term complications in insulin-dependent diabetes mellitus. *N Engl J Med*, **329**, 977–86.

Frier, B.M. (1997) Hypoglycaemia in diabetes mellitus, in *Textbook of Diabetes*, 2nd ed, (eds J. Pickup and G. Williams), Blackwell Science, **40**, pp. 1–22.

Hanas, R. (1998) *Insulin Dependent Diabetes*. Uddevalla Sweden, 1st edition. Service F.J. (1995) Hypoglycemia. in *Endocrine Emergencies*, The Medical Clinics of North America, **79**(1), 1–9.

6

Diabetic coma

Ioannis Ioannidis

CASE STUDY 1 – DIABETIC KETOACIDOSIS

A 25 year old young woman came to the hospital with fever and mild confusion. During the previous few weeks she had experienced polydipsia, polyphagia and polyuria, with significant weight loss (12 kg). She reported pain in her left flank area, with dysuria, for the previous 48 hours. Her mother reported that her daughter's breath had a peculiar, uncommon smell, and that her breaths were more frequent.

A physical exam was remarkable for evidence of dehydration. She had a low supine blood pressure (85/60 mmHg), with increased pulse rate (120 per min) and respiratory rate (32 breaths per min). Her breath had an acetone smell. There was mild clouding of sensorium, but without focal neurological signs. She had fever (37.9 °C [100.2 °F]) and tenderness on percussion of the left flank area (positive Giordano sign). A capillary blood glucose measurement showed a very high level: 484 mg/dl (26.9 mmol/L). At the same time, ketone bodies measured in the capillary blood with a portable meter (Medisense Xtra) were also very high: 4.5 mmol/L (note: these strips measure only β-hydroxybutyrate [b-HB] and not acetoacetate in the blood; levels > 3 mmol/L are considered a sign of ketosis). Arterial blood gas analysis showed the following: pH 7.08 (7.35–7.42); pCO_2 8 mmHg (35–45); pO_2 120 mmHg (80–100); and HCO_3^- 6 mmol/L (24–32).

The diagnosis of diabetic ketoacidosis (DKA) was made. An ECG, a chest X-ray and further laboratory tests were done. The results were:

Blood glucose:	525 mg/dl (29.1 mmol/L)	(75–110 mg/dl [4.2–6.1 mmol/L])
Sodium:	124 mmol/L	(132–144)
Potassium:	3.8 mmol/L	(3.4–4.8)
Chloride:	88 mmol/L	(93–108)

Diabetes in Clinical Practice: Questions and Answers from Case Studies. Nicholas Katsilambros *et al.*
© 2006 John Wiley & Sons, Ltd.

Urea:	92 mg/dl (15.3 mmol/L)	(18–36 mg/dl [3.0–6.0 mmol/L])
Creatinine:	3.2 mg/dl (282.9 μmol/L)	(0.7–1.2 mg/dl [61.9–106.1 μmol/L])
Urinalysis:	Urine cloudy and foul smelling, glucose: ++++, ketone: +++, many WBCs, abundant microorganisms, many RBCs.	
CBC:	Haematocrit: 44%, WBC: 22,000/μl (polymorphonuclear 88%).	

What is diabetic ketoacidosis and what is the cause of DKA in this young woman? What are the therapeutic targets and our immediate priority?

DKA is characterized by the triad:

1. Plasma glucose > 250 mg/dl (13.9 mmol/L)
2. Plasma ketone bodies (b-HB) > 3 mmol/L [or ketone bodies in plasma measured with Acetest strips > 2+])
3. Acidosis: pH < 7.3 or/and HCO_3^- < 18 mEq/L

Severity of DKA can be categorized as follows:

Mild: pH: 7.25–7.30

HCO_3^-: 15–18 mEq/L

Anion gap: > 10 mmol/L

Moderate: pH: 7.00–7.24

HCO_3^-: 10–15 mEq/L

Anion gap: > 12 mmol/L

Severe: pH: < 7.00

HCO_3^-: < 10 mEq/L

Anion gap: >14 mmol/L

(**Note**: Anion gap is calculated using the formula: $[Na^+] - [Cl^- + HCO_3^-]$ and has a normal value of around 10 mmol/L. If this value is > 10 mmol/L, this implies the presence of non-measurable anions in the blood, such as ketone bodies or lactic acid. Apart from DKA, other causes of metabolic acidosis with a high anion gap are lactic acidosis, renal failure and drug poisoning with acids).

DKA is due to lack of insulin, which leads to excessive production of ketone bodies, resulting in acidosis (metabolic acidosis with large decrease of bicarbonate) and compensatory hypocapnia. Lack of insulin also leads to a large increase in blood glucose levels, causing osmotic diuresis-polyuria and consequently a large loss of water and electrolytes. The final result is dehydration, with the clinical signs of hypovolaemia and significant electrolyte disturbances. Increased concentrations of compensatory hormones (glucagon, cortisol, catecholamines and growth hormone) contribute to the development of DKA as well.

The causes of DKA are: initial manifestation of Type 1 DM (insulin-dependent), omission of an insulin dose (accidental or deliberate) in a person with insulin-dependent DM, serious infections in a diabetic person (this refers to both types of diabetes), whereas in a certain percentage of patients the cause remains unknown. In the woman in our case, DKA was the first manifestation of Type 1 DM, and the urine infection (fever, significant increase in WBCs and positive urinalysis) contributed to its onset.

Clouding of sensorium and coma are associated with an increase in plasma osmotic pressure (intracellular osmolality is also altered and is usually associated with severe intracellular dehydration). Osmotic pressure or tonicity (osmolality) is calculated from the formula:

$$\textbf{Osmotic pressure or Osmolality (mOsm/kg)} = \textbf{2[Na}^+ \textbf{ (mEq/L)}$$
$$+ \textbf{ K}^+ \textbf{ (mEq/L)]} + \textbf{Glucose (mg/dl)/18} + \textbf{Urea (mg/dl)/6}$$

(Note: $BUN = Urea/2.14\,mg/dl$)

If increase in plasma osmolality is greater than $340\,mOsm/kg\,H_2O$, lethargy or coma is justified. Despite this, many people with lower osmolality values have clouding of sensorium, to which other factors seem to contribute as well: hyperketonaemia (alters brain oxygen consumption) and the frequently underlying disease (sepsis, etc.) are the most common.

The aims of therapy are:

1. Immediate priority: Rehydration – restoration of intravascular volume, aiming at restoring blood pressure, pulse rate and diuresis
2. Control of blood glucose (with insulin)
3. Replenishment of potassium losses
4. Correction of severe acidosis

First priority is replenishment of water deficit, since it can cause potentially dangerous hypovolaemia. Consequently, initial therapy should include the intravenous infusion of NaCl isotonic solution, at a rate of 1000 ml in the first hour (15–20 ml/kg/h). In hypovolaemic shock, this rate is continued further. Usually, another 1000 ml are infused in the following two hours (4–14 ml/kg/h) and then 1000 ml in four hours (4–14 ml/kg/h). If the patient is in hypovolaemic shock, an infusion of a colloidal solution or plasma will probably be needed. A total of 6–12 L of fluids may be needed in the first 24 hours.

Apart from fluids, insulin is infused, in the following way: initially a bolus injection of 10 IU regular insulin is given intravenously (0.15 IU/kg), and an intravenous infusion of 5–10 IU/hr is started at the same time (12.5–25 ml/h of a solution containing 100 IU regular insulin in 250 ml NaCl). This rate is achieved by using the special pumps of intravenous fluid administration or with a microdroplet infusion system. Blood glucose is measured hourly and the infusion rate is promptly adjusted (desirable decrease of glucose by 50–70 mg/dl/h [2.8–3.9 mmol/L/h]). Thus, if blood glucose does not decrease by at least 50–70 mg/dl (2.8–3.9 mmol/L) in one hour, the infusion rate should be doubled. When plasma glucose drops to 250 mg/dl (13.9 mmol/L), the infusion solution is converted to dextrose in water 5 percent (DW5 percent) at a rate of 150–250 ml/h (+0.45 percent NaCl) with simultaneous continuous insulin iv infusion (2–4 IU/h). Blood glucose target is 150–250 mg/dl (8.3–13.9 mmol/L), until metabolic control is stabilized.

It should be noted that although the various protocols of fluid and insulin infusion can vary in different hospitals, they are virtually similar regarding their basic principles and therapeutic targets.

For example, there are protocols that do not include a continuous insulin infusion, but only repeated bolus injections of insulin iv. Other protocols call for repeated administration of insulin, both intravenously and subcutaneously.

It should be emphasized that usually in DKA there is a significant shortage of potassium (as is the case with the other electrolytes as well), regardless of the initial serum potassium concentration. The causes of potassium shortage are as follows:

- Metabolic acidosis and decreased glycolysis result in exit of potassium from the cells and this can lead to hyperkalaemia (despite the fact that total potassium content of the body is low). A significant contributor to the exit of potassium from the cells is protein catabolism in the muscles, due to insulinopenia.

- Osmotic diuresis and secondary aldosteronism (hypovolaemia due to dehydration) lead to significant kaliuresis and potassium shortage.
- When there is hypokalaemia, the shortage is very large and usually prolonged vomiting or diuretic treatment is also involved.

Potassium shortage is usually large, and the initially high concentration in the blood, due to acidosis, can be misleading. Very soon, with volume restoration and insulin infusion, potassium concentration drops precipitously. For this reason, **it is imperative to monitor K$^+$ levels very closely and to administer adequate quantities promptly to replenish the low levels**.

Thus, if serum K$^+$ concentration is < 5.5 mEq/L, we do not add any potassium in the infusion fluids, but we recheck the level in two hours. If K$^+$ concentration is 3.5–5.5 mEq/L, we add 20–30 mmol K$^+$ in each L of fluids and if it is < 3.5 mEq/L, we add 40 mmol K$^+$ in each L of fluids per hour, until K$^+$ concentration is normalized. (Hypokalaemia can be directly dangerous for the life of the patient and should be given priority in its management.)

As regards hyponatraemia in DKA, this is due to various reasons:

- osmotic shift of water in the extracellular space;
- loss of sodium in the urine as a result of osmotic diuresis and as an accompanying kation of the excreted ketone bodies;
- accompanying vomiting;
- decreased intake due to nausea and vomiting;
- factitious (due to an increase in triglycerides or glucose) corrected sodium is calculated by the formula: measured Na + [(glucose/18) − 5.6]/2.

Bicarbonate (HCO$_3^-$) administration for management of acidosis is advised only when blood pH is < 7.0. When pH is between 6.9–7.0, 44 mmol HCO$_3^-$ is adequate (infused over 30 minutes) and when pH is < 6.9, 88 mmol HCO$_3^-$ is infused. When bicarbonate is administered, potassium needs are increased, and thus some authors suggest a separate additional potassium infusion.

How should this patient with DKA be monitored afterwards?

The following monitoring protocol is proposed (and may vary in different hospitals):

Clinical	Interval
Vital signs	20–30 minutes
(blood pressure, diuresis, respirations, pulse)	
Glascow scale (if in coma)	20–30 minutes
Laboratory	
Glucose	every hour (at the bedside)
Na^+, K^+, pH (venous)	0, 2, 6, 10, 24 hours
HCO_3^-, pCO_2, osmolality	every 2–4 hours
Urea	0, 12, 24 hours
Ketones (urine)	0, 4, 8, 12, 18, 24 hours
Ketones (plasma)	0, 6, 12, 24 hours

The great significance of the close monitoring of the patient by the treating physician is obvious. Joslin noticed long ago (1925) that 'recovery of the patients with diabetic coma is a result of the hard and incessant work, day and night, of usually young doctors, who practice the most up-to-date therapeutic methods'.

Close monitoring of the patient helps also in the potential discovery of the rare but serious complications of DKA: overhydration, ARDS, cerebral oedema, thromboembolic episodes.

When the patient is stable (lack of ketosis, improvement of metabolic acidosis, stabilization of vital signs, lack of gastroparesis – it is often seen in severe DKA and may need nasogastric tube insertion) feeding and hydration by mouth can start. Rapid-acting subcutaneous insulin can be administered every six hours, based on the measurements of blood sugar levels. Discontinuation of insulin iv infusion is done 30–60 minutes after the subcutaneous administration of the first dose of insulin.

After 1–2 days the patient can be treated with a classical insulin regimen, consisting of isophane insulin or long-acting insulin analogue (for example, insulin glargine) combined with rapid acting insulin or insulin analogue before meals.

CASE STUDY 2 – HYPEROSMOLAR NON-KETOTIC HYPERGLYCAEMIC COMA (HNKHC)

A 75 year old woman with a history of residual left hemiparesis due to a stroke, is transferred to the Emergency Room of the hospital. Recently, the patient has had intense polyuria and complained of profound thirst, the result of consuming of large quantities of juices. During the previous week she had experienced a decrease in her level of consciousness, with gradual clouding of sensorium, slowly deteriorating until she fell into a coma.

Physical examination revealed signs of dehydration, with blood pressure of 110/80 mmHg and pulse rate of 110 per min. The patient was deeply comatose, with bilateral positive Babinski sign, unresponsive even to painful stimuli and with decreased deep tendon reflexes. Initial impression was that she was suffering from a very severe stroke, probably in the medulla.

A stat-computed tomography of the brain showed an ischaemic area of the right hemisphere, compatible with the history of left hemiparesis, but no signs of haemorrhage of recent thromboembolic lesion. The patient had a temperature of 36 °C (96.8 °F) (37.2 °C [98.9 °F] rectally). Laboratory results were: Na^+ 138 mmol/L; K^+ 3.6 mmol/L; Cl^- 105.0 mmol/L; HCO_3^- 30 mmol/L; urea 92 mg/dl (15.3 mmol/L); creatinine 2.2 mg/dl (194.5 µmol/L). Blood glucose was 1,235 mg/dl (68.5 mmol/L)!! Urinalysis showed 4+ glucose and 1+ ketones.

What is the diagnosis and where is it based?

This is a case of hyperosmolar non-ketotic hyperglycaemic coma (HNKHC), because the following criteria are fulfilled:

1. significant hyperglycaemia (usually > 600 mg/dl [33.3 mmol/L]);
2. absence of or minimal ketosis (1+ or 2+ in the urine, < 3 mmol/L in the blood), pH > 7.30;
3. large increase of blood osmolality (usually > 320 mOsm/kg): hypernatraemia is frequently present (but not always).

What are the circumstances during which HNKHC develops?

HNKHC usually occurs in elderly Type 2 DM patients and is characterized by partial (not complete) lack of insulin. Hyperglycaemia is extremely high and ketosis is minimal to negligible. Characteristic hyperosmosis causes mild confusion initially, followed by lethargy and then coma. Frequently the clinical picture is mistaken for a cerebral stroke (hemiplegia, convulsions, choreioathetotic movements, Babinski sign, etc.). Mortality is high (up to 40 percent) with the old age and underlying diseases (severe infections, strokes, myocardial infarctions, pulmonary emboli, etc.) contributory factors.

Impaired renal function contributes to the intense osmolality seen in the syndrome (increase of renal glucose excretion threshold, resulting in inability of significant glucosuria). Furthermore, decreased feelings of thirst and decreased ability of these patients to drink water contributes as well.

The cause of absent ketosis is not quite clear. The most possible explanation is that insulin levels are sufficient to inhibit lipolysis but not gluconeogenesis and decreased intake of glucose by the muscles. Decreased perfusion of adipose tissue seems to contribute to impaired lipolysis as well. Finally, it seems that insulin levels are also sufficient to suppress ketogenesis in the liver.

What treatment will you offer to the patient?

Treatment of the patient includes the following:

1. **Fluid administration and restoration of electrolyte disturbances.** Mean fluid deficit amounts to 9–10 L. The administered fluid is isotonic solution of NaCl (0.9 percent) and only when Na^+ concentration is > 155 mmol/L is hypotonic solution of NaCl (0.45 percent) preferred (if this is not readily available, it can be prepared by adding four ampoules of NaCl in one L of water for injection).

   Generally, it is essential to monitor urine output, vital signs and cerebral function. In elderly people it is also useful to monitor central venous pressure (to avoid fluid overload).

   The frequently high Na^+ values subside with hydration and administration of hypotonic solutions (when the value is very high). The frequently normal K^+ values decrease with hydration and insulin administration. For this reason **K^+ should be administered very early** (with the first litres of administered fluids), on condition that diuresis is adequate. The concentrations in the blood should be monitored with repeated measurements.

2. **Correction of hyperglycaemia** with insulin administration (lower doses than needed in DKA). The dose of insulin is proposed at 3–5 units per hour, aiming at a gradual drop of plasma glucose (not more than 150 mg/dl [8.3 mmol/L] per hour) for avoidance of cerebral oedema or peripheral shock.

3. **Management of underlying diseases** (septicaemia is common, as well as strokes, cardiac episodes, etc.).

4. **Prevention of thromboembolic episodes.** Thromboembolic episodes are frequent, due to the hyperglycaemia and dehydration and can even be fatal, as is the case in thrombosis of superior mesenteric artery. For this reason administration of anticoagulants in small doses is usually proposed.
5. **Close monitoring in an intensive care unit.** The patient under discussion died four days later, despite her admission to an Intensive Care Unit. Her metabolic disturbances were successfully managed, but her brain function deteriorated.

CASE STUDY 3 – LACTIC ACIDOSIS

A 74 year old woman presents to the hospital with complaints of recent high blood glucose levels and a feeling of progressively deteriorating fatigue. Her family members report episodes of lethargy and intense sleepiness, as well as confusion during the previous week. The patient suffers from DM (for 12 years), hypertension, coronary heart disease, dyslipidaemia, heart failure and atrial fibrillation. An echocardiogram done three months before showed left ventricular hypertrophy, mitral regurgitation and an ejection fraction of 35 percent. Her medications include: glimepiride, 6 mg/day; digoxin, 0.125 mg/day; ramipril, 10 mg/day; furosemide, 20 mg twice a day; aspirin, 325 mg/day; and for the last two months metformin, with a gradual increase of the dose to 1700 mg/day. She does not smoke or drink alcohol.

Physical examination reveals a heart rate of 100/min, blood pressure of 168/72 mmHg, respiratory rate of 18/min and temperature of 36.8 °C (98.2 °F). An electrocardiogram shows presence of atrial fibrillation with a ventricular rate of 100 beats/min. Laboratory results are as follows: glucose 268 mg/dl (14.9 mmol/L); urea 48 mg/dl (8.0 mmol/L); creatinine 0.9 mg/dl (79.6 μmol/L); HbA$_{1c}$ 11.5 %; WBC 8600/μl; Na$^+$ 138 mEq/L; K$^+$ 4.4 mEq/L; Cl$^-$ 95 mEq/L. A chest X-ray is normal, without signs of cardiac overload or inflammatory infiltrates.

Blood gas analysis shows pH 7.20 (7.35–7.42), pCO$_2$ 28 mmHg (35–45), pO$_2$ 105 mmHg (80–100) and HCO$_3^-$ 15 mmol/L (24–32). Anion gap is calculated at 32 mmol/L (increased). Ketone bodies (measured with the portable meter Medisense Xtra) are 1.6 mmol/L. Given the history of metformin ingestion and the presence of metabolic acidosis with a high anion gap, lactate levels are measured in the blood and found to be 6.1 mEq/L (normal values are 0.7–2.1 mEq/L). Metformin is discontinued and the patient started on insulin treatment with a twice a day injection of medium duration insulin. Twenty-four hours later, lactate levels are 1.9 mEq/L. After a few days the patient returns home.

Lactic acidosis is a severe form of metabolic acidosis (pH < 7.3) with a high anion gap and serum lactate levels more than 5.0 mmol/L. It occurs more frequently in diabetic persons, is a serious condition and often fatal. There are two forms of lactic acidosis.

Type A lactic acidosis is characterized by severe tissue hypoxia (as, for example, in states of shock). In diabetic persons with severe DKA, co-existence of relatively high levels of lactate may aggravate metabolic acidosis (lactate levels are usually high in DKA due to hypovolaemia and tissue hypoxia). Furthermore, in these persons correction of DKA with insulin administration may transiently induce an increase of lactate level due to inhibition of hepatic gluconeogenesis. This increase is transient and without clinical significance.

Type B lactic acidosis is not characterized by tissue hypoxia (the case under discussion above) and is seen in diabetes, renal and hepatic insufficiency, leukaemia, vitamin B_{12} and B_1 deficiency, as well as in starvation.

Furthermore, the cause can sometimes be medicines, such as fenformin, isoniazid, salicylates, methanol and ethylene alcohol.

Biguanides, and mainly fenformin, increase lactate production. Frequently, however, manifestation of lactic acidosis requires the additional presence of some other disease or condition, such as renal failure, cardiopulmonary insufficiency, hepatic insufficiency, serious infections, severe anaemia, alcoholism, surgeries or shock.

Lactic acidosis is a dangerous condition and requires correction of the microcirculatory abnormalities, dealing with the aetiologic factors, treatment of the possibly coexistent infection or other aetiologic factor, and judicious administration of bicarbonate with the intent to raise pH above 7.2.

Bicarbonate administration has been among other things implicated in the deterioration of myocardial function (it causes increased production of CO_2 that easily enters myocardial cells and results in decrease of pH). Thus, alternatively, the use of Carbicarb has been proposed (a mixture of sodium bicarbonate and sodium carbonate).

In resistant cases dichloroxic acid is administered (decreases lactate production), although its usefulness is questionable.

Often, in severe and dangerous cases of lactic acidosis due to biguanide administration, haemodialysis helps in the removal of the biguanide. It should be emphasized that metformin administration is contraindicated when plasma creatinine concentration is > 1.5 mg/dl

(132.6 µmol/L) for men and >1.4 mg/dl (123.8 µmol/L) for women. In elderly people though, it is useful, despite the seemingly normal plasma creatinine concentrations, to calculate creatinine clearance using the Cockroft formula:

$$\text{Creatinine clearance (ml/min)} = \frac{(140 - \text{age}) \times \text{body weight (kg)}}{\text{plasma creatinine (mg/dl)} \times 72}$$

In women this should be multiplied by 0.85.

For the woman under discussion, who weighed 60 kg, calculating her creatinine clearance in this way found it to be 52 ml/min, which represents a moderate degree of renal impairment (despite a normal plasma creatinine level).

Therefore, when we intend to prescribe metformin in elderly persons, it is prudent to calculate creatinine clearance with this simple formula and avoid its prescription when values are <60 ml/min.

Further reading

Kitabchi, A.E. and Wall, B.M. (1995) Diabetic Ketoacidosis, in *Endocrine Emergencies*, Medical Clinics of North America, **79**, pp. 9–38.

American Diabetes Association (2004) Hyperglycemic Crises in Diabetes. *Diabetes Care*, **27**(Suppl 1), S94–S102.

Lorber, D. (1995) Nonketotic Hypertonicity in Diabetes Mellitus, in *Endocrine Emergencies*, The Medical Clinics of North America, (ed. K.P. Ober), pp. 39–52.

Kreisberg, R.A. (1998) Diabetic Ketoacidosis in Adults, in *Current Therapy of Diabetes Mellitus* (eds R. A. Fronzo, Mosby, pp. 20–30.

Salpeter, S.R., Greyber, E., Pasternak, G.A., Salpeter, E.E. (2003) Risk of fatal and non fatal lactic acidosis with metformin use in type 2 diabetes mellitus. *Arch Intern Med*, **163**, 2594–2602.

7

Surgery in diabetes

Ioannis Ioannidis

CASE STUDY 1

A 54 year old man is referred to the urologist by his primary physician, because of intense dysuric symptoms during the last six months and three episodes of urinary tract infections. He was examined by the urologist and had an ultrasound examination of the kidneys, ureter and prostate. A significant hypertrophy of the prostate gland was found, accompanied by an appreciable amount of residual urine in the bladder after urination. A transurethral prostatectomy was suggested.

The patient has been suffering from Type 2 DM for the previous six years, treated with metformin 850 mg tablets, twice a day and nateglinide 120 mg tablets, thrice a day, before meals. His glycaemic control is satisfactory, as depicted in his SMBG measurements and his HbA_{1c} level (6.7 percent). The urologist refers the patient back to his primary physician, so that pre-operative instructions for optimal control of his blood glucose before surgery are given.

Can the patient be directly operated on, and if yes, should he be admitted to the hospital before the surgery?

The patient has satisfactory glycaemic control and could be directly operated on. He does not even need to be admitted to the hospital before the operation.

It is estimated that about 50 percent of diabetic patients will need to undergo at least one surgical procedure during their lifetime. Around 17 percent will have a complication from the surgery. Complications and potential poor outcome of surgery depend on the presence of chronic complications of DM, such as renal insufficiency, cardiovascular diseases, widespread atherosclerosis, proliferative retinopathy, neuropathy of the autonomic nervous system, and so forth. Hyperglycaemia during the

Diabetes in Clinical Practice: Questions and Answers from Case Studies. Nicholas Katsilambros *et al.*
© 2006 John Wiley & Sons, Ltd.

perioperative period also contributes to the adverse outcomes of surgery, since it promotes infections, electrolyte abnormalities, dehydration, acidosis, poor wound healing and thrombotic complications.

Why should hyperglycaemia be avoided in the surgical diabetic patient?

Hyperglycaemia predisposes to dehydration and electrolyte abnormalities, decelerates the occlusion and healing of the surgical wound, and predisposes to infections or even to ketoacidosis (especially in Type 1 DM sufferers). A desirable target is to maintain blood glucose levels around 150–200 mg/dl (8.3–11.1 mmol/L) during surgery, a level that is protective against hypoglycaemia.

The most common complications of diabetic patients during surgery, anaesthesia and in the post-operative period are as follows:

- **Metabolic:**
  Diabetic ketoacidosis
  Hyperosmolar coma
  Hypoglycaemia
  Electrolyte disturbances (frequently hyperkalaemia or hypokalaemia)
- **Cardiovascular:**
  Hypotension (associated with diabetic neuropathy)
  Postoperative infarction
  Thrombotic phenomena
  Arrhythmias
- **Renal:**
  Acute renal failure
  Fluid overload
  Infections

What does the preoperative evaluation of this patient include?

The preoperative evaluation of a diabetic patient includes evaluation of his cardiac, renal and respiratory function, as is the case with all patients anyway, as well as management of possible anaemia.

Cardiac examination is very important because it is well known that, very frequently, coronary heart disease in diabetic people is 'silent'.

Furthermore, the presence of cardiovascular autonomic neuropathy significantly increases the risk of vascular complications and should be diagnosed preoperatively. Usually a recent cardiovascular history, a physical examination and an ECG are sufficient. Depending on findings from these, further tests may be needed.

Patients with well-controlled arterial hypertension can undergo a surgical procedure without excess risk. If β-adrenergic blockers are used in the patient's regimen, he or she can have hypoglycaemia without warning symptoms, and so should be closely monitored. These patients frequently exhibit an increased risk for thromboses. Unless there are contraindications, they should be treated prophylactically with low-molecular-weight heparin subcutaneously and elastic stockings during surgery and postoperatively.

The use of vasoactive agents to treat the hypotension that frequently accompanies large decreases of intravascular volume or sepsis, causes severe peripheral vasoconstriction. Patients with underlying poor peripheral perfusion (for example, those with non-palpable peripheral pulses) can develop critical ischaemia or even gangrene with the use of such agents.

Evaluation of renal function is also essential. Plasma creatinine measurement is not enough, because it increases only in advanced stages of diabetic nephropathy. Measurement or calculation of creatinine clearance is recommended (with 24-hour urine collection or the Cockroft formula) as well as measurement of 24-hour urine protein excretion. Pursuit of the presence of microalbuminuria is essential, when the above results are normal.

Renal function evaluation is very important because patients with impaired renal function are at higher risk for acute renal failure. Nephrotoxic agents should be avoided in these people (intravenous dye, aminoglycoside antibiotics, etc.) as well as decreased renal perfusion (avoidance of hypotension, low cardiac supply, etc.). Albuminuria is known to increase cardiovascular mortality in these people, and so they should be closely monitored and cared for.

Neurologic evaluation

Diabetic sufferers can possibly have impaired gastrointestinal motility, which increases the risk of aspirations and also delays onset of patient feeding postoperatively.

Possible presence of urinary bladder dysfunction frequently leads to urine retention, which is also facilitated by the postoperative use of strong opiate-containing analgesics. The doctor should be aware of the presence of gastrointestinal and bladder dysfunction, and so should exert extreme diligence in monitoring fluid balance and using medicines that affect them during surgery.

The anaesthesiologist should be aware of the possible presence of orthostatic hypotension (which is commonly associated with neuropathy), so that he or she can predict possible haemodynamic alterations during anaesthesia.

What hormonal changes occur during anaesthesia and surgery?

During anaesthesia and surgery a series of hormonal changes (as a response to stress) can significantly affect the diabetic patient's metabolic control. The most important changes are:

- increased secretion of compensatory hormones (they promote hepatic glucose production and decreased clearance of glucose from peripheral tissues);
- decreased secretion of insulin;
- decreased activity of insulin (increased insulin resistance).

These alterations result in hyperglycaemia, ketosis and increase in metabolic rate and catabolism of the body.

How can metabolic control of this patient be achieved?

General principles for achieving metabolic control in diabetic patients who are going to be operated on are as follows:

1. Metabolic control should be evaluated and its improvement optimized on an outpatient basis for non-urgent surgeries. Chronically hyperglycaemic patients are often dehydrated. This dehydration is accompanied by electrolyte abnormalities and low intravascular volume, which lead to haemodynamic instability.
2. Admission to the hospital is recommended 12–16 hours prior to surgery (for small surgeries) for all patients with Type 1 DM and for Type 2 DM patients with poor metabolic control (the patient under

discussion had Type 2 DM with good metabolic control and therefore admission before the surgery was not indicated).

For this specific patient – as well as for every patient with insulin-treated Type 2 DM (1–2 injections daily) or Type 2 DM treated with pills or diet only – the following steps are recommended:

- Surgery is planned early in the morning.
- If the patient is treated with metformin or sulfonylureas, they are discontinued at noon of the previous day before the operation. Glitazones are not discontinued.
- If it is a *minor* surgery (as was the case described above) the usual diet and treatment is followed. If the patient is already in the hospital, blood glucose is measured every 4–6 hours and insulin is administered subcutaneously based on an empiric sliding scale, on condition that after insulin administration small meals are offered, mainly containing carbohydrates.
- If it is a *major* surgery (abdomen, thorax, transplantation, arterial bypass, etc.), and regardless of the type of diabetes (1 or 2), one of the schemes described below is followed.

The authors of the present book frequently use continuous intravenous infusion of a glucose solution 5 percent (more rarely 10 percent) with the necessary electrolytes, depending on each patient's needs. In every litre of fluids, 8 to 16 units of rapid-acting insulin are added. Capillary blood glucose is measured with the use of portable meters every six (sometimes four) hours and supplemental rapid-acting insulin is injected subcutaneously, based on an individualized sliding scale. When the patient is able to receive solid food by mouth, the intravenous infusion is discontinued, while the six-hourly subcutaneous injections are continued with small meals.

Various other schemes and protocols are reported in the literature. An especially popular one is the so-called GIK (glucose, insulin, potassium [K]). According to this scheme, glucose, insulin and potassium are administered together in the same solution. The fluid is dextrose 10 percent in 500 ml and contains 10 mmol K^+ as well as 15 units of rapid-acting insulin.

The infusion rate is 100 ml/h. The necessary insulin quantity varies to some degree, depending on the state of the patient and the coexistent conditions. For these reasons, the above-mentioned proposals are an initial approach and later insulin quantity (per gram of glucose) is adjusted as follows:

	i.u. of insulin per g of glucose
Patient of normal weight	0.25–0.35
Obesity	0.4
Liver disease	0.4–0.6
Corticosteroid administration	0.4–0.5
Septic conditions	0.5–0.7
Cardiopulmonary bypass	0.9–1.2

If on the morning of the surgery, blood glucose level is more than 270 mg/dl (15.00 mmol/L) the surgery is cancelled, or – if absolutely needed – a 10 percent dextrose solution with 60 i.u. insulin per litre is administered. Alternatively one could administer insulin in a continuous intravenous infusion (4–6 i.u. per hour). Usually this regimen is started in the morning of the planned operation. Occasionally, it may be necessary for some patients to measure a blood glucose level at 3 a.m. before the surgery. If the level at that time is > 200 mg/dl (11.1 mmol/L) it is recommended to administer rapid-acting insulin subcutaneously at a dose 25–50 percent lower than the usual pre-prandial dose. The GIK system requires very frequent measurements of blood glucose: immediately before surgery, during (if the duration of the operation is > 2 hours), immediately after and at regular intervals after the surgery (usually every 1–2 hours and every 4 hours later). For blood glucose levels of 120–180 mg/dl (6.7–10.0 mmol/L), the glucose solution remains stable. For levels < 120 mg/dl (6.7 mmol/L), insulin concentration in the solution is decreased by 5–10 units, whereas for blood glucose levels > 180 mg/dl (10.0 mmol/L), insulin concentration is increased by 5–10 units. Administration of the GIK solution is discontinued when the patient is able to eat satisfactorily.

Some authors, especially in Intensive Care Units, prefer to administer rapid-acting insulin with an intravenous infusion pump (1 i.u./ml). This is achieved by diluting 50 i.u. of rapid-acting insulin in a 50 ml syringe and glucose is administered as in GIK solutions. The insulin infusion rate is per hour 1/24th of the previously total daily need in subcutaneous insulin. Blood glucose is measured every hour and the glucose infusion rate is adjusted so that its level will range from 120 mg/dl (6.7 mmol/L) to 180 mg/dl (10.0 mmol/L). If the previous insulin dose is unknown, we start the infusion at 0.3 i.u. per gram of intravenously administered glucose.

CASE STUDY 2

A 42 year old man comes to the hospital because of fever and intense abdominal pain. He has an increased WBC count of 18,000/µl and a toxic clinical picture (he has the face of a sick person, tachycardia, hypotension and high fever). Hydrops of the gallbladder is detected from radiological examinations. A decision was made to take the patient immediately to surgery. He is suffering from Type 1 DM, being treated with an intensive insulin regimen, with 10–12 units of rapid-acting insulin before meals and 36 units of basal insulin (glargine) before bedtime. His blood glucose level is 283 mg/dl (15.7 mmol/L), and electrolytes, urea, and creatinine concentrations are within normal limits. How can this patient be managed so that urgent surgery can be performed?

Since this is an urgent situation for surgery, but at the same time the patient has intense hyperglycaemia, a period of 12–16 hours of stabilization is proposed, if possible. In patients with serious metabolic derangement (ketoacidosis or hyperosmosis) who need emergency surgical treatment, an intensive management of blood glucose for 6–8 hours significantly improves the metabolic state and the general condition. Further management is based on one of the previously mentioned schemes.

Furthermore, when they are going to undergo a major surgery (see above), the administration of an insulin and glucose solution is recommended preoperatively in all Type 1 diabetic patients, in insulin-treated Type 2 diabetics and in patients with Type 2 diabetes with poor metabolic control.

Were this patient (with Type 1 DM) to undergo a minor surgical procedure, how should he be managed?

For well-controlled patients who are going to have minor surgery under local anaesthesia, surgery is usually planned early in the morning, with frequent measurements of blood glucose (every two hours). The patient should be given a third to a half of the morning isophane (intermediate-acting) insulin dose (the rest of the dose is administered after the surgery), whereas for people using glargine insulin, the dose remains unchanged.

If needed, subcutaneous rapid-acting insulin can be administered based on a sliding-scale (an example is given in the table below).

Blood glucose (mg/dl – mmol/L)	Units of insulin
< 140 (7.8)	0
140–180 (7.8–10.0)	2–4
180–220 (10.0–12.2)	4–8
220–260 (12.2–14.4)	8–10
260–300 (14.4–16.7)	10–12
> 300 (16.7)	10 subcutaneously and 10 iv bolus

Alternatively, the Joslin clinic proposes the administration of rapid-acting insulin subcutaneously every 4–6 hours or every 2–4 hours for rapid-acting insulin analogues, as is depicted in the following table (if blood glucose is > 250 mg/dl [13.9 mmol/L], more frequent measurements are recommended).

	Body weight I (< 80 kg [176.4 lb])	Body weight II (81–99 kg [178.6–218.3 lb])	Body weight III (> 100 kg [220.5 lb])
Capillary blood glucose, mg/dl (mmol/L)	Insulin (units)	Insulin (units)	Insulin (units)
< 150 (8.3)	0	1	2
150–200 (8.3–11.1)	1	2	4
201–250 (11.2–13.9)	2	4	6
251–300 (13.9–16.7)	4	6	8
301–350 (16.7–19.4)	6	8	10
351–400 (19.5–22.2)	8	10	12
> 400 (22.2)	Insulin infusion	Insulin infusion	Insulin infusion

Further reading

Amiel, S.A. and Alberti, K.G.M.M. (2005) Diabetes and surgery, in: *The diabetes Mellitus Manual*, (ed. S.E. Inzucchi), McGraw-Hill Co. Inc., pp. 231–42

Gavin, L.A. (1992) Perioperative Management of the Diabetic Patient. *Endocrinology and Metabolism Clinics of North America*, **21**, 457–75.

Hall, G. (1999) *Diabetes and Hospital Management*. London, England, BMJ Books, 102–21.

Hemmerling, T.M., Schmid, M.C., Schmidt, J. *et al.* (2001) Comparison of a continuous glucose-insulin-potassium infusion versus intermittent bolus application of insulin on perioperative glucose control and hormone status in insulin-treated Type 2 diabetics. *J Clin Anesth*, **13**, 293–300.

Jacober, S. and Sowers, J. (1999) An Update on Perioperative Management of Diabetes. *Arch Intern Medicine*, **159**, 2405–11.

Marks, J. (2003) Perioperative Management of Diabetes. *Am Fam Physic*, **67**, 93–100.

Queale, W.S., Seidler, A.J., Brancati, F.L. (1997) Glycemic control and sliding scale insulin use in medical inpatients with diabetes mellitus. *Arch Intern Med*, **157**, 545–52.

Schade, D.S. (1998) Surgery and diabetes. *Med Clin North Am*, **72**, 1531–43.

8

Acute illness in diabetes

Stavros Liatis

What instructions should be given to a diabetic person with an acute illness at home?

Instructions in this case are individualized and depend on a variety of factors, including the type of DM, the kind of therapy (pills or insulin, scheme of insulin therapy), the presence of complications and the type of the acute illness. Diabetic persons, just like non-diabetic ones, frequently have common infections, mild or more serious, during which many questions regarding the treatment of blood glucose arise. It is essential that appropriate instructions be given beforehand, so that patients do not panic and treatment of the acute condition is timely, appropriate and effective. It should always be kept in mind that possible inappropriate management can lead to a significantly poor metabolic control that could increase the risk of an acute complication, such as diabetic ketoacidosis or hyperglycaemic hyperosmolar coma.

General instructions for an acute illness at home are as follows:

1. Insulin should not be omitted. Even when there is a feeding problem (nausea, vomiting), it is more likely that additional insulin will be needed (due to the stress that the acute illness has caused) rather than reduction of insulin. This rule is more relevant to persons with Type 1 DM.
2. Frequency of capillary blood glucose measurements is recommended to increase (at least every 3–4 hours).

Diabetes in Clinical Practice: Questions and Answers from Case Studies.   Nicholas Katsilambros *et al.*
© 2006 John Wiley & Sons, Ltd.

3. People with Type 1 DM should check their urine (or capillary blood) for ketones every 4–6 hours (also depending on blood glucose levels).
4. Ample intake of water is advised (at least ½ a glass [100–150 ml]) every hour. Food should be light.
5. Rest is advised. Exercise should be avoided.
6. Good communication between the patient and his or her treating physician is essential, so that proper instructions for coping with any special situation can be given at any time.

What changes should be made in the insulin regimen during periods of an acute illness?

Basically, the intensive insulin regimen is followed, as it is, provided the patient is normally fed. If needed, the doses of 'prandial' and basal insulin are increased. Sometimes it may be necessary to administer rapid-acting insulin (or even better a rapid-acting insulin analogue) between meals. In this case, small doses are preferred. If the patient is unable to receive food, the dose of basal insulin is administered normally and, if needed, rapid-acting insulin is administered every 4–6 hours, or a rapid-acting analogue every 3–4 hours. At the same time, intake of carbohydrates in the form of liquid or semi-solid food (i.e., juice, refreshments, soups, purée, etc.) is recommended. Insulin dose is empirically determined each time as 1/10th of the usual total daily dose when blood glucose is > 150 mg/dl (8.3 mmol/L) and as 1/5th of the total daily dose when blood glucose is > 200 mg/dl (11.1 mmol/L) or urine ketones are present.

When insulin is administered as a twice a day regimen (intermediate acting or a mixture of rapid-acting (or analogue) and intermediate-acting, in the morning and evening), and if the patient eats normally, this scheme is initially preserved and additional rapid-acting (or rapid-acting analogue) insulin is possibly administered in between, based on blood glucose measurements. If the patient is unable to eat (for example due to nausea or vomiting), a decrease in the insulin dose by 30–50 percent is recommended initially, as well as close monitoring of the blood glucose levels, intake of carbohydrates in the form of liquid or semi-solid food and possibly administration of rapid-acting (or analogue) insulin. If the condition persists, it may be necessary to admit the patient to hospital (see below).

How is an acute illness managed in patients who receive antidiabetic pills?

When diabetes is under good control and small doses of pills are received (monotherapy or combination), no significant problem usually arises. During the period of the acute illness, blood glucose can have a mild or moderate increase and later return to the previous levels. In people who receive maximum doses of oral antidiabetic medicines, a problem of poor glycaemic control can ensue, and in this case a temporary period of insulin treatment may be needed.

When is admission into hospital recommended?

Admission to hospital is recommended in the following cases:

1. when poor glycaemic control is accompanied by an alteration in the level of conscience;
2. ketonuria or ketonaemia are present and persist for more than six hours, despite the administration of insulin, carbohydrates and fluids;
3. blood glucose levels are > 400 mg/dl (22.2 mmol/L) in more than two repeated measurements, despite the administration of rapid-acting insulin.
4. inability to get hydration by mouth.

CASE STUDY 1

A 30 year old man with Type 1 DM is under treatment with isophane insulin (NPH), 10 units in the morning and 14 units in the evening, as well as insulin Aspart before each meal (at a dose determined based on the carbohydrate content of the meal and the pre-prandial blood glucose level). The usual daily dose of insulin Aspart is 20–24 units). His glycaemic control is very good (recent HbA$_{1c}$: 6.9 percent). The patient called his primary physician in the morning because during the previous night he had four episodes of vomiting, abdominal pains and three episodes of diarrhoea. His blood glucose level in the morning was 320 mg/dl (17.8 mmol/L). He continued to feel intense nausea and when attempting to drink water, he vomited again.

The doctor initially asked the patient to check his urine for ketones with a special urine stripe (which the patient had been instructed in the past to have at home) and call him back.

A few minutes later the patient informed the doctor that the urine test was positive for ketones (semi-quantitative determination: ++). Based on the guidelines analysed above, the doctor recommended the injection of eight units of insulin Aspart subcutaneously (20 percent of the total daily dose – see previous paragraphs) and repeat blood glucose measurement and ketones in 2–3 hours. At the same time, the doctor asked the patient to drink tea with some sugar (one teaspoon – 30 g per glass) slowly (at least one glass every 30–45 minutes). Furthermore, he gave additional instructions to the patient (see relevant questions of the present chapter) and asked him to call again if urine ketones still persisted in six hours (or earlier if they increased) or if blood glucose level was persistently higher than 300 mg/dl (16.7 mmol/L), despite the administration of insulin.

Two and a half hours later the patient had a blood glucose level of 237 mg/dl (13.2 mmol/L) and urine ketones had decreased to (1+). The sugar beverage had been well tolerated. Nausea had subsided but there had been two additional diarrhoeal bowel movements. Eight units of insulin Aspart subcutaneously were administered and the tea beverage continued. Three hours later the patient felt much better, despite again having diarrhoea; his blood glucose level was 173 mg/dl (9.6 mmol/L) and ketones were no longer detected in the urine. He had a light meal (soup with chicken broth and some rice with a piece of toast) and calculated the pre-prandial Aspart dose as usual with an addition of five units (10 percent of total daily dose – see relevant questions of the present chapter). In the afternoon he felt weak, but diarrhoeas had significantly decreased. Blood glucose level was 135 mg/dl (7.5 mmol/L) and no more insulin was administered. After his (light) dinner he returned to his regular schedule.

CASE STUDY 2

A 70 year old woman with Type 2 DM for 10 years, smoker, with mild chronic obstructive pulmonary disease (COPD), is being treated with oral antidiabetic medicines (glibenclamide 15 mg daily and metformin 850 mg daily). Her glycaemic control is moderate (last HbA$_{1c}$: 7.9 percent). She urgently called her treating physician because 24 hours ago she developed fever (up to 38.6°C [101.5°F]), cough and a moderate degree of dyspnoea, which did not improved despite use of inhaled bronchodilators. Her blood glucose levels were persistently higher than 400 mg/dl (22.2 mmol/L) for the previous 12 hours, despite the fact that she 'does not eat nearly anything' and despite the fact that she took the initiative to take one extra pill of glibenclamide 5 mg and one of metformin 850 mg. She has a dry mouth, intense polydipsia and polyuria. She is asking for help with management of the high blood glucose levels.

This patient should receive insulin. Her blood glucose level is exceptionally high (despite the high dose of antidiabetic medicines); it aggravates the patient's condition, causing dehydration and electrolyte disturbances, and also increases the risk of a hyperosmolar coma. Furthermore, metformin administration, albeit in small doses, at times of hypoxemia (due to exacerbation of the underlying mild COPD) is contraindicated. Insulin administration will be difficult at home, since the patient has no education and training for this. In addition, the degree of existent dehydration will probably require intravenous fluid administration. Finally, the administration of corticosteroids may be necessary to manage the COPD exacerbation, which would further aggravate the metabolic control.

For all these reasons, admission to hospital was recommended, even though the severity of the infection alone was not serious enough to require admission.

Further reading

American Diabetes Association (2004) Standards of medical care in diabetes. *Diabetes Care*, **27**(Suppl 1), S15–S35.

Bolli, G.B. (2003) Insulin treatment and its complications, in (eds. J. Pickup and G. Williams) *Textbook of Diabetes*, 3rd edn, Blackwell Science Ltd, Oxford, **43**, 1–38.

Mellinger, D.C. (2003) Preparing students with diabetes for life at college. *Diabetes Care*, **26**, 2675–8.

9

Diabetes and exercise

Konstantinos Makrilakis

What is the definition of exercise and what are its characteristics?

Exercise (physical or muscular activity) is defined as every physical movement produced by skeletal muscles, resulting in energy consumption. It is divided into two types: aerobic and anaerobic.

In aerobic exercise, consumed energy concerns the oxidation of glucose through the Krebs cycle and the respiratory chain, as well as of free fatty acids (aerobic endurance exercise). In this type of exercise, many groups of muscles contract at the same time, for example during walking, running, swimming, cycling, playing football, etc.

In anaerobic exercise, consumed energy is derived from anaerobic glycolysis and lactate production (anaerobic resistance training). In this type of exercise, only small groups of muscles or solitary muscles contract, for example in weightlifting, resistance exercises, muscle strengthening exercises, etc.

In addition to the type of exercise (aerobic or anaerobic), other characteristics of exercise with clinical significance are duration and intensity. Exercise is defined as *short* when its duration is up to 30 minutes, *intermediate* when it lasts 30–60 minutes and *prolonged* when it lasts more than 60 minutes. Intensity grading is based either on the percentage of maximal oxygen consumption ($VO_{2max}[\%]$) or on the percentage increase of heart rate at the time of peak muscular effort (maximal heart rate %). Maximal heart rate (HR_{max}) depends on the age of the person and is

Diabetes in Clinical Practice: Questions and Answers from Case Studies. Nicholas Katsilambros *et al.*
© 2006 John Wiley & Sons, Ltd.

Table 9.1. Grading of exercise intensity

Intensity	VO$_{2max}$(%)	HR$_{max}$(%)
Very mild	< 20	< 35
Mild	20–39	35–54
Moderate	40–59	55–69
Heavy	60–84	70–89
Very heavy	> 85	> 90
Maximal	100	100

VO$_{2max}$ = maximal oxygen consumption
HR$_{max}$ = maximal heart rate (220−age)

calculated by the formula: HR$_{max}$ = 220 − age. Table 9.1 depicts grading of exercise intensity based on VO$_{2max}$ (percent) and HR$_{max}$ (%).

What are the acute metabolic and hormonal effects of exercise on the body?

At rest, the main metabolic energy substrate for the muscles is derived from oxidation of blood free fatty acids (FFAs). Muscles have stored glucose inside them, in the form of a polysaccharide, called glycogen. This is the main energy source for the muscles during the first 5–10 minutes of exercise. Anaerobic degradation and metabolism of glycogen produces lactate. This then quickly supplies energy (ATP) to the exercising muscle. It should be noted that muscular glycogen (represents around 1100 kcal in a 70 kg man) differs from hepatic glycogen (around 400–500 kcal for a 70 kg man) in the sense that the muscles lack the enzyme glucose-6-phosphatase and thus cannot liberate the glucose phosphate that is derived from glycogen degradation into the circulation. In this way muscle glycogen is trapped inside the muscle and can be used only as a source of energy for the muscle and not for contributing to the increase of blood glucose pool. As exercise continues and muscular glycogen is depleted, blood glucose and FFAs assume an increasingly more pronounced role as energy substrates for the exercising muscles. Blood glucose is derived from the degradation of hepatic glycogen (glycogenolysis) or production of glucose by other non-carbohydrate sources (amino-acids, lactate or glycerol) via the process of gluconeogenesis. If exercise persists for several hours, glucose contribution decreases and FFAs (derived from degradation of fat stored in the adipocytes) comprise the main fuel for energy supply to the exercising muscles.

During moderate intensity exercise in non-diabetic people, blood glucose levels remain essentially stable. This is due to the fact that hepatic glucose production (through glycogenolysis and gluconeogenesis mentioned above) increases 2–4 fold, to compensate for the increased needs of the exercising muscles. Hepatic glucose production during and after the exercise session is under the direct control of glucagon and insulin and is mainly determined by the molecular relationship of glucagon/insulin in the portal vein circulation. If moderate intensity exercise continues for several hours, hepatic glucose production can no longer compensate for the increased muscular utilization and plasma glucose levels tend to decrease. This, in conjunction with the increased insulin sensitivity that exercise produces, leads to a decrease in insulin secretion by the pancreas. In contrast, glucagon levels increase (which promotes glycogenolysis and gluconeogenesis in the liver and lipolysis in the adipose tissue). If exercise is more prolonged, secretion of other compensatory hormones in addition to glucagon (epinephrine, norepinephrine, growth hormone and cortisol) starts to play an increasingly primary role. These hormones promote lipolysis and stimulate hepatic glucose production. Adipose tissue triglycerides are hydrolyzed to FFAs and glycerol, used as fuel in the muscles and as glucose production substrate in the liver, respectively. Consequently, prolonged exercise (for several hours), accompanied by a reduction in insulin secretion and increased secretion of compensatory hormones, ultimately results in a decrease of glucose utilization and increase of FFA utilization by the exercising muscles.

What are the long-term effects of exercise in the body?

Regular, repeated muscular activity has significant beneficial effects in muscular function, leading to an effective utilization of energy substrates. At the same time it promotes an increase in the quantity and activity of mitochondrial enzymes, the number of muscle fibres and the number of newly synthesized capillary vessels. Furthermore, it promotes the translocation of glucose transporters (GLUT4) from intracellular stores to the cellular membrane, which facilitates glucose uptake (this is considered to be the main mechanism by which exercise increases insulin sensitivity). This increase in insulin sensitivity is generally lost after 48–72 hours, which demonstrates the great importance of regularly performed, repeated muscular activity for the achievement of beneficial effects on the body. Regular physical activity is also associated with beneficial effects on the lipid profile (increase in HDL-cholesterol, decrease in triglycerides and small decrease in LDL-cholesterol), decrease in arterial hypertension and contribution – in combination with proper nutrition – towards a decrease of body weight and mainly towards the maintenance of weight loss and free-fat-mass in obese persons.

Regular physical activity has also been proven to decrease cardiovascular morbidity and mortality in the general population. This protective role of exercise has been attributed to various mechanisms: i) the beneficial effect of exercise on the traditional cardiovascular risk factors (hypertension, dyslipidaemia, obesity, insulin resistance); and ii) the beneficial effect of muscular activity to the heart itself (increased oxygen supply, decreased myocardial oxygen needs, formation of lateral coronary circulation, electrical stabilization of the myocardium, etc.). Physical activity is also associated with a multitude of psychological and socio-economical beneficial effects, which promote feelings of energy and vitality, increased self-esteem, decreased depressive feelings and optimism, enthusiasm and productivity in daily life.

What are the effects of exercise in a diabetic person?

Physical activity has both acute and chronic effects in the diabetic person, which differ depending on the type of DM (Type 1 or 2).

During exercise in normal persons, pancreatic insulin secretion decreases (as already mentioned) in response to the increased insulin sensitivity brought about by exercise. In persons with Type 1 DM, however, that use insulin injections for their treatment, this physiological decrease in insulin secretion cannot happen, because insulin has been exogenously administered. Circulating insulin suppresses the expected rise of hepatic glucose production and, on the contrary, aggravates the exercise-induced glucose uptake by the exercising muscles. This hyperinsulinaemia also hinders the normal mobilization of triglycerides from the adipose tissue during exercise, which results in a decreased supply of FFAs for use as a fuel from the muscles.

Metabolic and hormonal response to exercise in Type 1 DM varies to a great extent and depends on multiple factors, including intensity and duration of exercise, glycaemic control before exercise, the kind and dose of insulin administered before the exercise session, the injection site and the temporal relation of the insulin injection with the last (before exercise) meal. Consequently, blood glucose levels can increase, decrease or remain unchanged. Specifically, plasma glucose tends to decrease if there is hyperinsulinaemia during the exercise session, if the exercise is prolonged (> 30 minutes) and if carbohydrates are not consumed before or during the exercise. Hyperinsulinaemia during exercise can be due to the fact that peak action of the administered insulin (short or medium duration) can coincide with the time of the exercise or because insulin injection was administered to an exercising part of the body, resulting in faster absorption. Blood glucose levels usually remain stable when exercise is of short duration and mild to moderate intensity and the appropriate quantity of carbohydrates is administered before or during a moderate intensity exercise session. Finally, blood glucose levels tend to increase if there is hypoinsulinaemia during exercise, the exercise is very intense or an excessive quantity of carbohydrates is consumed before exercise. The final result is hyperglycaemia, with increased mobilization of lipids and increased hepatic ketogenesis. The practical conclusion, therefore, is that in Type 1 DM glucose control during exercise is very complex and dependent on multiple factors.

Despite this complexity, a well-informed diabetic individual can participate in exercise programmes, even competitive ones (marathon running, etc.), successfully and without complications provided they follow some rules of good glycaemic control before the exercise session (the usual desirable blood glucose limits for avoidance of hypo- or hyperglycaemia are 100–250 mg/dl [5.6–13.9 mmol/L], respectively). It is essential that they also regularly check their blood glucose levels (especially in the cases of prolonged exercise, every 30–60 minutes) and consume extra carbohydrates if needed (usually an additional 10–15 g of carbohydrates are required for each hour of moderate intensity exercise, in a 70 kg person). It is important that after a bout of prolonged exercise, these patients monitor their blood glucose levels for possible occurrence of hypoglycaemia several hours later (usually 3–15 hours) or even the next day, owing to the increased uptake of glucose from the exercised muscles for replenishment of the exercise-induced depleted glycogen stores. Table 9.2 shows general instructions for safe exercise in Type 1 diabetics. It should also be emphasized that most intervention

Table 9.2. Instuctions for safe exercise in Type 1 DM

- Adequate metabolic control before starting the exercise programme
- Self monitoring of blood glucose is essential
- Avoidance (or delay) of exercise when blood glucose level is < 100 mg/dl (5.6 mmol/L) or > 250 mg/dl (13.9 mmol/L) with ketosis or > 300 mg/dl (16.7 mmol/L) even without ketosis
- Carbohydrate intake should increase before exercise, depending on blood glucose levels before its initiation, and for the duration and intensity of exercise. Generally, 10–15 g of carbohydrates should be consumed one hour before or after a moderate intensity exercise session. Further carbohydrates should be consumed when blood glucose levels are < 100 mg/dl (5.6 mmol/L) before exercise
- Be prepared for possible hypoglycaemia a few hours after the exercise (usually 3–15 hours, until even the following day)
- A relatively prolonged exercise session may require decrease in the insulin dose in order to avoid hypoglycaemia
- Injection site should preferably be away from an exercising part of the body
- Consumption of fluids is very important and should be encouraged
- All people with DM should carry an identity card and carbohydrate-containing food when they exercise

physical activity studies in Type 1 diabetes have not shown an improvement of glycaemic control with exercise. The main reason for this is possibly the excessive decrease in the insulin dose or the excessive carbohydrate intake before exercise, in an attempt to avoid hypoglycaemias. Type 1 diabetics who participate in competitive sports may observe that their glycaemic control deteriorates, possibly due to the irregular intense exercise schedules, the decrease of insulin doses and the increased carbohydrate consumption. Nevertheless, the long-term benefits of regular physical activity regarding cardiovascular morbidity and mortality that apply to the general population, and those with Type 2 DM (examined below), are applicable to these patients as well.

In Type 2 diabetics (characterized by hepatic and peripheral insulin resistance and hyperinsulinaemia during the initial stages), peripheral glucose utilization during moderate intensity exercise increases more than its hepatic production, resulting in a tendency for blood glucose levels to decrease. At the same time, however, plasma insulin levels decrease, and thus hypoglycaemia risk in these patients (who do not use exogenous insulin) is relatively small. Despite that, for patients who use insulin or insulin secretagogues (sulfonylureas or meglitinides), the risk of hypoglycaemia is real (albeit less than in Type 1 DM).

Physical activity (together with proper nutrition) represents the cornerstone of Type 2 DM treatment. Exercise improves insulin sensitivity, which is accompanied by improvement in glycaemic control (decrease in HbA_{1c} by 0.7 percent in a meta-analysis) and all the other atherosclerotic risk factors already mentioned for non-diabetic people (hypertension, dyslipidaemia, obesity) that very frequently accompany Type 2 diabetes as part of the metabolic syndrome. These improvements are reflected in the amelioration of morbidity and mortality of Type 2 diabetics that exercise regularly, compared with those diabetic persons who do not exercise. During the last few years several prospective and retrospective studies have proven the reverse relationship between muscular activity level and cardiovascular morbidity and mortality in diabetic patients (Type 1 and 2). Selection of timing of exercise may be an especially important parameter for Type 2 diabetics. Exercise late in the evening has been shown to decrease hepatic glucose production and fasting plasma glucose levels the following morning. Furthermore, postprandial exercise can be beneficial since it decreases the frequently observed postprandial hyperglycaemia. Apart from this beneficial effect of exercise in treating DM, well planned clinical studies during the last few years have proven that physical activity programmes, with or without dietary interventions, decrease the risk of developing Type 2 DM in high-risk people (for example, persons with impaired glucose tolerance). Specifically, in two of the best studies performed (one in the USA. and one in Finland) the risk of developing Type 2 DM was decreased by 58 percent in the exercise and diet group compared to the control group (see also Chapter 30 'Prevention of diabetes mellitus').

The type and intensity of exercise necessary for cardiovascular protection has not been definitely elucidated. The American College of Sports Medicine (Albright, *et al.*, 2000) recommend that all diabetic persons should strive to expend at least 1000 kcal/week in leisure time physical activities, at a moderate intensity level (40–70 percent VO_{2max}), 3–5 times per week, with a minimum duration of at least 30 minutes per day. Higher intensity exercise does not seem to contribute to a further decrease in cardiovascular risk and is accompanied by a higher chance of complications. The value of anaerobic exercise (resistance training) – for example weightlifting – in healthy people of any age, regarding cardiovascular benefits, has been recognized in the last 10–15 years.

Traditionally there has been a reluctance to recommend anaerobic exercise, especially in elderly diabetics, due to the fear of abrupt increases in blood pressure. Lately, however, many studies have shown that anaerobic exercise is quite safe and effective in improving glycaemic control, even in elderly diabetic people.

What are the risks of exercise in diabetic persons?

Despite the beneficial effects that were mentioned above, physical activity may also be accompanied by unwelcome effects and incur risks for the exercising person, especially if certain conditions and safety rules are not fulfilled. These risks (apart from the already mentioned hypoglycaemia), are sudden death, serious arrhythmias, myocardial infarction etc., especially in those with underlying heart disease (very common in diabetic persons). In diabetic patients specifically, certain diabetic complications can restrict physical activity levels or even preclude some forms of muscular activity. For example, patients with neuropathy should avoid long-term walking and exercises that entail jumping (risk of musculoskeletal trauma); those with nephropathy should be advised to avoid intense exercises (risk of increase in proteinuria); and persons with proliferative retinopathy should avoid weightlifting and very heavy exercises with a chance of hurting themselves (risk of intraocular haemorrhage or retinal detachment). Table 9.3 succinctly depicts the risks associated with exercise in diabetic persons.

What tests should precede an exercise programme in diabetic persons?

Prior to the initiation of an exercise programme, diabetic patients (especially those with long-standing DM or other atherosclerotic risk factors) are advised to undergo an ECG stress test, to better delineate possible cardiovascular risk. This is especially recommended for people older than 35 years, or those older than 25 years with Type 2 DM of > 10 years' duration or Type 1 DM of more than 15 years' duration. Presence of suspicious ECG abnormalities at rest or during exercise should be further investigated (with a thallium stress test, echocardiogram, coronary angiography, etc.). Presence of peripheral occlusive vascular disease, hypertension, nephropathy,

Table 9.3. Risks of exercise in DM

---

1. Hypoglycaemia during treatment with insulin or insulin secretagogues
  a) exercise-induced
  b) late hypoglycaemia several hours after the exercise
2. Hyperglycaemia
  a) with ketosis, due to uncontrolled diabetes (insulinopenia)
  b) after a short, exhausting exercise session
3. Deterioration of silent heart disease
  a) angina
  b) myocardial infarctionc)
  c) sudden death
4. Deterioration of diabetic complications
  a) Proliferative retinopathy
    – vitreous haemorrhage
    – retinal detachment
  b) Nephropathy
    – increase in albuminuria
  c) Peripheral neuropathy
    – soft tissue and joint injuries
5. Autonomic nervous system neuropathy
  a) unexpected hypoglycaemia (disappearance of adrenergic responses)
  b) decreased cardiovascular adaptation to exercise
  c) decreased maximal oxygen consumption (VO_{2max}), resulting in easy fatiguability
  d) poor adaptation to dehydration
  e) orthostatic hypotension

---

retinopathy and neuropathy (peripheral or autonomic) should also be investigated with appropriate tests (clinical and laboratory), because their presence may necessitate alteration in the exercise programme.

The diabetic person should also be informed about the correct way to exercise. The best and easiest exercise is walking. A period of 10–15 minutes warm up should always precede and a period of 10–15 minutes gradual decrease of physical activity should follow at the end of an exercise programme, so that musculoskeletal and cardiovascular complications are avoided. Use of proper footwear, regular inspection of the lower extremities after or even before an exercise session, proper hydration and taking of all the necessary precautions mentioned in Table 9.2 will help the diabetic person to profit from all the benefits of exercise, while minimizing the risks.

CASES STUDY 1

A 37 year old man with Type 1 DM since the age of 14, comes to the diabetes clinic for a routine visit. He is treated with an intensive insulin regimen, consisting of three injections of rapid-acting insulin analogue before main meals (dose based on pre-prandial glucose measurements and carbohydrate food counting) and one injection of long-acting insulin glargine at bedtime. He consumes three main meals and 2–3 snacks daily. His glycaemic control has generally been quite good for many years (fasting blood glucose: 80–110 mg/dl [4.4–6.1 mmol/L], postprandial < 140 mg/dl [7.8 mmol/L], HbA_{1c}: 5.7 percent), with relatively few hypoglycaemic episodes, of which he is always aware. During the last month the patient has started participating in an exercise programme with some friends, playing tennis three times a week, late in the afternoon (7–8 p.m.). He observed that on the days of tennis playing he had severe hypoglycaemic episodes during the following night. Indicative measurements of the last five days are shown in Table 9.4 (the units of rapid-acting insulin analogue administered are in parenthesis).

Table 9.4. Blood glucose values (mg/dl [mmol/L]) for the patient in Case study 1). Other numbers in parentheses represent units of rapid-acting (regular) insulin administered at that time

Day of exercise	Morning		Noon		After-noon	Evening		Before bedtime	Night
	Before break-fast	2 hrs after	Before lunch	2 hrs after	Before exercise (7 p.m.)	Before dinner	2 hrs after	12 mid-night	3 a.m.
No	88 [4.9] (3)	96 [5.3]	112 [6.2] (8)	120 [6.7]		122 [6.8] (5)	130 [7.2]	136 [7.6] (glargine 20)	
Yes	92 [5.1] (3)	98 [5.4]	110 [6.1] (8)	124 [6.9]	142 [7.9]	135 [7.5] (5)	138 [7.7]	130 [7.2] (glargine 20)	**38 [2.1]**
No	**192 [10.7]** (7)	144 [8.0]	118 [6.6] (8)	132 [7.3]		128 [7.1] (5)	142 [7.9]	120 [6.7] (glargine 20)	
Yes	100 [5.6] (3)	102 [5.7]	108 [6.0] (8)	122 [6.8]	135 [7.5]	128 [7.1] (5)	135 [7.5]	126 [7.0] (glargine 20)	**42 [2.3]**
No	**216 [12.0]** (9)	132 [7.3]	130 [7.2] (8)	136 [7.6]		134 [7.4] (5)	126 [7.0]	120 [6.7] (glargine 20)	

The problems immediately evident are the night-time hypoglycaemias during the days of exercise (38 mg/dl [2.1 mmol/L] and 42 mg/dl [2.7 mmol/L]), and the subsequent morning hyperglycaemias (192 mg/dl [10.7 mmol/L] and 216 mg/dl [12.0 mmol/L]), which are reactive to night-time hypoglycaemias (Somogyi phenomenon). For several hours after a bout of exercise, muscles take up glucose from the blood in order to replenish stored glycogen that was consumed during exercise, resulting in a gradual decrease in blood glucose levels. If these amounts are not replenished, it is not uncommon to have a hypoglycaemic episode even many hours after the exercise, especially in people who use insulin. Therefore, the solution would be that the patient decrease his evening insulin dose before dinner (maybe by one unit) and eat a larger snack before bedtime. Continuing to monitor blood glucose levels will show if this practice is effective or whether other alterations are needed in his therapeutic regimen (for example, decrease of insulin glargine dose at days of exercise, etc.).

CASE STUDY 2

A 34 year old man with well controlled diabetes receives six units rapid-acting (regular) insulin and six units isophane insulin before breakfast (9 a.m.), four units rapid-acting insulin before lunch (1 p.m.) and four units rapid-acting insulin with six units isophane insulin before dinner (8 p.m.). He exercises daily (walks around 5 km [3.1 miles] every morning before breakfast). For the previous two days he felt a bit sick, with mild fever and cough, but decided not to abandon his daily exercise programme. He woke in the morning (8 a.m.) with blood glucose level 298 mg/dl (16.5 mmol/L) and decided to take his usual walk and administer his morning insulin afterwards, before breakfast. He noticed he was much more tired today after walking and was surprised to see his blood glucose level had climbed up to 355 mg/dl (19.7 mmol/L) after walking. Urine ketones were positive.

The evening dose of isophane insulin at 8 p.m. sometimes does not last until the next morning. Furthermore, insulin needs are higher in the early morning hours (6–7 a.m.) due to the circadian rhythm of compensatory hormone secretion (cortisol, growth hormone), which increases insulin resistance (Dawn phenomenon). The presence of the mild upper respiratory tract infection aggravates his insulin needs even more. The high fasting blood glucose level (298 mg/dl [16.5 mmol/L]) clearly shows the patient has hypoinsulinaemia. It would be best not to exercise that day. Not only does exercise under conditions of low blood insulin levels and increased insulin resistance not decrease blood glucose levels, infact it causes their increase and fast tiredness of the muscles, which will work under conditions of insulin shortage (despite hyperglycaemia). Insulin shortage can even lead to ketone-body production by the liver and to ketosis. The patient should not have exercised that day or, if re insisted, he should have delayed exercise initiation. He should have first taken a small dose of rapid-acting insulin (for example, 4–5 units subcutaneously) and have rechecked his blood sugar an hour later. He should have exercised only if his levels had been within the desirable range of 100–250 mg/dl (5.6–13.9 mmol/L).

Further reading

Albright, A., Franz, M., Hornsby, G., Kriska, A., Marrero, D., Ullrich, I. *et al.* (2000) American College of Sports Medicine position stand. Exercise and Type 2 diabetes. *Med Sci Sports Exerc,* **32**, 1345–60.

American Diabetes Association (2004) Physical activity/Exercise and diabetes. *Diabetes Care,* **27**(Suppl 1), S58–S62.

Batty, G.D., Shipley, M.J., Marmot, M., Smith, G.D. (2002) Physical activity and cause-specific mortality in men with Type 2 diabetes/impaired glucose tolerance: evidence from the Whitehall study. *Diabet Med,* **19**, 580–88.

Boule, N.G., Haddad, E., Kenny, G.P., Wells, G.A., Sigal, R.J. (2001) Effects of exercise on glycemic control and body mass in Type 2 diabetes mellitus: a meta-analysis of controlled clinical trials. *JAMA,* **286**, 1218–27.

Duncan, G.E., Perri, M.G., Theriaque, D.W., Hutson, A.D., Eckel, R.H., Stacpoole, P.W. (2003) Exercise training, without weight loss, increases insulin sensitivity and postheparin plasma lipase activity in previously sedentary adults. *Diabetes Care,* **26**, 557–62.

Makrilakis, K., Panagiotakos, D.B., Pitsavos, C., Chrysohoou, C., Ioannidis, I., Dimosthenopoulos, C., Toutouzas, P., Stefanadis, C., Katsilambros, N. (2004) The association between physical activity and the development of acute coronary syndromes in diabetic subjects (The CARDIO2000 II Study). *Eur J Cardiovasc Prev Rehabil,* **11**, 298–303.

Sigal, R.J., Kenny, G.P., Koivisto, V.A. (2003) Exercise and diabetes mellitus, in *Textbook of Diabetes,* 3rd edn, (eds J. Pickup and G. Williams) Blackwell Science Ltd, Oxford, **37**, pp. 1–19.

Steppel, J.H. and Horton, E.S. (2004) Exercise in *Therapy for Diabetes Mellitus and Related Disorders* 4th edn, American Diabetes Association, (ed. H.E. Lebovitz), pp 149–56.

Tanasescu, M., Leitzmann, M.F., Rimm, E.B., Hu, F.B. (2003) Physical activity in relation to cardiovascular disease and total mortality among men with Type 2 diabetes. *Circulation,* **107**, 2435–39.

10

Diabetes and pregnancy

Panagiotis Tsapogas

Diabetes mellitus during pregnancy is a very serious health problem and requires a lot of effort from the physician and the pregnant woman to cope with it. Apart from the possibility of preexisting known Type 1 DM (more rarely Type 2) before the pregnancy, another alternative is the occurrence of DM for the first time during the period of pregnancy (gestational diabetes, see below).

What is the definition of gestational diabetes?

Every degree of glucose impairment that occurs (or is detected) for the first time during pregnancy is called gestational diabetes, regardless of the persistence of the condition after delivery and regardless of the need of diet only or insulin to treat it.

What is the classification of gestational diabetes?

Gestational diabetes is classified as a separate form of DM. It is not uncommon, following the occurrence of gestational diabetes, for the condition to continue after delivery, either in the form of Type 2 DM or even as a first occurrence of Type 1 DM.

It should be noted that during the course of a normal pregnancy there is resistance to the action of insulin which causes increased circulation of glucose and free fatty acids, so that adequate supply of these nutrients is available for the foetus. This condition is compensated for by an

Diabetes in Clinical Practice: Questions and Answers from Case Studies. Nicholas Katsilambros *et al.*
© 2006 John Wiley & Sons, Ltd.

increased secretion of insulin. In 2–4 percent of pregnancies, however, insulin production is inadequate and gestational diabetes occurs.

How is gestational diabetes diagnosed?

Diagnosis is carried out in one or two phases. The first phase is a 50 g oral glucose tolerance test at the 24–28th week of gestation, which the pregnant woman receives regardless of prior food ingestion. Venous plasma glucose values above 140 mg/dl (7.8 mmol/L) one hour after glucose ingestion are considered abnormal, although some authors suggest a lower level (130 mg/dl [7.2 mmol/L]). When a cut-off point of 140 mg/dl (7.8 mmol/L) is used, around 80 percent of gestational diabetic women are detected, whereas with 130 mg/dl (7.2 mmol/L) as cut-off, around 90 percent are detected. At the same time, however, the false positive rate is increased, i.e. women wrongly considered to have gestational diabetes. This particular glucose tolerance test is not accepted by all, though it is easy and cheap, as it includes only one blood glucose measurement, regardless of food intake.

If an abnormal result is found in the 50 g oral glucose tolerance test, a second oral glucose tolerance test follows, either with 100 g glucose (three hours) or with 75 g glucose (two hours). There is no unanimous agreement whether an increased intake of carbohydrates for three days should precede the test, although this has been proposed. Diagnostic criteria for gestational diabetes, depending on the method used, are shown in Table 10.1.

It should be noted that there is disagreement over whether to screen all pregnant women without exceptions for gestational diabetes or only those at high risk. The same disagreement applies over the methods and diagnostic criteria. Most authors, however, insist on screening all pregnancies without exceptions, given the fact that hyperglycaemia management during gestation protects from a series of complications, whereas during selection some risk factors may be missed.

CASE STUDY 1

A 35 year old healthy woman, with a history of an unexplained miscarriage six months ago, wishes to become pregnant again. Is there a chance that this woman will develop gestational diabetes and how will the diagnosis be made?

Table 10.1. Oral glucose tolerance test during pregnancy

---

100 g oral glucose tolerance test (adapted from O'Sullivan, 1964)

For diagnosing gestational diabetes mellitus, at least two abnormal values are required:

Fasting plasma glucose	$\geq$ 95 mg/dl (5.3 mmol/L)
1 hour	$\geq$180 mg/dl (10.0 mmol/L)
2 hours	$\geq$155 mg/dl (8.6 mmol/L)
3 hours	$\geq$140 mg/dl (7.8 mmol/L)

75 g oral glucose tolerance test

American Diabetes Association Criteria

At least two values higher than the following:

Fasting plasma glucose	$\geq$ 95 mg/dl (5.3 mmol/L)
1 hour	$\geq$ 180 mg/dl (10.0 mmol/L)
2 hours	$\geq$ 155 mg/dl (8.6 mmol/L)

World Health Organization Criteria

Fasting plasma glucose	$\geq$ 125 mg/dl (6.9 mmol/L)
or	
2 hours	$\geq$ 140 mg/dl (7.8 mmol/L)

The chance that a woman will develop gestational diabetes mellitus is large when at least one of the following applies:

1. family history of DM, especially in first degree relatives;
2. body weight before pregnancy larger than ideal body weight, at least by 10 percent;
3. age more than 25 years;
4. history of impaired glucose tolerance;
5. a member of an ethnic group with high prevalence of diabetes (black race, etc.);
6. a previous unexplained perinatal interruption of pregnancy or intrauterine death or birth of a neonate with congenital abnormalities or with a body weight of more than 4 kg (8.82 lb);
7. multiparous (more than four pregnancies).

Some authors have added more risk factors.

Regardless of the above situations that require greater vigilance from the clinician and possibly indicate the need for screening from the first clinic visit, screening for gestational diabetes should be performed, according to most authors, in all apparently normal pregnancies at the 24–28th week of gestation.

Could development of gestational diabetes represent the first manifestation of Type 2 DM?

It is very possible that several cases of gestational diabetes represent preexisting undiagnosed Type 2 DM. Occurrence of Type 2 DM in pregnancy is considered to have increased in recent years, since this type of diabetes can now be diagnosed at younger ages with increasing frequency. Insulin usage in pregnancy does not allow the easy and precise evaluation of Type 2 DM and this problem is bigger in peoples with a high prevalence of Type 1 DM, such as in Scandinavia. Correspondingly, in peoples with a high prevalence of Type 2 DM, maybe half of all diabetic cases at pregnancy are Type 2.

It should also be noted that complications of pregnant women with Type 2 DM have been recorded, such as diabetic retinopathy and pre-eclampsia as well as foetal complications, at percentages similar to those of Type 1 DM. The increase in Type 2 DM prevalence in developing and developed countries is expected to increase the percentage of pregnant women with Type 2 DM in the near future.

CASE STUDY 2

During prenatal screening, a young woman with diagnosed Type 1 DM monitored at the Diabetes Outpatient Clinic, is enquiring about safety of her pregnancy.

Although complications in neonates of mothers with gestational diabetes are usually minimal, Type 1 DM pregnancies incur a high risk for teratogenesis in the neonate due to hyperglycaemia and other difficulties, especially if the mother suffers from nephropathy, retinopathy or heart disease.

Gestational complications affect prognosis. Pre-eclampsia, the frequency of which is double in pregnant diabetics compared to non-diabetics, is associated with premature births.

The White classification (Table 10.2) is used for pregnancy prognosis and the risks of DM to the foetus. This classification is based on age at onset and duration of DM, as well as on the presence of complications.

Table 10.2. The White classification of diabetes in pregnancy

Category		Description
A		Impaired glucose tolerance, at any age, treated only by diet therapy
B		Onset of diabetes at age 20 years or older and duration of less than 10 years
C		Onset of diabetes at age 10–19 years and duration of 10–19 years
D		Onset before 10 years of age, duration over 20 years, benign retinopathy, or hypertension (not preeclampsia)
	D1	Onset before age 10 years
	D2	Duration over 20 years
	D3	Calcification of vessels of the leg (macrovascular disease)– formerly called Class E
	D4	Benign retinopathy (microvascular disease)
	D4	Hypertension (not preeclampsia)
R		Proliferative retinopathy or vitreous haemorrhage
F		Nephropathy with over 500 mg/day proteinuria
RF		Criteria for both classes R and F
G		Many pregnancy failures
H		Evidence of arteriosclerotic heart disease
T		Prior renal transplantation
Classes B through T require insulin treatment		
Gestational diabetes		
A1		Diet-controlled gestational diabetes
A2		Insulin-treated gestational diabetes

How do metabolic disturbances of a pregnant woman with DM affect the foetus?

Impaired insulin action in the diabetic pregnant woman is not adequate to compensate for the increased needs of pregnancy. This can possibly lead to congenital malformations of the foetus, miscarriages, macrosomia and neonatal hypoglycaemia. These conditions are part of the general entity of the so-called foetopathy.

When hyperglycaemia of the mother occurs early in the course of the pregnancy, it can more frequently cause spontaneous miscarriages and major malformations (embryopathy). For this reason, strict glycaemic

Table 10.3. Perinatal complications of a diabetic pregnancy

Perinatal mortality	0.6–4.8%
Caesarean section	32–45%
Prematurity	
< 37 weeks of gestation	24–33%
< 34 weeks of gestation	14–16%
Congenital anomalies	1.7–9.4%
Perinatal asphyxia	9–28%
Macrosomia	9–28%
Intrauterine growth retardation	2–8%
Respiratory distress syndrome	2–6%
Hypoglycaemia	5–25%
Hypocalcaemia	4%
Polycythemia	5–33%
Hyperbilirubinaemia	11–29%
Cardiomyopathy	5–10%
Symptomatic	
Asymptomatic	30–50%

The lower complication rates occur when there is strict glycaemic control

control of women with Type 1 DM, prior to conception and then during the course of the pregnancy, is really essential to decrease the risk of congenital malformations.

Perinatal complications (Table 10.3) of a diabetic pregnancy should also be considered, since they tend to appear in high frequency (from 0.6 to 4.8 percent), despite the fact that intensive insulin therapy has significantly decreased them.

How is macrosomia defined and how is it caused?

Macrosomia is defined as the condition during which the neonate's body weight at birth is higher than the 90th percentile for gestational age or higher than 4 kg (8.82 lb). Macrosomia occurs in every type of diabetic pregnancy unless there is angiopathy. Neonates are large and corpulent, with an excessive accumulation of fat in the abdomen and shoulders. Furthermore, visceral enlargement occurs. Macrosomia predisposes to trauma during delivery, especially shoulder dystocia, which is prevented by caesarian section.

The proposed mechanism for the abnormal foetal conditions (foeto-pathy) includes hypertrophy of the β-cells of the pancreatic islets and hyperinsulinaemia of the foetus, due to the mother's hyperglycaemia. A result of this hyperinsulinaemia is an increased synthesis and storage of fat. The foetus is big for its gestational age (macrosomia). This condition is the result of poor glycaemic control of the mother, especially during the last two trimesters of pregnancy. Good glycaemic control minimizes the risk for this complication.

Furthermore, macrosomia causes hypoxaemia due to increased oxygen needs, as well as polycythemia, catecholamine overproduction, hypertension and cardiomegaly.

Apart from macrosomia, how can other conditions harm the foetus of a pregnant woman with DM?

Excessively strict glycaemic control can lead to intrauterine growth restriction as well as to small-for-gestational age neonates. Angiopathy (White stage H) and pre-eclampsia can also cause intrauterine growth restriction.

Congenital malformations account for nearly a half of perinatal deaths in diabetic pregnancies. There is no specific congenital anomaly that specifically connects to diabetic pregnancies. The majority of cases, however, involve caudal agenesis (caudal regression syndrome, 200 times more frequent compared to non-diabetic pregnancies).

Induced labour is more common in diabetic pregnancies, especially when pre-eclampsia occurs.

Infant respiratory distress syndrome is also more common in infants of diabetic mothers for every gestational age, possibly owing to delayed maturation of surfactant factor, due to pneumonia, hypertrophic cardio-myopathy or other conditions.

Hypoglycaemia (blood sugar level below 40 mg/dl [2.2 mmol/L]) frequently occurs during the first hours of life, especially in macrosomic babies, due to the hyperinsulinaemia of the neonate, which is now taken away from the hyperglycaemic environment of the mother. Furthermore, premature or small-for-gestational age infants may have restricted hepatic glycogen stores. This complication, which requires very strict monitoring of the infant, can be minimized by the strict glycaemic control of the mother during the perinatal period.

Hypocalcaemia (total serum calcium level < 7 mg/dl [1.75 mmol/L] or ionized calcium < 4 mg/dl [1.0 mmol/L]) is a common complication, especially in low birth weight infants of diabetic pregnancies. The extent of hypocalcaemia is related to the severity and duration of maternal diabetes. It is thought to be caused by the lower parathyroid hormone (PTH) concentrations after birth in infants of diabetic mothers compared to normal infants. It is combined with hyperphosphataemia and is usually asymptomatic, as is hypomagnesaemia.

Polycythemia (haematocrit > 65 percent) and *hyperviscosity syndrome* have also been observed, with resultant ischaemia and infarcts of various organs of the neonate.

Hyperbilirubinaemia and *jaundice* are also more frequently observed in macrosomic infants, especially when glycaemic control is poor. The mechanism most likely involves glycosylation of red blood cells membranes, which predisposes to increased haemolysis.

Also, transient *hypertrophic* (and more rarely *restrictive*) *cardiomyopathy* has been described, due to the hyperinsulinaemia.

Should a woman with Type 1 DM be counselled regarding future pregnancies, and why?

The primary physician should counsel the woman with Type 1 DM mellitus regarding a future pregnancy from the time of puberty. Programming of the pregnancy, so that at its initiation and evolution the best possible glycaemic control has been achieved, is essential for the prognosis.

The diabetic woman who wants to become pregnant should know that pregnancy can have detrimental effects on already existent microvascular diabetic complications, can cause hypoglycaemia or ketoacidosis, hypertension or aggravation of preexistent hypertension, polyhydramnios, premature birth or be complicated by acute pyelonephritis or other infections.

Hyperglycaemia seems to be the most significant risk parameter for the foetus of a diabetic woman. It is however clear, that when maternal blood glucose levels are within normal levels both before and during the course of the pregnancy, spontaneous abortions, congenital malformations and macrosomia are reduced to proportions similar to those of non-diabetic mothers.

Are retinopathy and nephropathy in a woman with DM contraindications for her pregnancy?

Pre-existent diabetic retinopathy can be exacerbated by strict glycaemic control, which is necessary, however, for foetal development and normal progression of the pregnancy. Strict glycaemic control can decrease plasma volume and thus accelerate the closure of small retinal blood vessels that were narrowed but still clear. The deterioration has been associated with presence of hypertension, hypoglycaemias and smoking but not with presence of retinopathy in previous pregnancies. For protection from this complication, ideal control before conception is pursued, preferably with laser therapies, if indicated. Photocoagulation or vitrectomy can also be performed during pregnancy, under strict, regular monitoring of the woman. In conclusion, diabetic retinopathy is not a contraindication for pregnancy, regardless of stage.

Severe gastroparesis that will be aggravated by heperemesis gravitarum should be seriously considered, because it renders strict glycaemic control impossible.

Pregnancy does not seem to increase future risk of nephropathy. However, possible preexistent nephropathy or microalbuminuria are associated with increased rates of premature delivery, due mainly to pre-eclampsia occurrence, which can lead to intrauterine growth retardation and more rarely to death of the infant or even of the mother. During diabetic pregnancy the glomerular filtration rate is reduced, even with strict glycaemic control. When there is established proteinuria, urinary protein excretion can increase significantly and decrease after delivery, without permanently affecting the kidney function, unless there is concomitant hypertension. Pre-eclampsia and premature labour are observed at rates above 60 percent in women with creatinine clearance less than 80 ml/min or urinary protein excretion more than 1 g/24 hs. Women, however, with plasma creatinine levels more than 2 mg/dl (176.8 µmol/L) are at increased risk for these complications and so this creatinine level, as well as the presence of proteinuria above 2 g/24 hs, is considered a relative contraindication for pregnancy. The same applies to protein excretion rates of > 300 mg/24 hs when there is concomitant hypertension. Creatinine clearance less than 50 ml/min is associated with the development of a significant degree of hypertension and a large infant death rate, so pregnancy is allowed only after a renal transplantation has been performed.

CASE STUDY 3 – MANAGEMENT OF A WOMAN WITH GESTATIONAL DIABETES

A pregnant woman in the 25th week of gestation is subjected to a three-hour oral glucose tolerance test with 100 g glucose. The following results are obtained: fasting plasma glucose: 90 mg/dl (5.0 mmol/L); one hour 198 mg/dl (11.00 mmol/L); two hours 160 mg/dl (8.9 mmol/L); and three hours 115 mg/dl (6.4 mmol/L). What advice should she be given and how should she be monitored during pregnancy after these results?

This woman is suffering from gestational diabetes, since two glucose values are higher than the cut-offs recommended for this test (see Table 10.1).

Insulin action changes in pregnancy. During the 12–14th week of gestation insulin sensitivity is slightly high, but then it decreases for the rest of the pregnancy, especially during the last trimester. Gestational diabetes is typically manifested at the end of the second trimester.

At the first visit, the treating physician should examine the patient thoroughly, explain to her the possible complications of gestational diabetes, discuss issues of follow-up and educate her in the special issues of diabetes (body weight, nutrition, physical exercise, glycaemic control targets, self monitoring of blood glucose, urine ketone monitoring, clinic visits, blood pressure, lower extremity swelling, etc.).

This woman should receive individualized nutritional guidance, depending on her weight and height. Ample calories for the needs of the pregnancy should be administered. If the woman is obese (BMI > 30 kg/m^2), calories should be decreased to about 25 per kg body weight per day, since it has been shown that in this way triglycerides and glucose levels are better controlled without increased ketonuria. Ketone body determination in the urine is useful to detect insufficient intake of carbohydrates.

Moderate physical exercise possibly decreases glucose concentration.

The pregnant woman should be trained to measure her blood sugar level regularly every day (at least four times a day). At the clinic visit strict glycaemic targets should be set (see below). If these targets cannot be achieved with diet and exercise, insulin should be started.

What is the role, and what are the principles, of a proper diet in pregnancy?

A well-balanced diet concerning nutrients is always of great importance for the health of the mother and for the successful completion of the pregnancy. Chosen foods comprise the nutritional substrate for the development of the foetus. For women with gestational diabetes, it is not uncommon that proper nutrition alone, can preserve blood glucose levels in the normal range, and thus this is the generally the first step for the management of gestational diabetes, before insulin initiation. Care must be taken about the total number of calories that the mother consumes, the avoidance of foods that increase blood glucose levels and the preference of nutrients that preserve them in normal levels. The help of a dietitian is essential and usually necessary, so that every pregnant woman can individually programme her diet. An effective nutritional approach results in good blood glucose control, avoidance of ketosis (which has detrimental effects to the foetus), adequate weight gain and normal foetal development. It should be noted that when, despite proper nutrition, a strict glycaemic control is not achieved, the chance of macrosomia is relatively large. Insulin therapy is required in this case.

Blood glucose levels normally fall during pregnancy by around 20 percent. Consequently, the targets of a good glycaemic control are stricter in pregnancy (see below). Furthermore, postprandial glucose concentration has actually been associated more closely with complications of the pregnancy and especially neonatal macrosomia.

Weight gain of the mother is a crude indication of foetal nutrition. Desired gain depends on pre-conception weight and is determined based on the body mass index. A large weight gain frequently means an increase in body fat, insulin resistance and blood glucose levels. Loss of weight or weight gain less than expected, due to excessively strict diet, can also be detrimental (can cause premature labour). The weekly rate of body weight increase is also monitored and varies in each trimester.

Special catalogues with foods, calories and included nutrients give the necessary information for planning of the diet. In general, the daily calorie intake is calculated based on the ideal body weight at the beginning of pregnancy and is shown in Table 10.4. Energy needs

Table 10.4. Recommended calories at pregnancy, based on body weight

Percentage of ideal body weight at onset of pregnancy	Recommended daily caloric intake (kcal per kg body weight)
< 80%	40
80–120%	30
120–150%	24
> 150%	12–15

increase by 300 kcal per day during the second and third trimesters of pregnancy, as do protein needs.

Allocation of calories generally consists of 50 percent carbohydrates, 20 percent protein and 30 percent fat. Most dietary programmes recommend three main dishes and three snacks a day, with individualization of the needs based on blood sugar measurements. Complex carbohydrates, such as those in vegetables, legumes and fruit, as well as foods rich in dietary fibres, are preferred because they cause less postprandial hyperglycaemia. Foods with a low fat content should also be encouraged due to their lower calorie content and consequent lower tendency towards obesity.

For well-known reasons, unsaturated fats and especially olive oil are preferred.

A snack at bedtime, which contains proteins and carbohydrates, is recommended, because during the night there can be lower insulin production resulting in fat oxidation (if no carbohydrates have been consumed) and ketone-body production (detected in the morning urine). Ketoacidosis of the mother has been associated with decreased intelligence index of the child later in life. Furthermore, women who use insulin should receive a snack at bedtime to avoid possible night-time hypoglycaemia.

Avoidance of alcoholic beverages is also recommended, since there is evidence that even moderate alcohol consumption can be associated with foetal growth retardation, miscarriages and birth of small-for-gestation infants, as well as poor control of the mother's diabetes (hypoglycaemias, etc.).

Vitamins, iron and folate needs are usually similar to those of a non-diabetic pregnancy. Avoidance of overloading with vitamin A supplements is emphasized because hypervitaminosis A is associated with congenital malformations of the face, eyes, ears and soft palate, whereas folate supplements (5 mg per day) are usually necessary for prevention of foetal neural tube defects. Given the fact that the foetal neural tube closes around 18–26 days after conception, it is obvious that addition of folate supplements should start, if possible, even before the day of conception. Smoking should also be avoided, due to its multiple detrimental effects both for the mother and the embryo.

During the last trimester there may be fluid retention (oedemata) and weight gain. Restriction of salt intake with the food is recommended during this period (and not restriction of calories of the food), together with rest. Blood pressure and urinary protein excretion of the mother should be monitored, to exclude the possibility of preeclampsia.

Regular physical activity is recommended as well, especially in pregnant women with Type 2 or gestational diabetes, to decrease the insulin resistance that accompanies these types of diabetes and to achieve the desirable weight.

What are the targets regarding blood glucose levels and how is a woman with gestational diabetes monitored?

The treating physician will set the blood glucose targets for the pregnant woman. These targets, according to the American Diabetes Association, are: fasting blood glucose < 95 mg/dl (5.3 mmol/L), and one hour and two hours after a meal ≤ 140 mg/dl (7.8 mmol/L) and ≤ 120 mg/dl (6.7 mmol/L), respectively.

The pregnant woman should measure her blood glucose levels several times a day, record the results and discuss with her physician the progress of glycaemic control at a regular basis.

When does a woman with gestational diabetes need to start insulin treatment and what regimens are followed?

As mentioned above, when diet is not enough to achieve therapeutic targets, insulin therapy is required, usually after a period of a few days of self blood glucose monitoring with levels above these desired. It is usually postprandial blood glucose levels that are higher than accepted cut-offs.

The mother should be told that injected insulin does not cross the placenta and does not affect the foetus. In contrast, increased blood glucose crosses the placenta and is responsible for possible diabetic complications to the foetus (macrosomia, etc.).

Initiation of insulin treatment can be done with small doses of rapid-acting insulin before meals. However, an intensive insulin regimen with multiple injections may also be needed (combination of rapid-acting insulin before meals with medium-acting insulin for regulation of pre-meal blood glucose values) or the use of an insulin pump. Intensive insulin regimen requires self blood glucose monitoring and adjustment of insulin doses accordingly. The pregnant woman should be educated and trained in the use of insulin and the problems of hypoglycaemias (awareness, prevention, treatment).

Usually, 0.6–1.0 units of insulin per kg body weight are required, depending on the age of gestation. Insulin needs increase with progression of pregnancy, whereas at labour they decrease significantly and discontinuation of insulin treatment may be required.

Should women with gestational diabetes give birth by caesarian section?

According to the American Diabetes Association recommendations, labour should be performed within the 38th week of gestation, since prolongation of pregnancy has been frequently associated with macrosomia of the infant. Generally normal vaginal delivery is preferred, but the decision should be individualized and a caesarean section may be suitable if significant complications exist (preeclampsia, non-vertex presentation, foetal distress, shoulder-pelvis disproportion, etc.). A previous caesarean section is not an absolute indication for a second. An emergency caesarean section has the same indications in the diabetic pregnancy as in the non-diabetic one.

Nevertheless, caesarean section rates in Type 1 diabetic pregnancies are double that of the general population. According to one study, this rate in the USA from 1975–1985 was 47 percent for diabetic women. In 1996, in the same country, the caesarean section rate was 21 percent in the general population.

Will a woman with gestational diabetes need antidiabetic treatment after delivery?

Usually not. During labour, antidiabetic treatment is discontinued and the woman is monitored with blood glucose measurements while in the hospital. One to two months later the woman is reevaluated, and if there is no indication of diabetes, a glucose tolerance test is recommended six months later.

It is noteworthy that women with gestational diabetes are at high risk of developing diabetes in the future, especially if their body weight increases

(50–70 percent of obese women after delivery develop Type 2 DM within five years, compared to 25 percent of women with normal weight after delivery). The risk of future development of diabetes is also definitely higher when impaired glucose tolerance is detected after delivery (12 percent of pregnant women with normal glucose tolerance develop diabetes 6–8 weeks after birth, compared to 84 percent of those with impaired glucose tolerance). Also, 30–60 percent of women with gestational diabetes will manifest gestational diabetes again in a next pregnancy. The risk is higher following multiparous births by older women as well as for those who gained lots of weight between pregnancies. Around 20 percent of pregnant women with gestational diabetes will develop impaired glucose tolerance after delivery. These women should be regularly followed for possible development of Type 2 DM in the future and receive proper dietary advice for avoidance of obesity and 'diabetogenic' medicines. For these reasons, recommendations after delivery are: i) achievement and maintenance of a normal body weight; ii) increase in muscular activity; and iii) periodic monitoring of fasting blood glucose levels and performance of a glucose tolerance test.

MONITORING OF PREGNANT WOMEN WITH PRE-EXISTING TYPE 1 DM

What preparation is required for a Type 1 diabetic woman so that she can have a successful and safe pregnancy?

- Strict glycaemic control targets. Fasting blood glucose, as well as during the night: 60–90 mg/dl (3.3–5.0 mmol/L); and two hours after a meal; < 120 mg/dl (6.7 mmol/L) (women with Type 2 DM should discontinue pills and start insulin therapy).
- Control of possible hypertension. Discontinuation of angiotensin converting enzyme (ACE) inhibitors.

What care is required from the physician for a Type 1 diabetic pregnant woman without chronic complications?

If the woman belongs to either B or C categories in the White classification (see Table 10.2), the following steps are required:

- Intensive self monitoring of blood glucose (4–7 measurements a day).
- Intensive insulin regimen using the classic rapid-acting insulins or insulin analogues and possibly continuous insulin infusion pumps.
- Glycaemic control targets: Fasting blood glucose 60–90 mg/dl (3.3–5.0 mmol/L) and two hours postprandially < 120 mg/dl (6.7 mmol/L).
- Regular clinic visits so that the doctor can adjust treatment and control blood glucose. Visits should be at the most every 15 days up to the 34th week of gestation and then weekly.
- HbA_{1c} measurements every month.
- Regular ophthalmologic examinations at intervals depending on findings.
- Determination of 24-hour urinary protein excretion and creatinine clearance at initial visit and then quarterly.
- At labour, glucose level should be maintained below 90 mg/dl (5.0 mmol/L) with NaCl infusion together with insulin or/and glucose, based on blood glucose measurements every hour.

The American Diabetes Association also recommends the following obstetric monitoring:

- Level 2 ultrasound during the 18–22nd week and then every 4–6 weeks.
- Non-stress test at 32–34th week and then every week.

Is a pregnant woman allowed to take antihypertensive medicines and which ones? Which particular hypertensive problem exists for pregnant women with Type 1 DM?

All antihypertensive medicines should be discontinued if hypertension is under control (< 130/80 mmHg) with restriction of table-salt and proper nutrition. These levels should be maintained during the whole course of the pregnancy.

ACE inhibitors and inhibitors of angiotensin receptors are contraindicated in pregnancy due to a nephrotoxic action on the foetus and should be discontinued before a woman becomes pregnant. If during the course of the pregnancy hypertension develops, rest is recommended and frequently prescription of various medicines is required, such as methyldopa, labetalol, clonidine or hydralazine or even beta-blockers, with the provision that they can mask the early symptoms of hypoglycaemia.

According to some studies women with Type 1 DM have more frequent rates of pre-eclampsia than the general population (16 versus 5 percent) and this rate is thought to surpass 50 percent when nephropathy coexists. Women with long-standing DM under poor control, who are on their first pregnancy and have proteinuria > 190 mg/24 hours or have nephropathy are at the highest risk.

The 130/80 mmHg blood pressure target refers to the duration of pregnancy, as well as before it.

When do we recommend use of contraceptive methods in a woman with DM?

Pre-existing vascular heart disease is associated with high maternal mortality, and so presence of severe ischaemic heart disease is a contra-indication to pregnancy.

Furthermore, when a woman has poor glycaemic control it is advisable to avoid pregnancy. No specific type of contraceptive method is contraindicated or specifically recommended in diabetic women. Newer contraceptives administered in lower doses are usually safe in regards to metabolic control (blood glucose, lipids, coagulability) and control of blood pressure. Nevertheless, the American College of Obstetricians and Gynaecologists recommend these medicines be prescribed only to those diabetic women with no micro- or macro-vascular complications or hypertension and who do not smoke. Unless there is macroangiopathy, long-acting medroxyprogesterone acetate injections (depot) can be used, but not in older women, since their chronic use can affect serum lipids and promote atherosclerosis. Intrauterine devices are safe and effective as in non-diabetics.

What are the chances of an infant of a diabetic mother also developing DM later in life?

The answer depends on the type of DM (see also Chapter 2).

The chances that the child of a Type 1 diabetic mother will develop DM amount to 1.3–2 percent and are higher than a child with negative family history of diabetes (0.4 percent). If the father suffers from Type 1 DM, the risk for the child is much higher, up to 6 percent.

The risk of a child whose father has Type 1 DM also developing Type 1 DM is 6 percent. When a sibling has Type 1 DM, the risk is 5 percent and if a monozygotic twin sibling has Type 1 DM, then the risk is up to 30–50 percent.

The life-long chances for the development of Type 2 DM in a child with first degree relatives with Type 2 DM are 5–10 times higher than for persons of similar age and weight with a negative family history. Diabetes development is influenced by genetic factors as well as metabolic derangements during intrauterine life. It should be noted, however, that development of Type 2 DM occurs at a relatively older age.

According to observations from Pima Indians, Type 2 DM develops more frequently in children of diabetic pregnancies (45 percent) than in children of pre-diabetic (8.6 percent) or non-diabetic (1.4 percent) mothers. Also, children of diabetic mothers have higher weight for their height (at ages 5 to 19 years) compared to children of non-diabetic or pre-diabetic mothers.

Hyperglycaemia and hyperinsulinaemia during intrauterine life can affect adipose tissue and β-cell development, resulting in obesity and glucose metabolism disturbances in the future.

It is also noteworthy that children of mothers with gestational diabetes develop obesity mainly at the ages of 4–7 years. In another study of offspring of diabetic mothers, it was found that increased concentrations of amniotic fluid insulin are associated with impaired glucose tolerance (36 percent).

Impaired glucose tolerance and disturbances in insulin secretion have also been observed in adult offspring of diabetic mothers, regardless of genetic predisposition.

Further reading

American Diabetes Association (2000) Report of the Expert Committee on the Diagnosis and Classification of Diabetes Mellitus (Committee Report). *Diabetes Care*, **23** (Suppl 1), S4–S19.

American Diabetes Association (2004) Gestational Diabetes Mellitus. *Diabetes Care*, **27** (Suppl1), S88–S90.

Buchanan, T.A. (2004) Gestational diabetes mellitus, in *Therapy for diabetes mellitus and related disorders*. American Diabetes Association 4th Edn (ed H.E. Lebovitz) pp. 20–8.

Feig, D.S. and Palda, V.A. (2002) Type 2 diabetes in pregnancy: a growing concern. *The Lancet*, **11**, 1690–2.

Girling, J. and Dornhorst, A. (2003) Pregnancy and diabetes mellitus in (eds J. Pickup and G. Williams) *Textbook of Diabetes*, 3rd edn, Blackwell Science Ltd, Oxford, **65**, pp. 1–39.

Hanna, F.W.F. and Peters, J.R. (2002) Screening for gestational diabetes; past, present and future. *Diabetic medicine*, **19**, 351–8.

Kitzmiller, J.L., Buchanan, T.A., Kjos, S., Combs, C.A., Ratner, R.E. (1996) Preconception care for diabetes, congenital malformations, and spontaneous abortions (Technical review). *Diabetes Care*, **17**, 1502–13.

O'Sullivan, J.B. and Mahan, C.B. (1964) Coiteria for oral glucose tolerance test in pregnancy. *Diabetes*, **13**, 278.

Reece, E.A., Homko, C., Jovanovic, L. (2004) Management of pregnant womaen with diabetes, in *Therapy for Diabetes Mellitus and Related Disorders*. American Diabetes Association 4th Edn (ed. H.E. Lebovitz), pp. 29–37.

Ryan, E.A. (2003) Hormones and insulin resistance during pregnancy. *The Lancet*, **362**, 1777–8.

Sacks, D.A. (2004) Antepartum and intrapartum obstetric care, in *Therapy for Diabetes Mellitus and Related Disorders*. American Diabetes association 4th Edn (ed. H.E. Lebovitz) pp. 37–50.

11

Diabetes and the young

Ioannis Ioannidis

CASE STUDY 1

A 12 year old boy has lost 6 kg (13.2 lb) over the last six months. At the same time he exhibited intense polydipsia and polyuria. His paediatrician ordered some laboratory tests and found that he was suffering from Type 1 DM. Information about the disease brought up many queries for the child and his parents. The child was not initially receptive to talking about the problem or getting trained for insulin injections and self monitoring of blood glucose. Is this anticipated? What is the reaction of a young person and his or her family to the onset of Type 1 DM?

The diagnosis of a chronic disease, especially at a young age, causes initial many difficulties to the child or adolescent as well as to his or her family.

Adaptation to a new way of life usually requires time. Four different phases to the crisis caused by diagnosis of the disease are described below.

The first phase is *the phase of 'shock'*. During this phase it is difficult for someone to think clearly. Everything is tangled and hazy in the mind. Everything looks false: 'This cannot have happened, it is not true'. During this phase the young patient is not able to assimilate any information. The physician should talk, explain and give hope for the future while emphasizing the need for education and training in insulin administration and self monitoring of blood glucose. The young patient, and frequently the parents, look at the doctor talking and moving and although they realize the seriousness of the condition, are not able to understand what they are being told. There are many questions, but thoughts cannot be put in order at this point.

Diabetes in Clinical Practice: Questions and Answers from Case Studies.   Nicholas Katsilambros *et al.*
© 2006 John Wiley & Sons, Ltd.

The phase of reaction follows. During this phase there is sorrow and anger. The young patient displays aggressiveness and anxiety and frequently cannot even fall asleep (intense insomnia). Support is essential and must be sincere. Phrases such as 'You shouldn't be sorry' are not effective. Everybody is entitled to feel sorry for themselves in a situation like this! Sorrow and anger become even more intense when someone 'healthy' tries to persuade the young patient that the problem is not significant. This interference seems ironic and life in the eyes of the young patient looks even more unfair. Support should be silent until sorrow is slowly followed by acceptance.

The next phase is *the phase of compensation*. The patient starts thinking that something must be done for the management of the disease. Now is the time for passing on knowledge. This is the phase to teach everything needed about insulin and injections, self monitoring of blood glucose, hypoglycaemias and their management and about proper nutrition. The small pieces of knowledge and information that the patient and the family gather, gradually help in building a new reality.

The last phase is *the phase of reorientation*. At this phase diabetes is now an important part of the young patient's life, but not his or her whole life. Life is no longer the same, but nevertheless includes once again small daily routines, such as going out with friends, school chores, excursions, parties, etc. Fear and anger frequently cross the mind of the patient but rarely stay there.

CASE STUDY 2

A 15 year old girl is suffering from Type 1 DM. She is treated with four injections of insulin per day. During the last two days she had vomiting and intense polyuria and polydipsia. She was admitted to the hospital with diabetic ketoacidosis. The cause, as the patient herself admitted, was that she had neglected her injections lately, in an attempt to lose weight. Is this frequent? What are appetite disturbances in young persons with DM?

Unfortunately many young girls are afraid of gaining weight. This fear frequently becomes an obsession and leads to dangerous behaviour. Young girls with Type 1 DM frequently neglect their insulin injections in an attempt to lose weight. This is a frequent cause of poor glycaemic control and diabetic ketoacidosis in these patients.

Anorexia nervosa, the extreme form of this behaviour, can lead these young girls, diabetic or not, to intense emaciation, which is accompanied by menstrual disturbances. Apart from minimal consumption of food, the condition is also characterized by induced vomiting and intense physical exercise, for consumption of calories.

Anorexia nervosa is most common in young diabetic girls. The percentage is, according to some reports, up to 7 percent in diabetic persons 16–25 years old.

Sometimes the same people can develop bulimia, which leads to over-consumption of food and especially sweets. Frequently, this over-consumption of food causes feelings of remorse and leads to induced vomiting.

Most of the time, however, young diabetic women display relatively mild disturbances and simply miss doses or more frequently inject less of the required units of insulin. Family support and support from the health care team are very useful. More difficult cases require the help of a psychologist or psychiatrist.

CASE STUDY 3

Mrs Anna is 38 years old and is the mother of a 16 year old girl who suffers from Type 1 DM. During the last two years, the daughter has had very poor glycaemic control and continues to be extremely disobedient. The mother wants to discuss the problem with the physician and look for solutions.

Poor glycaemic control in adolescence, apart from other problems encountered in all ages, can be due to the following:

1. Episodes of nocturnal polyphagia, especially sweets, seen in young girls. These episodes can co-exist with other appetite disturbances, as mentioned above.
2. Avoidance of insulin injections (mentioned above).
3. Fear of hypoglycaemia, leading to avoidance of desirable blood glucose levels. This fear sometimes leads to injection of insulin after and not before the meal.
4. Diabetic control ranks low in the priorities of many adolescents. Insulin administration in these persons is frequently done only to avoid the symptoms of hyperglycaemia.
5. Use and abuse of alcohol in this age contributes to occurrence of hypoglycaemias or ketoacidosis.

Management of many of these problems is difficult and requires the cooperation of the family with specialists. Above all, however, patience and sympathy are needed.

CASE STUDY 4

A 7 year old boy is suffering from Type 1 DM. His parents are anxious and want to ask the physician and the treating health care team what they should know themselves and what the child should know.

One of the first things the parents and child should be educated and trained about is the correct administration of insulin. This is immediately necessary because it involves the life of the child. Later, and gradually, the parents and child are going to learn all the small and big secrets of the disease. They should not try to learn everything immediately. It is impossible!

They should therefore learn:

1. **Insulin injections** – the technique of aspiration and injection (when a syringe is used) or the technique of insulin pen preparation and injection (when an insulin pen is used).
2. **Hypoglycaemias** – how to recognize, prevent and treat them.
3. **High blood glucose levels** – how to recognize, prevent and treat them.
4. **Monitoring** – how to measure glucose concentration correctly in the blood of the child and ketones in his or her urine when needed.
5. **Nutrition** – what kind of food to prepare, how much food to serve and how often.
6. **Physical exercise** – how to adjust insulin and food when the child exercises.
7. **Rules for days of acute illness** – how to treat the child on days when he or she is sick.

As regards informing the child, that depends on his or her age and maturity. Children older than 12 years are usually able to measure their blood sugar levels and inject their insulin themselves. Parents should oversee the treatment and share with their children the responsibility of a correct treatment, until at least completion of puberty. At older ages (15–16 years) children increase their self medication, bringing the associated need of strict, daily control by the parents.

At younger ages, as in our example (7 years old), the greatest responsibility for the care of the child lies with the parents. Depending on the child's age and level of maturity, the parents gradually transfer some of their responsibilities to the child. They should also quickly recognize hypoglycaemia symptoms and be trained in their quick treatment.

Close and frequent follow-up, clear and individualized targets, understanding of personal problems and multifactorial support (psychological support of the patient and his or her environment) are some of the significant key points in the management of the young diabetic patient.

CASE STUDY 5

A 16 year old boy is suffering from Type 1 DM. His glycaemic control is poor and his parents are worried because he eats lots of sweets and has started smoking. Is there reason for worry? Can the problem be dealt with?

An adolescent should be promptly informed about the tremendous risks that smoking entails especially for diabetic persons.

One out of two persons who smoke finally dies from a cause that is related to this habit. Nicotine causes vasospasm, adversely affecting insulin absorption. At the same time it increases insulin resistance leading to a need for an increase in the injected doses. Information should be given in plain and clear scientific terms, without the characteristics of admonition and criminalization that are frequently counter-productive at this age. The association of smoking cessation with beneficial effects, both in daily life and long-term, can have an effect. Even if smoking cessation is not achieved, repeating this information at every clinic visit can ultimately work.

As regards consumption of sweets, ice-cream and other 'forbidden' foods, management should be realistic. The general information for avoidance of such foods should be repeated, but the adolescent should be counseled to 'handle' such glycaemic loads with the proper rapid-acting insulin administration so that postprandial hyperglycaemia is controlled. Usually 1–2 units of insulin are enough for the metabolism of 12–15 g of carbohydrates. Since carbohydrates of such foods are very readily digestible, administration of very rapid-acting insulin analogues, like lispro or Aspart, are preferred.

Further reading

Greene, S.A., Newton, R.W. (1997) Diabetes mellitus in childhood and adolescence, in (*Textbook of Diabetes*, 2nd edn (eds J. Pickup and G. Williams) Oxford, pp. 37.1–37.18.

Hanas, R. (1998) Insulin dependent diabetes in children, adolescents and adults. Uddevalla Sweden.

12

Diabetes and old age

Konstantinos Makrilakis

What is the frequency of DM in old age?

The main form of DM in old age (above 65 years) is essentially Type 2 DM. The ageing of the population, sedentary lifestyles and obesity (factors that promote development of Type 2 DM) mean that the frequency of this type of DM increases with age. According to an extensive study of the First Department of Propaedeutic Medicine Clinic (Katsilambros, 1993) in an urban part of the Greek population, the prevalence of diagnosed Type 2 DM at ages 40–49 years was around 1.8 percent, at ages 50–59 years it was 7.7 percent, increasing to 13.6 percent between 60 and 69 years, and much higher at ages above 70 years. There is thought to be a large number of undiagnosed cases at all age groups. Among frail persons of old age living in nursing homes, it is estimated that the prevalence of DM is > 20 percent.

What is the aetiology of DM development in old age?

The pathogenesis of Type 2 DM in old age is essentially the same as in younger ages (see Chapter 3). The combination of resistance to insulin action and impaired insulin secretion from the pancreas lead to the gradual development of impaired glucose tolerance and finally to DM. Increase in body adipose tissue with ageing, the simultaneous decrease in physical activity and the use of various potentially diabetogenic medicines (thiazide diuretics, beta-blockers, corticosteroids, etc.) most likely contribute to DM.

Diabetes in Clinical Practice: Questions and Answers from Case Studies. Nicholas Katsilambros *et al.*
© 2006 John Wiley & Sons, Ltd.

What are the consequences of DM in the elderly?

The consequences of DM can be more serious in elderly patients due to functional disabilities, frequent presence of other comorbidities (renal, hepatic, cardiac impairment, etc.) and polypharmacy. Both acute and chronic complications can have catastrophic consequences in elderly diabetic patients.

Poor metabolic control in DM with excessive hyperglycaemia is accompanied by glucosuria and weight loss. It is a catabolic condition that predisposes diabetics to the development of various acute abnormal conditions, mainly infections. Also, the symptoms of decreased vision and mental dysfunction that often accompany dehydration caused by hyperglycaemia may frequently be erroneously attributed to old age or be mistaken for a stroke. The most extreme example of poor metabolic control is the hyperglycaemic hyperosmotic non-ketotic syndrome, which is more frequent in elderly diabetics and is associated with high mortality (see Chapter 6: 'Diabetic coma'). Among the frequent causes of hyperglycaemia in elderly persons are infections, myocardial infarction, stroke, insufficient antidiabetic therapy or the use of diabetogenic medicines (corticosteroids, thiazide diuretics, beta-adrenergic blockers, etc.). Coexistence of renal and/or hepatic dysfunction frequently aggravates the condition.

Nevertheless, hypoglycaemias are also very common in elderly diabetic people and can have catastrophic consequences, because they can lead to a decrease in mental function and vision as well as falls resulting in fractures. Furthermore, hypoglycaemia symptoms may not be readily recognized by the elderly, either due to insufficient education or hypoglycaemia unawareness (a consequence of multiple factors, such as autonomic nervous system neuropathy, insufficient compensation to hypoglycaemia mechanisms, etc.), resulting in an increased risk, perhaps even of death, for the diabetic person. The frequent coexistence of renal and/or hepatic dysfunction in old age causes an increased tendency towards hypoglycaemias in diabetics who use sulfonylureas or insulin (their action is prolonged).

What are the chronic complications of DM in the elderly?

The chronic complications of DM in the elderly are similar to the well known ones in younger patients (micro- and macro-vascular).

For example, the prevalence of retinopathy in DM increases with ageing. The same applies to the prevalence of cataract and glaucoma. Consequently, elderly diabetic patients should be regularly examined by an ophthalmologist (at least once a year if everything is normal) because poor vision can lead to social isolation, aggravation of depressive manifestations, increased risk of accidents and deterioration of metabolic control (due to difficulty with intake of necessary medicines or insulin administration). Early diagnosis of retinopathy can be vision-saving with proper treatment.

Old age itself can also cause impairment of renal function. However, in the vast majority, diabetics do not develop nephropathy unless it occurs by the age of 65–70 years, since about a decade is needed for microalbuminuria to progress to renal insufficiency. Consequently, regular measurement of 24-hour urine albumin excretion rate is not recommended after the age of 70 years (measurement of serum urea and creatinine and urinalysis are usually sufficient). Furthermore, proteinuria in elderly diabetics is not always due to diabetic nephropathy (other causes such as multiple myeloma, glomerulonephritides, etc., are quite frequent).

Lower extremity problems are also quite frequent in diabetic persons, with a higher frequency in older age, due to more frequent vascular and neurologic disturbances. Ulcers in diabetic feet, with possible microbial infection, can lead even to the need for amputation of the extremity, with disastrous consequences for the quality and duration of life. The recommendation for all diabetics to check their feet frequently for the presence of calluses, ulcerations, minor trauma, etc., is even more imperative in older age. The help of relatives or friends if the old person is unable to examine his or her own feet (due to poor vision, mental problems, etc.) is crucial.

Erectile dysfunction is more frequent in elderly diabetics (around 55–95 percent of elderly diabetic men are affected compared with around 50 percent of elderly non-diabetics). Its causes comprise vasculopathy, neuropathy of autonomic nervous system, hormonal disturbances, endothelial dysfunction, psychological factors and various medications. Evaluation and treatment of this problem should not be neglected in elderly people, since it can have tremendously beneficial effects in the psychological well-being of the patients (see Chapter 19: 'Sexual function in diabetes').

The biggest problem by far, however, in this age group is cardiovascular disease. Its frequency increases and is aggravated by the presence of diabetes, hypertension, dyslipidaemia, obesity and smoking and it comprises the number one cause of death among elderly diabetic people. The spherical management of all the risk factors that contribute to its development is essential for the decrease of its frequency. 'Aggressiveness' of therapy in older age is individualized though, and depends on multiple factors (life expectancy, complexity of therapy, resources, coexistent diseases, etc. [see next question]).

What are the general therapeutic principles for DM in elderly persons?

The appropriate targets for the management of DM and its various complications in old age are not the same for all patients. Since there are no specific studies for glycaemic targets in elderly people with DM, these have to be individualized. For example, in a 70 year old diabetic who is, in all other aspects healthy and has a life expectancy of more than five years, the HbA_{1c} target could be > 7.0 percent (the same as in younger diabetic persons), with a fasting blood glucose target between 110–150 mg/dl (5.6–8.3 mmol/L) and post-prandial < 180 mg/dl (10.0 mmol/L). Achievement of these targets will maintain a satisfactory glycaemic control, with a relative decrease in the risk of microvascular complications. To avoid, however, the dangerous risk for this age-group of hypoglycaemia, a more realistic target could be HbA_{1c} < 8.0–8.5 percent. When life expectancy is shorter, HbA_{1c} target could be a bit higher (> 8.5 percent).

Arterial hypertension should also be treated in the elderly, with a target of $> 140/90$ mmHg or less than 20 mmHg from the initial blood pressure level (if this were > 180 mmHg). It is noteworthy that isolated systolic hypertension is common in the elderly and this should also be treated and not considered a physiologic consequence of ageing.

Dyslipidaemia should also be treated, by diet or/and medicines, with therapeutic targets not different from those of younger diabetics (LDL-cholesterol < 100 mg/dl [2.6 mmol/L]).

Generally, however, the therapeutic strategy for an elderly diabetic person should take into consideration many factors, including:

- The life expectancy of the patient.
- The ability and willingness of the patient and his or her family to comply with and follow the healthcare team's advice. For this reason

therapeutic targets should be realistic and the regimen simple, clear and feasible.

- Financial and other resources.
- The presence of other coexistent medical problems (psychiatric or mental disturbances, diabetic complications, functional insufficiencies, etc.).
- The frequency and type of DM follow-up appointments.

What are the types of therapeutic management of DM in elderly persons?

All therapeutic means that are used in the management of DM in younger persons can be used in the elderly as well, with some provisions and alterations.

Proper nutrition and physical activity are generally the cornerstones of therapeutic management of Type 2 DM. Their usefulness is also invaluable in elderly diabetic persons. However, often these persons not are obese, but infact very thin, so that hypocaloric diets are not suitable for them. A less restrictive diet can frequently improve the quality of life of these people, without significant aggravation of the glycaemic control. If, however, obesity is present, weight loss will definitely have beneficial effects on glycaemic control, just as in younger diabetic patients. Furthermore, physical activity has the same beneficial effects in elderly diabetics as in younger ones. Its level and intensity should depend on the physical condition and possible coexistent problems of the patient. The commonly present silent cardiac ischaemia, movement problems due to arthritis, mental dysfunction, etc., render physical activity programmes relatively difficult in elderly diabetic people and require special attention (for example, with performance of an exercise stress test before starting a physical activity programme).

If therapeutic targets are not achieved with diet and exercise within 6–8 weeks, it is usually necessary to start medicines. All available categories of oral antidiabetic medicines, and even insulin, can be used for the achievement of glycaemic control in elderly diabetic patients (see Chapters 27 and 28), but of course under certain provisions, as previously emphasized.

Sulfonylureas are frequently used because they are generally well tolerated. Hypoglycaemia risk is, however, especially high in these age groups, due to the frequent coexistence of renal, hepatic or cardiac dysfunction, which leads to prolongation of their action. Glibenclamide especially has been associated even with deaths in some studies (maybe due to presence of active metabolites), although not in all. Meglitinides (nateglinide and repaglinide) can also be used successfully in these age-groups.

Metformin is very effective, both in obese and lean diabetic persons, and with the exception of gastrointestinal problems and the relative risk of lactic acidosis in renal or hepatic dysfunction, it is generally well tolerated. It should be emphasized, however, that evaluation of renal function in old age should not be solely based on measurement of plasma creatinine (it is often deceptive) but instead, creatinine clearance should be calculated (based on the simple formula of Cockroft and Gault):

$$\text{Creatinine clearance} = \frac{(140 - \text{age}) \times (\text{body weight})}{(\text{plasma creatinine}) \times 72}$$

(age in years, body weight in kg, and plasma creatinine in mg/dl).

The above number is multiplied by 0.85 in women, and the dose of administered medicines is promptly adjusted.

Acarbose has mild hypoglycaemic actions and its use is often restricted by gastrointestinal complications.

Glitazones (pioglitazone, rosiglitazone) decrease insulin resistance and improve glycaemic control, without causing hypoglycaemias. They can sometimes, though, cause weight gain and fluid retention. For this reason they should be administered carefully in heart failure (they are contraindicated in advanced heart failure or their co-administration with insulin, for the same reason).

If proper metabolic control of DM is not achieved with oral antidiabetic medicines, it is a mistake to consider that insulin is not appropriate for therapy of elderly diabetic persons. Depending on the circumstances and selected therapeutic targets, it is possible to use all insulin combinations, from the very simple regimens with only one basal insulin injection per day (with or without pills) to intensive regimens (see Chapter 28). It is implicit that insulin use requires the cooperation of diabetic patients or their families, with self monitoring of blood glucose at home. In this way, both acute hyperglycaemic states (e.g. hyperosmotic conditions, etc.) and hypoglycaemias can be avoided. Furthermore, in acute situations (e.g. after a myocardial infarction, stroke, infections, etc.) it is mandatory to use insulin for some time, even provisionally.

Generally, it should be emphasized once more that it is a mistake to consider old age as a mandatory obstacle to the proper evaluation and therapeutic management of diabetes in any way. Many elderly people are functionally very active and are entitled to the full attention and understanding of their problems by the treating physician.

CASE STUDY 1

An 85 year old man with Type 2 DM for 20 years, hypertension and dyslipidaemia, presents with a stroke, that causes left hemiparesis and severe restriction in his mobility (he can transfer from the bed to the chair only with help, he can dress with help, he can eat alone but cannot walk alone). His DM is treated with a combination of oral antidiabetic medicines (metformin at noon) and two doses of a mixture of insulin (70 percent isophane and 30 percent rapid-acting) in the morning and night before meals. His glycaemic control prior to the stroke was moderate (HbA$_{1c}$ 7.5 percent, fasting blood glucose 150–200 mg/dl [8.3–11.1 mmol/L], though very rarely did he measure post-prandial blood glucose levels, usually > 200 mg/dl [11.1 mmol/L]). Before the stroke he lived alone, but now he lives with his daughter, who works during the day and has hired a helper to care for her father during her absence. The daughter reports that her father has become more insular since the stroke and 'seems to have declined: he frequently doesn't eat his food, shows no interest in anything and sleeps all the time'. She is worried about his glycaemic control, whether it could lead to a second stroke. She also has difficulties with insulin injections (in the morning she leaves for work early, before her father eats his breakfast; the helper comes later). She is asking for the doctor's advice.

It is obvious that the stroke has dramatically changed the life of the patient and his environment. Quality of life has dramatically deteriorated (dependence on others for simple activities of daily life), something that has definitely produced symptoms of depression. The therapeutic regimen for diabetes control (especially with the two injections of insulin) has also become problematic. Use of rapid-acting insulin in a mixture, in a person who is not guaranteed to eat adequately, definitely entails the risk of hypoglycaemia (it may be possible that even the sleepiness symptoms that the daughter describes are an expression of some mild hypoglycaemia and not only depression). If it is not possible to measure post-prandial blood glucose occasionally (the helper could be trained to do this), the insulin regimen should definitely be changed. Quality of life and realistic targets now have priority over very strict glycaemic control. The daughter should understand that the risk of a second stroke is high after a first one, but there is no reason for very strict control of blood glucose that increases the risk of hypoglycaemia. Anyhow, insulin is not being properly administered. It would be simpler and more realistic to set looser glycaemic control targets (HbA$_{1c}$: 8.0–9.0 percent). The insulin mixture could be substituted with isophane insulin twice a day or with insulin glargine (see Chapter 28) once every evening, at a dose that maintains a fasting blood glucose level close to 120–150 mg/dl (6.7–8.3 mmol/L) and at an acceptable level for the rest of the day. Physiotherapy would also be very helpful, to help the patient become independent in his daily chores and improve his psychological well-being. Use of antidepressant medications might also be of assistance.

CASE STUDY 2

A 76 year old woman with Type 2 DM for 15 years comes to the diabetic clinic for a routine visit. She is treated with maximal doses of sulfonylureas and metformin. Her blood pressure is 130/80 mmHg and her weight 82 kg (180.8 lb, BMI: 27 kg/m^2). She occasionally measures her blood sugar at home (3–4 times per week, usually in the morning or more rarely at noon after lunch – she says that's how her doctor instructed her). Her measurements are usually high (in the morning 180–220 mg/dl [10.0–12.2 mmol/L], post-prandially at noon always > 200 mg/dl [11.1 mmol/L]). Her HbA$_{1c}$ is 8.2 percent. She also receives a statin every night and an ACE inhibitor/ thiazide diuretic combination antihypertensive tablet. She has no complaints except for nocturia (once or twice a night) and is generally very active. She has mild benign retinopathy (the ophthalmologist has recommended quarterly follow-ups for the time being) and no microalbuminuria. What is the proper further management of this patient?

The glycaemic control of this patient is not satisfactory (HbA$_{1c}$ 8.2 percent), despite maximal doses of two oral antidiabetic medications. The long duration of diabetes (15 years) combined with the poor metabolic control despite two oral antidiabetic medicines, raises a high suspicion that insulin stores of this patient are nearly depleted – this is the natural progress of Type 2 DM, where β-cell secretory capacity gradually declines with time and is obviously genetically predetermined (see Chapter 3). The majority of Type 2 diabetic patients, after 10–15 years with the disease, are going to need insulin for effective manage-ment of the blood glucose. The UKPDS study showed that up to 70 percent of Type 2 diabetic patients with known duration of the disease of 7–8 years will need insulin for achievement of good glycaemic control. This can be objectively evaluated by performing a glucagon stimulation test, where insulin secretory reserves of the pancreas are evaluated (see Chapter 1), or by treating the patient with maximal doses of oral antidiabetic medications for a few months and confirming the inability to control blood glucose levels. In the case under discussion, the patient uses two categories of oral antidiabetic medicines in maximal doses (sulfonylureas and metformin). It is doubtful whether the addition of a third category will lead to the achievement of therapeutic targets, if pancreatic insulin stores have been depleted – acarbose has mild hypoglycaemic action (decreases HbA_{1c} by 0.5–1 percent) whereas glitazones (rosiglitazone was recently approved for triple therapy) decrease HbA_{1c} by 1–1.5 percent.

This situation is explained to the patient and initiation of insulin therapy, together with oral antidiabetic medicines, is advised. The patient refuses, saying she does not want to start insulin, which she considers as the last resort (she also reports the unpleasant experience she had with her mother, who 'needed insulin and finally died').

It is obvious that the patient has very poor information regarding diabetes (not rare, given the complexity of the disease) and needs ample time devoted to her for discussion and explanations. The fact that she refuses the proposed therapy does not mean she must be 'punished' and abandoned in her fate. It needs to be explained again that insulin is a substance that physiologically exists in our body and that in her particular case it is lacking and needs to be replaced. It is not insulin that causes problems or even death but uncontrolled diabetes. Insulin aims at preventing the complications of uncontrolled diabetes and ameliorating the metabolic condition. The delay of its initiation, when its use is necessary, can only cause deterioration of the problem. Nevertheless, the patient has the absolute right to decide for herself (after she is informed properly) and her wish should be respected.

The patient decides after extensive discussions to be educated in the use of insulin for the time being, but prefers to try further compliance with the diet and the addition of a third oral antidiabetic medicine to control her blood glucose ('since I feel alright, why should I start insulin?'). She is referred back to the dietitian for advice and glitazone is added to her regimen. Regular self monitoring of blood glucose at home is recommended, at various times during the day (pre-prandially and sometimes two hours after the meals). Three months later her HbA_{1c} was 7.9 percent and her weight had increased by 2 kg (4.4 lb). Nocturia persisted.

Glycaemic control continued to be unsatisfactory. Given the fact that the patient had no other obvious medical problem and her life expectancy was good, the attempts to persuade her into starting insulin continued. A glucagon stimulation test could objectively show her insulin reserves.

The glucagon stimulation test showed very small insulin reserves in the pancreas. The patient accepted she had to start insulin with a once a day basal insulin injection every night, together with metformin and sulfonylurea in the morning. Glitazone was discontinued (it has not been approved in combination with insulin in Europe and in the USA it is approved only when there is no heart failure). Adjustment of insulin dose can continue based on self monitoring of blood glucose by the patient at home and her willingness to control blood glucose levels as close to normal as possible (see also Chapter 28).

CASE STUDY 3

A 78 year old man with Type 2 DM for 30 years, and a history of coronary heart disease (myocardial infarction and coronary artery bypass surgery eight years ago), hypertension and dyslipidaemia, comes to the diabetic clinic for a routine follow-up. He uses a mixture of 70/30 insulin, 28 units in the morning and 18 units in the evening before meals and occasionally rapid-acting insulin before lunch (usually 5–6 units before meals) subcutaneously. He says he measures his blood sugar regularly (always twice and sometimes three times a day) and is unhappy that his glucose control is not very good (morning blood sugar levels 120–220 mg/dl [6.7–12.2 mmol/L], evening 180–240 mg/dl [10.0–13.3 mmol/L], noon 200–340 mg/dl [11.1–18.9 mmol/L]). The patient is in very good general health, walks daily for at least 30–45 minutes without any problems and is generally very active (he is a retired civil servant and likes to work in his garden). He reports very frequent hypoglycaemias, usually around noon. His HbA_{1c} is 8.4 percent, his weight 92 kg (202.9 lb, BMI: 30.1 kg/m^2) and his blood pressure under good control.

Despite his age and past medical problems the patient is quite fit now and essentially follows quite an intensive programme of self blood glucose monitoring at home (he measures 2–3 times a day and injects insulin 2–3 times a day). His poor glycaemic control is obviously due to the wrong timing of insulin injections during the day relative to his needs. Given the fact that he leads a very active life (he is engaged in gardening, walks every day), it is not appropriate that his insulin doses are stable every day, since his needs change. The fact that he is 78 years old with Type 2 DM does not necessarily mean that a more intensive insulin regimen is absolutely out of the question, as long as the patient wishes to have as good a glycaemic control as possible, is willing to follow a more intensive glucose monitoring programme (which he already does anyway) and has the cognitive ability to understand the requirements and responsibilities he is taking up. His noon time hypoglycaemias are more likely due to his morning physical activities (gardening, walking) with poor timing of insulin doses with his snacks. His hyperglycaemias before lunch-time are most likely due to over-correction of his previous hypoglycaemias or to insufficient morning insulin doses. In any case, an intensive insulin regimen (basal-bolus) would be appropriate for this patient. Addition of metformin would also help in ameliorating insulin resistance (the patient is obese) and would help not to increase insulin requirements too much.

It was proposed to the patient to start an intensive insulin regimen with one injection of insulin glargine, 22 units subcutaneously at bedtime (around 70 percent of the total isophane dose that he previously used: $[28 + 18 = 46$ units of the 70/30 mixture contain 32.2 units of isophane insulin]) together with a very-rapid-acting insulin analogue (lispro or aspart) three times daily, before meals, with doses adjusted depending on pre-prandial blood glucose measurements and food carbohydrate counting. He was referred to a dietitian for education regarding food carbohydrate counting and correct timing of insulin injections with his meals. Instructions were also given regarding very frequent self monitoring of blood glucose (especially in the beginning until insulin needs are determined with more accuracy) and especially before periods of physical activity. It was explained that due to the very rapid action of 'meal' insulin he did not need to delay his lunch any more after the injection. He seemed to understand the requirements of the programme and wished to try it.

After an initial adjustment period that required some telephone communication between the patient and his physician to clarify some queries, the patient was under much better control, with a significant decrease of hypoglycaemic episodes and improvement of his metabolic control (HbA_{1c} after 2.5 months: 7.2 percent).

Further reading

Cockroft, D., Gault, M.H. (1976) Prediction of creatinine clearance from serum creatinine. *Nephron*, **16**, 31–41.

Halter, J.B. (2004) Geriatric patients, in *Therapy for Diabetes Mellitus and Related Disorders*, 4th edn, American Diabetes Association, (ed. H.E. Lebovitz), pp. 259–65.

Katsilambros, N., Aliferis, K., Darviri, C., Tsapogas, P., Alexiou, Z., Tritos, N., Arvanitis, M. (1993) Evidence for an increase in the prevalence of known diabetes in a sample of an urban population in Greece. *Diabet Med*, **10**, 87–90.

Meneilly, G.S., Hards, S., Tessier, D. *et al.* (1996) NIDDM in the elderly. *Diabetes Care*, **19**, 1320–75.

Sinclair, A.J. (2003) Diabetes in old age, in Textbook of Diabetes, 3rd edn, (eds J. Pickup and G. Williams) Blackwell Science Ltd, Oxford, **67**, pp.1–18.

Shorr, R.I., Ray, W.A., Daugherty, J.R. *et al.* (1997) Incidence and risk factors for serious hypoglycemia in older persons using insulin or sulfonylureas. *Arch Intern Med*, **157**, 1681–6.

UKPDS Study Group (1990) UK Prospective Diabetes Study 6. Complications in newly diagnosed Type 2 diabetic patients and their association with different clinical and biochemical risk factors. *Diabetes Research*, **13**, 1–11.

13

Diabetic retinopathy

Evanthia Diakoumopoulou

What is diabetic retinopathy (DR)?

Diabetic retinopathy (DR) is a form of microvascular disease that affects the pre-capillary arterioles, the capillaries and the post-capillary venules of the retinal vascular net. It is characterized both by increased capillary permeability as well as microvascular obstruction. DR is divided into *non-proliferative* (NPDR or background DR) and *proliferative* (PDR), depending on the presence or not of neovascularization in the retina (in the optic disk area or in the periphery), and it can be also accompanied by *diabetic maculopathy* at any stage.

During the first two decades of suffering from diabetes, nearly all Type 1 diabetic patients and more than 60 percent of Type 2 ones, suffer from DR.

DR is the most common cause of blindness among 20–74 year old adults, and especially when the macula is affected, blindness risk is higher.

What is the frequency of DR occurrence?

The frequency of DR occurrence is closely associated with the duration of diabetes. Based on existing statistics, when diagnosis of diabetes is done at an age below 30 years, after 10 years, 50 percent of the patients will suffer from DR. After 30 years, this rate increases to 95 percent of patients.

Diabetes in Clinical Practice: Questions and Answers from Case Studies.   Nicholas Katsilambros *et al.*
© 2006 John Wiley & Sons, Ltd.

Which factors affect progression of DR?

- *The type of diabetes:* in Type 1 DM proliferative retinopathy is more common, whereas in Type 2 DM diabetic maculopathy prevails.
- *Age:* the frequency of DR increases with Age.
- *Diabetes duration:* (see previous question).
- *Blood glucose control:* good glycaemic control has a beneficial effect on DR progression, despite an initial deterioration (Oslo group, 1992).
- *Dyslipidaemia and arterial hypertension* are associated with DR and diabetic nephropathy (DN) and also cause a deterioration of macular oedema. Furthermore, there is a strong correlation between proliferative DR, hypertension and hypercholesterolaemia (EURODIAB, 2001).
- *Diabetic nephropathy* and diabetic retinopathy have a parallel course, especially during the first 12–15 years of the disease.
- *Pregnancy* can aggravate DR or cause its occurrence.
- *Smoking* aggravates DR in young patients with Type 1 DM. It can also convert background DR into proliferative DR.
- *Alcohol abuse, oral contraceptive pills* (progesterone content may contribute to acceleration of DR) and *aspirin* (its use does not prevent the occurrence or progression of DR), can affect the progression of DR.
- Local factors (myopia) have a protective effect on DR progression, whereas others can aggravate it, such as cataract surgery with intraoperative complications.

How is increased capillary permeability explained in DM?

There is a decrease in pericytes in DM, i.e., the supportive cells of the capillary walls, which have myofibrils and regulate the volume of blood that passes through the capillaries. As a result, the capillary wall is locally dilated and microaneurysms form, with resultant fluid or cellular components leak. Furthermore, hyperglycaemia causes loosening of the junctions between endothelial cells, resulting in breakage of the retinal barrier and diffusion of cellular and non-cellular components of the blood. In this way *oedema* is formed due to the exit of fluid from the retina, *hard exudates* due to the release of lipoproteins and *haemorrhages* due to the release of red blood cells and platelets. Other factors that contribute to the increased vascular permeability are the increased production of free radicals from endothelial cells and white blood cells that accumulate in the region, leukotrienes production from white blood cells, LDL oxidation and release of IGF-1 (insulin-like growth factor-1), interleukin 1b, nitrous oxide and VEGF (vascular endothelial growth factor) from endothelial cells.

What is the cause of microvascular obstructions of the retina?

The thickness of the retinal basement membrane, activation and accumulation of leukocytes with local release of stimulatory factors and increase in adhesion molecules, comprise the basic aetiological factors. Furthermore, other factors that contribute are the proliferation of endothelial cells, alterations in red blood cells specific in DM (i.e., rigidity of red blood cell membrane, accumulation of red blood cells around macromolecules – fibrinogen and α_2 globulin, and the difficulty of oxygen dissociation to the tissues, that is conversion of haemoglobin to oxyhaemoglobin), as well as the increased aggregability of platelets. The above factors, together with increased levels of PAI-1 (plasminogen activator inhibitor-1) and von Willebrand factor, create a hypercoagulable state, resulting in microvascular obstructions, hypoxia and anoxia.

What damage is caused by hypoxia of the retina?

- Cotton wool (or soft) exudates (cotton wool spots): these comprise localized ischaemic oedema of the retinal neural layer, caused by capillary obstruction in the superficial layer of the neural fibres, resulting in interruption of the flow along the neuron axon and accumulation of the transfer substances in the neuron axon.
- Form and course of the veins, becoming like a string of beads in the early stages.
- Arteriovenous communications, referred to as intraretinal microvascular abnormalities (IRMA). They can be complicated by intraretinal neovascularization.
- Neovascularization of the optic disk or the periphery of the retina, resulting in haemorrhages or retinal detachment due to contraction.

- Neovascularization of the iris (rubeosis iridis) with a risk of secondary haemorrhagic glaucoma from the rupture of the newly synthesized vessels and the resulting haemorrhage.

How is the diagnosis of diabetic retinopathy made?

It is based on a comprehensive ophthalmologic evaluation, which should be performed by an ophthalmologist. As expected, some studies have shown that evaluation by an ophthalmologist has greater effectiveness and sensitivity in detecting retinal damage. However, the initial evaluation by the primary physician (general practitioner, diabetologist, endocrinologist), who should perform a minimal ophthalmologic exam, is also important. In this way, possibly serious damage that could go undetected can be prevented. A comprehensive ophthalmologic exam includes visual acuity evaluation, pupil reaction to light (myosis of the pupil on application of light on it), and fundoscopy. Monoocular examination with the direct ophthalmoscope is not always able to detect all possible retinal lesions, especially when the examiner is not very experienced. Furthermore, diagnosis of maculopathy with simple fundoscopy is difficult to detect in detail, even by very experienced ophthalmologists. For this reason, examination with a slit-lamp is essential. More specialized examinations, such as fundus photography for further evaluation and follow-up of the lesions, fluorescein retinal angiography, measurement of intraocular pressure and possibly fundus ultrasonography, should be performed by a specialist ophthalmologist if this is necessary. Fluorescein angiography includes the intravenous injection of a special substance, fluorescein, which is bound to serum albumin and accumulates in the retinal vessels, revealing their anatomy. Recently, the new technique of optical coherence tomography (OCT) of the macula (available in specialized centres) allows the diagnosis of macular oedema to be made objectively and with great precision and reliability, permitting the diagnosis of maculopathy much more easily than in the past.

What is diabetic maculopathy?

Diabetic maculopathy is characterized by the presence of microaneurysms, flame-like haemorrhages, cotton-wool like or even hard exudates

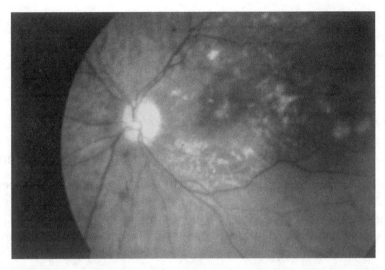

Figure 13.1. Photograph of the retina of the patient showing multiple exudates, micro-haemorrhages and micro-aneurysms on the macula area, as well as scars from previous Laser photocoagulation.

and oedema, at a distance of one disk diameter (1500 μm) from the centre of the macula (Figure 13.1). The possibility of macular damage is higher as the disease progresses and proportional to the stage severity (2–3 percent in background DR and 20–71 percent in proliferative DR). Depending on the lesions present and the mechanism of their production, the following types of diabetic maculopathy exist:

- *Focal or exudative maculopathy:* this is characterized by focal dye leakage during fluorescein angiography and by hard exudates circularly arranged.
- *Diffuse or oedematous maculopathy:* there is dilatation of the retinal capillaries and arterioles, with diffuse leakage of fluid. The increased vascular permeability and impaired function of the pigmented epithelium pump are implicated in the causation of these lesions. The absence of hard exudates and the presence of cystic retinal lesions in the area of the macula, when fluid accumulation increases a lot, are characteristic of this type of diabetic maculopathy as well.
- *Ischaemic maculopathy:* this is characterized by an intense aberration of the perimacular net architecture (extensive degradation – expansion).

Ophthalmoscopic features of ischaemia are the presence of muddy oedema, multiple cotton-wool like exudates and white obstructed arterioles. Prognosis is poor – no response to laser treatment – and there is significant reduction in visual acuity.

How does diabetic retinopathy evolve?

In increasing order of severity, the stages of diabetic retinopathy are:

1. **Non- proliferative diabetic retinopathy – background diabetic retinopathy (NPDR):** this is characterized by dilatation of retinal veins, microaneurysms, punctate or flame-like haemorrhages, and hard exudates, at a distance larger than one optic disk diameter from the macula. Depending on severity, it is divided into mild, moderate, severe and very severe.
2. **Pre-proliferative DR:** this includes all of the above and also smooth exudates, special lesions of the veins (loops, tortuous course, course like a string of beads, reduplication), arterial lesions (segmental stenosis, obstruction) and intraretinal abnormalities with formation of arteriovenous communications (IRMA).
3. **Proliferative DR:** this is characterized by neovascularization of the optic disk and the periphery of the retina and formation of connective tissue.
4. **Advanced diabetic disease:** there is extensive haemorrhage of the vitreous body, retinal detachment due to contraction and neovascularization of the iris (rubeosis iridis, with increased risk of neovascular glaucoma).

How is diabetic retinopathy treated?

- **Photocoagulation with LASER (Light Amplification by Stimulated Emission of Radiation) beams.** Depending on the element used there are various kinds of laser beams, which emit at different wave length: Argon, Krypton, Xenon, Diode. Photocoagulation aims at producing a tissue chemical burn at a predetermined retinal area, with the least possible damage to the neural retina. The ultimate aim of photocoagulation is therefore to convert hypoxic retinal areas to anoxic, so that the mechanism of neovascularization is inhibited. Photocoagulation is absolutely indicated in the following situations: i) in severe and very severe NPDR; ii) in diabetic maculopathy; iii) in proliferative DR. In diabetic maculopathy, focal or direct and the grid-pattern photocoagulation is applied. In proliferative DR, panretinal photocoagulation is applied with 3–4 laser sessions. The benefit of decrease in the risk of visual acuity loss with laser treatments is more than 50 percent.

A high risk of blindness exists in diffuse or oedematous maculopathy, ischaemic maculopathy, vitreal haemorrhage and retinal detachment, due to contraction, as well as in haemorrhagic glaucoma.

Complications of laser photocoagulation include pain, transient loss or decrease in vision immediately after a laser session (it returns after a few hours), decrease of the visual optic field and haemorrhage in the fundus.

- **Surgical treatment** is implemented in cases of secondary retinal detachment from contraction, which is a serious complication of proliferative DR, and especially when the area of the macula is threatened. Repeated haemorrhages of the vitreous cavity are also an indication for surgical treatment, i.e. vitrectomy, with satisfactory effects in 40 percent of cases. During this operation, the cataract lens and the haemorrhagic vitreous body are removed, retinal integrity is restored and the retina is transferred back to its original position, so that evolution of the disease is inhibited.

- **Medicines:** aspirin administration has been tried in various studies, without success, however, as regards to inhibition of DR progress. ACE inhibitors have also been used in proliferative DR. Furthermore, good control of diabetes, hypertension, nephropathy, heart failure and anaemia are indispensable for a good outcome of DR. Encouraging results have also been reported with the use of somatostatin products.

What is the relationship between cataract and DM?

Cataract is 30 percent more common in diabetic than in non-diabetic persons. Cataract development is a physiologic manifestation of ageing, but this process occurs earlier and more quickly in diabetic people. The mechanisms of cataract development in ageing and in diabetes are similar. The *polyol pathway* has been incriminated in cataract production in experimental models of diabetic animals, with resultant accumulation of sorbitol and galctitol (a product of galactose) in the lens. This view is strengthened by the beneficial effect that aldose reductase inhibitors have on inhibition of this process and cataract formation, on condition these medicines are used early in diabetic patients. Furthermore, the role of lack of myoinositol or special aminoacids has been discussed, as well as the detrimental effect of free radicals, a view supported by the beneficial effect of antioxidant substances on delay or even prevention of cataract formation. The current prevailing view, however, for the mechanism of cataract formation is the *enzymatic glycosylation of the lens contents* and especially of the crystalline protein fibres. This process evolves at an accelerating pace in diabetes. At the same time the glycosylated crystalline fibres are more susceptible to oxidative damage, a process that is accelerated by their bipolar interaction with disulphide bonds. This leads to formation of molecular entities of higher molecular weight, resulting in the loss of the ability to diffuse light inside the lens. Similar phenomena have been observed with ageing.

It is also interesting that the enzymatic glycosylation theory can be connected to that of polyol formation, since it was proven that aldose reductase inhibitors inhibit not only the protein glycosylation but also the formation of pentosidine bonds, which is considered an index of long-term protein destruction.

Cataract removal can deteriorate existent maculopathy and proliferative DR if intraoperative complications occur. For this reason, cataract operation is decided only when the quality of the patient's life has been seriously affected from loss of vision or when the ability to detect and treat underlying DR is being hampered by the presence of the cataract lens. Disk oedema and proliferative DR should be treated with laser photocoagulation before the surgery, if possible. The process of the operation includes destruction of the cataract lens with the use of ultrasound (photocoemulsification), whereas the effect on vision can be worse than in non-diabetic subjects, due to possible deterioration of coexistent retinopathy and especially maculopathy. Finally, the possibility of postoperative inflammation is higher in diabetic people. The use of acrylic or heparin-eluted lenses is indicated, since they cause fewer inflammations or cellular deposits compared to silicone lenses. Silicone can be used during vitrectomy.

In which cases can the diabetic person manifest acute glaucoma?

The main causes of acute glaucoma in the diabetic patient are: i) erythrosis of iris after bleeding; and ii) neovascularization in the angle of the anterior chamber.

When can DM cause reversible haziness of the lens?

Multiple reversible haziness of the lens can occur rarely in patients with Type 1 DM (children or young adults) after severe hyperglycaemia and evolve over days or weeks ('snowflake cataracts'). This condition is gradually reversed with control of diabetes. Similar but less intense episodes can be seen in diabetic patients during periods of poor control of their diabetes. This happens more frequently, is manifested with transient refractive visual abnormalities – mostly myopia – which are primarily associated with electrolyte disturbances through the lens, and is reversible.

CASE STUDY 1

A 68 year old woman, with poorly controlled DM of 25 years duration, comes to the diabetes clinic for follow-up. Her fasting blood glucose is around 256 mg/dl (14.2 mmol/L) and her HbA$_{1c}$ is 11.2 percent. The patient complains of pricking pains, burning sensation and numbness in her lower extremities, as well as frequent cramps. Furthermore, she reports deterioration of her vision lately with decrease in her visual acuity and blurred vision. She has a history of operated cataract in the left eye. Physical examination is remarkable only for: BP 170/90 mmHg, a systolic murmur in the apex and abolition of Achilles tendon reflexes bilaterally. Her antidiabetic regimen includes: glibenclamide tablets 5 mg, 1 × 3, and metformin tablets 850 mg, 1 × 3 daily. Fundoscopy reveals diabetic maculopathy bilaterally, without obvious lesions in the rest of the retina. What would you recommend for this patient?

A complete blood count (CBC), urinalysis, biochemistry tests and a lipid profile were done. The patient was asked to monitor her blood glucose levels at home, both fasting as well as two hours postprandially. Furthermore, since most likely she has developed secondary failure to the oral antidiabetic medicines due to her long-lasting diabetes, it would be useful to confirm this by measuring fasting C-peptide and insulin levels, as well as six minutes after the intravenous administration of glucagon, which evaluates the maximal secretory capacity of the pancreas. Also, a complete ophthalmologic examination would be necessary for a more precise characterization of the ophthalmic disease and planning of the appropriate therapy by the specialist ophthalmologist.

A week later the patient returned to the clinic with the following diagnosis from the ophthalmologist: Oedematous diabetic maculopathy. Fundoscopy and fundus photography revealed multiple hard exudates, microhaemorrhages, and microaneurysms in the whole area of the macula, with diffuse oedema of the macula, in contrast to the rest of the retina which was unremarkable. Also, there was decolorization from optic disk atrophy (Figure 13.1). Findings were in both eyes, most prominent in the left eye fundus. Fluorescein angiography revealed masking of the normal macular appearance, due to multiple leakages from the capillaries and the microaneurysms of the perimacular vascular net. There was also masking of the optic disk due to atrophy(Figure 13.2). Laser treatments were recommended.

Laboratory evaluation showed the following: Ht = 36.1 percent, Hb = 12.2 g/dl, WBC = 7000/µl, (polymorphonuclears = 55 percent, lymphocytes = 37 percent, monocytes = 6 percent), Platelets = 164,000/µl, ESR = 23 mm/hr, glucose = 285 mg/dl (15.8 mmol/L), creatinine = 0.76 mg/dl (67.2 µmol/L), cholesterol = 161 mg/dl (4.16 mmol/L), HDL-cholesterol = 57 mg/dl (1.47 mmol/L), LDL-cholesterol = 87 mg/dl (2.17 mmol/L),

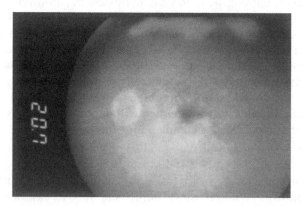

Figure 13.2. Fluorescein angiography of the left eye (before the application of Laser therapy): Oedema of the posterior pole from leakage of the capillaries and micro-aneurysms of the perimacular network.

triglycerides $= 98$ mg/dl (1.11 mmol/L), SGOT $= 16$ U/L, SGPT $= 24$ U/L, γGT $= 19$ U/L. Urinalysis: SG $= 1005$, urine protein $(-)$, urine glucose $(+)$, microscopic exam: normal.

The glucagon stimulation test revealed the following results: fasting C-peptide $= 0.14$ ng/ml (normal 0.09–4.38 ng/ml) and six minutes after iv administration of glucagon: C-peptide $= 0.33$ ng/ml.

How would you advise the patient now, based on these findings?

As already mentioned, diabetic retinopathy is divided into non-proliferative DR (NPDR or background DR) and proliferative DR (PDR) depending on the presence or not of neovascularization of the retina (in the area of the optic disk or the periphery), and it can, at any stage, be accompanied by diabetic maculopathy.

Studies in Type 1 diabetic patients (DCCT, 1995) showed that good glycaemic control based on intensive insulin therapy decreased the risk of DR by 76 percent, after the first 36 months of therapy. Also, in the group of secondary prevention, intensive insulin therapy decreased the risk of retinopathy progression by 54 percent, despite initial deterioration during the first year of therapy. Furthermore, in patients with Type 2 DM (UKPDS study), intensive therapy either with insulin or with oral antidiabetic medicines decreased microvascular complications risk by 25 percent compared to the group that was treated with conventional therapy.

It is also obvious that the patient has secondary failure to the oral antidiabetic medicines. Fasting blood glucose measurements in the morning, as well as two hours postprandially, were mostly higher than 200 mg/dl (11.1 mmol/L). Furthermore, C-peptide levels were especially low (see Chapter 1). Based on these findings, it was decided to start an intensive insulin regimen with slow-acting insulin combined with rapid-acting insulin before the three main meals. At the same time the patient was treated with laser photocoagulation (grid pattern). In this case photocoagulation is the treatment of choice with proven value in maintaining and possibly improving vision. The patient did not accept the recommended intravitreal injection of triamcinolone (0.4 mg/0.1 mm^3 normal saline). Fluorescein angiography of the fundus after the laser treatments is shown in Figure 13.3.

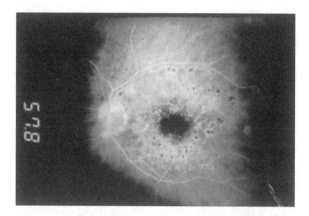

Figure 13.3. Late phase fluorescein angiography of the patient's fundus, showing the micro-aneurysms that fluoresce and the sites of previous Laser photocoagulation. On the optic disk there are hyperfluorescent foci due to probable early neovascularization.

During the next seven months the patient improved her blood glucose control dramatically (HbA$_{1c}$ = 6.7 percent). There are other treatments, however, that can still be recommended to the patient.

Apart from a good glycaemic control, attention needs to be paid to control of hypertension and serum lipids, and management of other coexistent complications, like diabetic nephropathy and albuminuria, heart failure and anaemia.

Strict control of blood pressure is therefore equally essential. The UKPDS study showed that good control of blood pressure in Type 2 diabetic patients decreased the risk of DR progression by 34 percent, irrespective of the kind of antihypertensive therapy (ACE inhibitor or beta-blocker). Also, the EUCLID study (EURODIAB Controlled Trial of Lisinopril in Insulin Dependent Diabetes) showed that therapy with lisinopril decreased the risk of DR progression, but this could be due to the lisinopril-induced decrease in blood pressure in patients with latent hypertension. According to the American Diabetes Association guidelines, the higher cut-off level for blood pressure control is 130/80 mmHg. Therefore, the use of an antihypertensive factor – preferably an ACE inhibitor – is absolutely indicated in this case.

Furthermore, the Early Treatment Diabetic Retinopathy Study (ETDRS, 1991) showed that aspirin (650 mg/day) had no effect – negative or positive – in the progression of DR.

Note: The case of this patient, although rare, is interesting, because it shows an example of oedematous maculopathy without coexisting DR in the rest of the retina.

Further reading

American Diabetes Association (2004) Retinopathy in diabetes. *Diabetes Care*, **27**(Suppl 1), S84–S87.

Brinchmann-Hansen, O., Dahl-Jorgensen, K., Sandvik, L., Hanssen, K.F. (1992) Blood glucose concentrations and progression of diabetic retinopathy: the seven year results of the Oslo study. *BMJ*, **304**, 19–22.

Chaturvedi, N., Sjolie, A.K., Stephenson, J.M., Abrahamian, H., Keipes, M., Castellarin, A., Rogulja-Pepeonik, Z., Fuller, J.H. (1997) Effect of lisinopril on progression of retinopathy in normotensive people with type 1 diabetes. The EUCLID Study Group. EURODIAB Controlled Trial of Lisinopril in Insulin-Dependent Diabetes Mellitus. *Lancet*, **351**, 28–31.

Early Treatment Diabetic Retinopathy Study Group (1991) *Effects of aspirin treatment on Diabetic retinopathy*, ETDRS Report No. 8. Ophthalmology, **98**, 757–65.

Knott, R.M. and Forrester, J.V. (2003) Pathogenesis of diabetic eye disease, in *Textbook of Diabetes*, 3rd edn, (eds J. Pickup and G. Williams) Blackwell Science Ltd, Oxford, **48**, pp. 1–17.

Porta, M., Sjoelie, A.K., Chaturvedi, N., Stevens, L., Rottiers, R., Veglio, M., Fuller, J.H. (2001) EURODIAB Prospective Complications Study Group. Risk factors for progression to proliferative retinopathy in the EURODIAB Prospective Complications Study. *Diabetologia*, **44**, 2203–9.

The Diabetes Control and Complications Trial (1995) The effect of intensive diabetes treatment on the progression of diabetic retinopathy in insulin-dependent diabetes mellitus. *Arch Ophthalmol*, **113**, 36–51.

Towler, H.M.A and Lightman, S. (2003) Clinical features and management of diabetic eye disease, in *Textbook of Diabetes*, 3rd edn, (eds J. Pickup and G. Williams) Blackwell Science Ltd, Oxford, **49**, 1–25.

UKPDS Study Group (1998) Intensive blood-glucose control with sulfonylurea or insulin compared with conventional treatment and risk of complications in patients with type 2 diabetes (UKPDS 33). *Lancet*, **352**, 837–53.

UKPDS Study Group (1998) Tight blood pressure control and risk of macro-vascular and microvascular complications in patients with type 2 diabetes (UKPDS 38). *BMJ*, **317**, 703–13.

14

Diabetic nephropathy

Evanthia Diakoumopoulou

What do we call diabetic nephropathy?

Diabetic nephropathy is the decline in renal function due to DM and manifests clinically with proteinuria, usually several years after the onset of hyperglycaemia. The earliest clinical indication of diabetic nephropathy is the appearance of a small quantity of albumin in the urine (albumin excretion rate ≥ 30 mg/24 h or ≥ 20 µg/min in a 4-hour or 8-hour urine collection or ≥ 30 mg/g creatinine in a spot urine sample). Specifically, microalbuminuria is defined as the excretion of 30–300 mg of albumin in a 24-hour period or 20–200 µg/min or 30–300 mg/g creatinine in a spot urine sample. When albumin excretion rate is higher than these cut-offs, we talk about macroalbuminuria or more precisely overt proteinuria (which corresponds to a total protein excretion rate of > 500 mg/24 hours).

It should be emphasized that it is wrong to use the term 'microalbumin' which is sometimes reported from some laboratories, since this does not exist. There is no 'small' or 'large' albumin. The term 'microalbuminuria' suggests an abnormally high excretion of albumin in the urine (> 30 mg/24 h), which is however still relatively low (< 300 mg/24 h), such that it cannot be detected from the dipstick examination of the urine in a urinalysis test.

What is the frequency of nephropathy in DM?

The cumulative incidence of diabetic nephropathy for both types of diabetes is around 30–35 percent. In Type 1 DM, microalbuminuria can

Diabetes in Clinical Practice: Questions and Answers from Case Studies. Nicholas Katsilambros *et al.*
© 2006 John Wiley & Sons, Ltd.

often occur more than 10 years after disease onset, whereas its prevalence is associated with the duration of diabetes and can reach 40–50 percent after 30 years of the disease. Unless certain therapeutic interventions are applied at the stage of persistent microalbuminuria, proteinuria develops in 80 percent of the patients with Type 1 DM after another 10–15 years, so that 25 percent of patients ultimately develop proteinuria after 25 years of the disease. Around 50 percent of Type 1 diabetic patients with overt nephropathy develop end stage renal disease within 10 years, and 75 percent within 20 years.

In Caucasians with Type 2 DM, the course of diabetic nephropathy is similar to that in Type 1 DM, with the exception that persistent microalbuminuria can already be present at the time of diagnosis of the diabetes in 10–48 percent of the patients; this reflects the existence of the disease several years before its clinical manifestation and suggests irreversible renal damage. Prevalence of microalbuminuria in Type 2 DM is 10–42 percent depending on the population and ethnicity. Higher prevalence is seen in Asians, Pima Indians, African American and the inhabitants of the Maori islands in the Pacific, compared to Europeans. The relation between microalbuminuria and duration of diabetes is not as strong as in Type 1 DM. Without treatment, 20 percent of the patients with microalbuminuria and Type 2 DM will develop overt nephropathy, but only 20 percent of these will end up in end stage renal disease. After 20 years of the disease, the cumulative incidence of proteinuria is 27 percent, similar to Type 1 DM.

Which factors participate in the pathogenesis of nephropathy?

Genetic predisposition, ethnicity, diabetes duration, smoking and degree of glycaemic control are the principal factors for development of diabetic nephropathy.

How is the diagnosis of diabetic nephropathy made?

Quantitative determination of albumin in the urine can be expressed in three ways:

1. with measurement of the albumin to creatinine ratio in a random or morning urine sample (normal values < 30 mg/g creatinine or

< 3.5 mg/mmol creatinine in women and < 2.5 mg/mmol creatinine in men);
2. with a 4-hour or 8-hour urine collection (overnight urine collection, normal values < 20 μg/min);
3. with a 24-hour urine collection, with simultaneous determination of creatinine clearance (normal values < 30 mg/24 h).

Owing to the well known variation of urine albumin excretion over a 24-hour period, a first morning urine sample or overnight collection is preferred. Determination of albumin in the urine is performed with a radioimmunoassay (RIA, the most reliable method), with ELISA (enzyme linked immunoassay), nephelometry, etc. Qualitative determination of albumin in the urine can also be performed using a special dipstick (microalbumin test, micral II), but the specificity is lower than that of RIA.

Which other conditions, except diabetic nephropathy, may be accompanied by microalbuminuria?

Transient increase in albumin excretion in the urine or even proteinuria can be due to poorly controlled diabetes, urine infections, uncontrolled hypertension, heart failure, febrile illnesses, physical activity, pregnancy and increased intake of protein with the food. Furthermore, variation of albumin excretion can be observed not only during a 24-hour period, but from day to day as well. Nephropathy from other causes also – albeit rare – should be considered, especially in cases of acute deterioration of renal function and proteinuria, without an obvious cause (vasculitides, collagen vascular diseases, glomerulonephritides, multiple myeloma, monoclonal gammopathies accompanying other diseases, etc.). This is particularly likely when nephropathy is not accompanied by retinopathy. When there is pyuria, urine culture is necessary for exclusion of urinary tract infection. Other recommended tests are erythrocyte sedimentation rate (ESR), C-reactive protein (CRP) and immunologic evaluation (rheumatoid factor, antinuclear antibodies, anti-DNA, protein electrophoresis, quantitative immunoglobulin determination). Consequently, nephropathy in a diabetic person does not necessarily always mean diabetic nephropathy. Coexistence of diabetic retinopathy strengthens the possibility of a diabetic aetiology of the nephropathy.

When should microalbuminuria be checked?

As mentioned earlier, microalbuminuria is present in 10–42 percent of Type 2 diabetic patients at diagnosis, since the disease has most likely been silently present for many years before its clinical manifestation. For this reason, measurement of albumin excretion rate is recommended at the initial diagnosis of diabetes, and then yearly, if it is within normal limits initially.

As regards Type 1 DM, a check of the albumin excretion rate is recommended five years after the initial diagnosis – since microalbuminuria is rare at shorter durations of the disease – and yearly thereafter, if the initial results are within normal limits. If the result is positive for microalbuminuria, given the great variation of albumin excretion from day to day, it is recommended to repeat the test another couple of times within the next 3–6 months. If two of the specimens are positive, microalbuminuria is considered present. At the same time it is essential to consider – depending on specific indications – and possibly treat, the other conditions that are associated with microalbuminuria/proteinuria mentioned above, before the condition is attributed to diabetes. Ophthalmoscopy is always necessary, since, as mentioned, it strengthens the diagnosis of diabetic nephropathy.

What is the significance of microalbuminuria in diabetics?

Apart from being an index of renal damage progression, microalbuminuria has been associated with a high frequency of cardiovascular events (for example, myocardial infarctions). For this reason it is considered an index of generalized atheromatosis and cardiovascular mortality, the determination of which is considered necessary, not only for evaluation of disease progression and its complications (renal, cardiovascular) but also for their prevention.

What is the natural history of diabetic nephropathy?

From the time of microalbuminuria appearance, progression of the disease is gradual and without warning signs or symptoms, until the patient ends up at an advanced stage (clinically overt nephropathy or clinical proteinuria). According to Mogensen the following stages of diabetic nephropathy are described in Type 1 DM:

1. **Hyperfiltration stage:** At this stage there is evidence of renal hyperfunction, characterized by increased glomerular filtration and increase renal size. This stage is synchronous to diabetes diagnosis and lasts about two years.

2. **'Silent stage':** This stage is characterized by the first appearance of pathologic lesions in renal biopsies, i.e. basement membrane thickness and mesangial expansion. There are no clinical manifestations, which is why it is considered silent. Glomerular filtration rate and renal size remain increased. These first two stages are considered reversible with good control of diabetes.

3. **Stage of incipient nephropathy:** This stage is divided into two phases, depending on albumin excretion in the urine, and lasts for 10–20 years. At the initial phase, microalbuminuria excretion rate is 20–70 μg/min and blood pressure is normal or minimally elevated. At the late phase of this stage, albumin excretion rate has increased (70–200 μg/min) and hypertension is persistent. Optimal control of diabetes, and even more important of arterial hypertension, while aiming at controlling intraglomerular pressure as well, is essential for the deceleration of renal function decline in this stage.

4. **Stage of clinically overt nephropathy (clinical proteinuria):** The main characteristic of this stage is macroalbuminuria or proteinuria (that is, an albumin excretion rate > 200 μg/min or > 300 mg/24 h and a total quantity of protein in the urine > 500 mg/24 h). In this stage the urinalysis is usually dipstick positive for protein in the urine. There are two evolutionary phases: **the early phase**, which is characterized by intermittent proteinuria and incipient decline in glomerular filtration and **the late or advanced stage**, where proteinuria is persistent and gradually increasing, there is a greater decline of renal function (greater decrease of glomerular filtration rate), while at the same time hypertension develops. Usually 10 years elapse from the stage of persistent proteinuria to the final stage of chronic renal failure (CRF), if patients are not treated properly. Glomerular filtration rate declines by about 8–12 ml/min/year, and coexistent hypertension plays a detrimental role as well. Complications are frequent at this stage, with echocardiographic findings of left ventricular hypertrophy, hypercholesterolaemia, retinopathy parallel to nephropathy,

peripheral and autonomic neuropathy, peripheral vascular disease and coronary artery disease. It should be noted that many Type 2 diabetic patients can die prematurely from cardiovascular diseases before they reach the final stage of chronic renal failure. Hypertension management with two or more antihypertensive medicines has a primary role at this stage, with glycaemic control playing a secondary role.

5. **Stage of chronic renal failure (CRF):** At the final stage of CRF the patient needs renal replacement therapy or kidney transplantation.

How is diabetic nephropathy treated?

Glycaemic control

Intensive DM treatment, aimed at achieving glucose values as close to normal as possible, was shown in large randomized studies to delay onset of microalbuminuria and its progression to macroalbuminuria, both in Type 1 (DCCT trial) and Type 2 diabetic patients (UKPDS study). Intensive treatment plays a primary role in the first two stages of the disease, with the possibility existing of complete reversal of damage. In the following stages, DM control has a secondary role with hypertension control gaining primary importance.

In Type 2 diabetic patients with incipientl nephropathy, it is wise to use sulfonylureas carefully, discontinue metformin administration and use insulin if needed. The risk of prolonged hypoglycaemias from sulfonylurea administration when CRF occurs is high. Specifically, metformin administration is interrupted when creatinine is higher than 1.5 mg/dl (132.6 μmol/L) in men and > 1.4 mg/dl (123.8 μmol/L) in women, due to the heightened risk of lactic acidosis.

Arterial hypertension

In Type 1 DM, hypertension is usually a result of diabetic nephropathy and manifests at the stage of microalbuminuria. In Type 2 DM, hypertension is present at the time of diagnosis of diabetes in a third of the patients and may coexist with other parameters of the metabolic syndrome X, a common pathogenetic mechanism which is insulin resistant. It may also be due to diabetic nephropathy, coexistent idiopathic arterial hypertension, renal vascular disease or other causes.

Systolic and diastolic hypertension promote diabetic nephropathy to a significant degree. Aggressive antihypertensive treatment in Type 1 diabetic patients with already overt diabetic nephropathy, not only decreases albumin excretion rate (AER) but may also essentially delay decline of glomerular filtration rate (GFR) and decelerate progression to end stage renal disease. The UKPDS study also showed that BP control in Type 2 DM may decrease nephropathy risk (by 29 percent) irrespective of the kind of antihypertensive regimen (with a beta-blocker or an inhibitor of angiotensin converting enzyme).

The target is to achieve BP values < 130/80 mmHg. When urinary protein excretion is larger than 1 g/24 h, then BP control target should be lower (< 120/75 mmHg).

Both types of medicines that block the rennin-angiotensin system (i.e., ACE inhibitors and angiotensin receptors blockers [ARBs]) can be used with priority in the treatment of albuminuria/nephropathy. This has been proven in many studies and is explained by the special action of these medicines in the renal glomerulus and from a wide range of other actions that will be mentioned later. If intolerance to one category develops, the other can be used instead.

In hypertensive and non-hypertensive Type 1 diabetic patients with microalbuminuria, it has been proven that ACE inhibitors delay progression of nephropathy (that is, they decrease albumin excretion rate and progression to macroalbuminuria).

Furthermore, in hypertensive and non-hypertensive Type 2 diabetic patients with microalbuminuria, the beneficial effect of ARBs on delay of nephropathy deterioration and progression to macroalbuminuria has been proven (IRMA II and MARVAL studies). In studies specifically performed on Type 2 diabetic patients with hypertension, macroalbuminuria (albumin excretion rate > 300 mg/24 h) and mild renal insufficiency, ARBs were proven to delay progression of nephropathy (IDNT and RENAAL studies).

The basic mechanisms through which ACE inhibitors cause a reduction in BP are as follows: i) inhibition of angiotensin II formation; and ii) inhibition of bradykinin degradation resulting in its accumulation, nitric oxide (NO) and prostacyclin formation and subsequent vasodilatation.

Renoprotective mechanisms of ACE inhibitors, apart from a decrease in systemic blood pressure – a common feature of all antihypertensives – include many other actions, the majority of which refer to the category of ARBs as well. These include:

- A decrease in intraglomerular hypertension due to relaxation of the constricted efferent glomerular arteriole. A characteristic pathologic lesion in DM is an increase in intraglomerular pressure through vasodilatation of the afferent arteriole (due to effects of prostaglandin, bradykinin, atrial natriuretic peptide, etc.) and transmission of pressure from systemic circulation. Furthermore, there is constriction of the efferent arteriole due to an angiotensin II effect, which apart from its known systemic vasoconstrictive effect, contributes to the progression of renal disease through a variety of mechanisms. These include an increase in the formation of various cytokines in the kidney, such as transforming growth factor-β (TGF-β), collagen type IV, laminin, fibronectin and others. Evolving intraglomerular hypertension is considered responsible for the excretion of albumin and increase in basement membrane thickness. Thus, medicines of this category are considered as first line treatment of diabetic nephropathy due to their selective action on renal glomerulus.
- An increase in renal perfusion.
- A decrease in glomerular membrane permeability and decrease in proteinuria.
- Natriuresis.
- A decrease in peripheral insulin resistance.
- A decrease in transforming growth factor-β (TGF-β) and other cytokines, resulting in a decrease in extracellular matrix deposition.

Therapy with ACE inhibitors has also been associated with a decrease in cardiovascular mortality and incidence of stroke and myocardial infarction, in patients with a high risk of cardiovascular disease, including patients with DM (HOPE study). In a recent comparative study of the renoprotective action of ACE inhibitors and ARBs (telmisartan versus enalapril) in Type 2 diabetic patients with incipient nephropathy, no clinical superiority of one versus the other was proven. This fact proves the equivalence of these two categories of medicines for use in diabetic patients at high risk of deterioration of renal function and cardiovascular events. A recent study in hypertensive Type 2 diabetic patients without nephropathy, showed that an ACE inhibitor or a combination of an ACE inhibitor with verapamil (a non-dihydropyridine calcium channel blocker) delayed onset of microalbuminuria compared with verapamil alone or placebo (that is, use of other antihypertensive medicines for blood pressure control). This is the first indication of a preventive renoprotective effect of ACE inhibitors compared to other antihypertensives in DM. These findings should be considered preliminary, however, and we need to wait for the results of other similar studies before a reliable conclusion for the use of ACE inhibitors as preventive renoprotective therapy in Type 2 DM can be drawn. It should be also noted that the group that received ACE inhibitor (or combination with verapamil) in that particular study, had a slightly better BP control (by 3 mmHg).

In the other categories of antihypertensive medications that have been used in diabetic nephropathy, dihydropyridine calcium channel blockers (nifedipine, etc.), when used in comparison to ACE inhibitors at doses that produced a similar antihypertensive result, had unpredictable effects on microalbuminuria (they can decrease, increase, or leave it unchanged). Furthermore, differences in the actions of the various calcium channel blockers have been observed. This denotes that they should not be considered as a uniform group regarding their action in diabetic nephropathy. Thus, in two studies, enalapril and captopril significantly decreased AER, whereas nitrendipine and nifedipine increased it, despite the fact that they had a similar antihypertensive effect to the ACE inhibitors. In other studies, verapamil and diltiazem (non-dihydropyridine calcium channel blockers) decreased AER regardless of their antihypertensive action.

As regards beta-blockers, they also inhibit renin secretion, resulting in a decrease in angiotensin II, relaxation of efferent arteriole and, consequently, an action similar to ACE inhibitors at the level of the kidney. If there is an indication, therefore (for example, ischaemic heart disease), they can be combined with other antihypertensive medicines for treatment of hypertension accompanying diabetic nephropathy.

The same is true for diuretics and the other antihypertensive categories (centrally acting, etc.) which have no proven selective action on the nephron. In advanced stages of CRF, however, the use of loop diuretics and calcium channel blockers (or another antihypertensive category) is preferred for BP treatment, while ACE inhibitors (or ARBs) are to be used carefully, with serum K^+ monitoring, due to the fear of hyperkalaemia.

Diet

At the stage of clinical proteinuria, a relative restriction of food protein at a level of 0.8 g/kg body weight per day is recommended, i.e. almost the usually recommended level of intake for adults (10 percent of daily caloric intake). At the stage of CRF, a further restriction of protein intake is recommended (to the level of 0.6 g/kg body weight per day), as well as of sodium and phosphorus, with administration of phosphorus binding medicines, if necessary.

Furthermore, cessation of smoking is recommended, due to its well known association with macro- and micro-vascular complications. At every stage of diabetic nephropathy, therapy is supplemented with strict lipid control (target an LDL-cholesterol level < 100 mg/dl [2.6 mmol/L], triglycerides < 150 mg/dl [1.7 mmol/L] and HDL-cholesterol > 40 mg/dl [1.03 mmol/L]), initially with hypolipidaemic therapy and then with antilipidaemic factors (preferably with statins aiming at LDL and total cholesterol decrease). Additionally, regular monitoring of the haematocrit should be performed (for the possibility of anaemia development), as well as monitoring of 24-hour urine protein excretion and serum electrolytes (sodium, potassium, calcium and phosphorus) which, due to the coadministration of diuretics and ACE inhibitors (or ARBs), can have many variations.

RENAL TRANSPLANTATION

When is renal transplantation desirable in persons with DM?

Renal transplantation is the treatment of choice for people with end stage renal disease. Peritoneal dialysis and haemodialysis are both deficient as regards quality of life and expected survival. Survival of people with renal transplantation is estimated at 95–98 percent in the first year, and respective survival of people on haemodialysis is around 75 percent.

According to American official sources, diabetic nephrosclerosis is the primary cause of end stage renal disease treated with transplantation (37 percent), followed by hypertensive nephrosclerosis (27 percent). Patients with severe heart failure, uraemic encephalopathy, active hepatitis, malignancy or bone marrow depression are unsuitable for transplantation, as are elderly persons. Chronic hepatitis is not a contraindication (as long as there is no active disease or cirrhosis) and neither is tuberculosis (if proper treatment is given).

In countries where it is available, renal transplantation is usually reserved for Type 2 diabetics, whereas for persons with Type 1 DM and renal failure (even before the need for haemodialysis) the treatment of choice is double transplantation (kidney and pancreas).

How does kidney transplantation differ in people with and without DM?

Patients with Type 2 DM are usually older than non-diabetics or Type 1 diabetics and many of them have had a myocardial infarction in the past. They frequently have multivessel disease, which makes the operation more difficult.

Furthermore, according to some studies, graft survival is 1–2 years shorter by compared to people without DM.

The perioperative period is managed with an intravenous infusion of an insulin solution together with frequent blood glucose measurements and prompt adjustment of the solution rate or small additional bolus rapid-acting insulin injections (see Chapter 7: 'Surgery in diabetes'). Preoperative problems include the need for hydration restriction, whereas postoperatively, when initially large quantities of fluids are needed, blood glucose should be hourly monitored and insulin administration accordingly adjusted. High blood glucose levels due to cortisol administration are initially treated with large intravenous doses of insulin, and later with an intensive insulin regimen or mixtures of rapid acting and intermediate acting insulin. Steroid-induced diabetes that sometimes occurs in persons without a previous history of diabetes can be managed with antidiabetic pills, provided it is mild. Decrease in steroid doses during the following months makes management easier.

More information on transplantation is provided on Chapter 29: 'New therapies in diabetes'.

CASE STUDY 1

A 64 year old woman without previous history of DM presents at the outpatient clinic with mild xerostomia, polyuria and polydipsia. She reports having dyslipidaemia and hypertension for a year, treated with cilazapril 5 mg and amlodipine 10 mg daily. She is a smoker, has a moderate alcohol consumption, is obese (weight: 80 kg [176.4 lb], height: 1.62 m [5 ft, 4 in], BMI: 31 kg/m^2), and has arterial pressure 170/80 mmHg; otherwise her physical condition is unremarkable. Laboratory findings: fasting blood glucose 112 mg/dl (6.2 mmol/L); urinalysis abundant WBCs and urine protein (+++). What would you initially recommend for the patient?

Initially, an oral glucose tolerance test (with 75 g glucose) and urine culture for diagnosis of possible asymptomatic bacteriuria would be appropriate. Routine chemistry examinations and measurement of 24-hour urinary protein excretion would be useful. At the same time, a hypocaloric diet and recommendations towards smoking cessation are appropriate.

One month later the patient returned to the clinic with the following results: fasting plasma glucose = 125 mg/dl (6.9 mmol/L), urea = 25 mg/dl (4.2 mmol/L), creatinine = 0.9 mg/dl (79.6 μmol/L), total cholesterol = 240 mg/dl (6.21 mmol/L), triglycerides = 220 mg/dl (2.49 mmol/L), HDL-cholesterol = 55 mg/dl (1.42 mmol/L), LDL-cholesterol = 141 mg/dl (3.65 mmol/L), SGOT = 16 IU/L, SGPT = 28 IU/L, γGT = 45 IU/L, alkaline phosphatase = 140 IU/L, HbA$_{1c}$ = 7.4 percent, uric acid = 8.8 mg/dl, Ht = 52 percent, WBC = 11,300/μl (polymorphonuclears = 60 percent, lymphocytes = 35 percent, monocytes = 2 percent, eosinophils = 3 percent), platelets = 337,000/μl. Urinalysis: SG = 1025, WBC = 0–2 per high power field, glucose = negative, protein = (+++), urine culture = sterile, 24-hour urine protein = 731 mg. Oral glucose tolerance test: fasting plasma glucose = 120 mg/dl (6.7 mmol/L), serum glucose two hours after 75 g glucose = 230 mg/dl (12.8 mmol/L).

We conclude that this is a patient with recent clinical occurrence of Type 2 DM and proteinuria. Proteinuria is due mainly to DM and pre-existing hypertension. The exact time of DM initiation cannot be precisely estimated, which is quite common in this type of diabetes mellitus.

What would you recommend to the patient at this stage?

A portable glucose meter for monitoring blood glucose levels at home and for determining the kind of diabetes therapy is necessary. Regular measurements of blood pressure at home could also be helpful. Despite the obvious diagnosis of DM and the negative urine culture, an exclusion of other causes of proteinuria (see theoretic section above) would be appropriate as well. For this reason, potentially useful tests would be determination of erythrocyte sedimentation rate (ESR), CRP and immunologic tests. Fundoscopic evaluation by an ophthalmologist is also absolutely necessary.

Two weeks later the patient brought the following laboratory results: ESR = 10 mm/h, CRP = 5 mg/L, ANA = (−), and complement (C$_3$ and C$_4$) and serum and urine protein electrophoresis were within normal limits. Self monitoring of blood glucose at home showed fasting values 90–130 mg/dl (5.0–7.2 mmol/L) and two hours postprandially 160–230 mg/dl (8.9–12.8 mmol/L). Blood pressure varied from 140–160/80–90 mmHg.

Diabetic nephropathy (stage of clinical proteinuria) and uncontrolled hypertension are most likely to be responsible for causing proteinuria in this patient. As mentioned earlier, good control of blood pressure is of paramount significance at this stage. Initiation of antidiabetic treatment with short-acting insulin secretagogues (nateglinide-repaglinide) before main meals and targeting at post-prandial glucose control could be a legitimate initial choice, provided fasting blood glucose values are within normal limits (see Chapter 27: 'Treatment of diabetes with pills').

What kind of antihypertensive medicine would you choose?

Since the administration of two kinds of antihypertensive agents (ACE inhibitor and calcium channel blocker) are not enough for controlling BP of the patient, the addition of a thiazide diuretic could be a good choice (thiazides have a synergistic action with ACE inhibitors and there are fix combinations in the market). The primary target is to achieve BP levels < 130/80 mmHg, necessarily using a medicine blocking the renin-angiotensin axis. Monitoring of the patient's BP and repeat of urine protein measurement will show if this target can be achieved in the next 3–6 months. If not, treatment should be intensified with the addition of a fourth antihypertensive medicine (ARB or other category; see Table 22.1 in Chapter 22 for a list of categories of antihypertensive medicines).

What other instructions will you give to the patient?

The already mentioned instructions for dietary protein restriction and management of dyslipidaemia are appropriate. The expected improvement of metabolic control with the antidiabetic treatment should also decrease triglycerides and improve dyslipidaemia.

Further reading

American Diabetes Association (2004) Nephropathy in diabetes. Clinical Practice Recommendations 2004. *Diabetes Care*, **27**(Suppl.1), S79–S83.
Barnett, A.H., Stephen, C.B., Bouter, P., Karlberg, B., Madsbad, S., Jervell, J. and Mustonen, J. (2004) Angiotensin-receptor blockade versus converting-enzyme inhibition in Type 2 diabetes and nephropathy. *N Engl J Med*, **351**, 1952–61.

Brenner, B.M., Cooper, M.E., De Zeeuw, D., Keane, W.F., Mitch, W.E., Parving. H.-H., Remuzzi, G., Snappin, S.M., Zhang, Z. and Shahinfar, S. (2001) (for the RENAAL Study Investigators). Effects of losartan on renal and cardiovascular outcomes in patients with Type 2 diabetes and nephropathy. *N Engl J Med*, **345**, 861–9.

Friedman, E.A. (2004) Chronic kidney disease, in American Diabetes Association. *Therapy for Diabetes Mellitus and Related Disorders*. 4th edn (ed. H.E. Lebovitz), Alexandria VA, USA, pp. 398–409.

Gnudi, L., Gruden, G. and Viberti, G.F. (2003) Pathogenesis of diabetic nephropathy, in *Textbook of Diabetes*, 3rd edn (eds J. Pickup and G. Williams), Blackwell Science Ltd, Oxford, **52**, pp. 1–21.

Lewis, E.J., Hunsicker, L.G., Clarke, W.R., Berl, T., Pohl, M.A., Lewis, J.B., Ritz, E., Atkins, R.C., Rohde, B.S., Raz, I. (2001) Renoprotective effect of the angiotensin-receptor antagonist irbersartan in patients with nephropathy due to Type 2 diabetes. *N. Engl. J. Med.*, **345**, 851–860.

Lewis, E.J., Hunsicker, L.G., Bain, R.P. and Rohde, R.D. (1993) The effect of angiotensin–converting enzyme inhibition on diabetic nephropathy. The Collaborative Study Group. *N Engl J Med*, **329**, 1456–62.

Marshall, S.M. (2003) Clinical features and management of diabetic nephropathy, in *Textbook of Diabetes*, 3rd edn (eds J. Pickup and G. Williams), Blackwell Science Ltd, Oxford, **53**, pp. 1–22.

Mogensen, C.E. (1990) Prediction of clinical diabetic nephrophaty in IDDM patients. Alternatives to microalbuminuria? *Diabetes*, **39**, 761–67.

Parving, H.H., Lehnert, H., Bröchner-Mortensen, J., Gomis, R., Andersen, S., Arner, P. (2001) The effect of irbersartan on the development of diabetic nephropathy in patients with Type 2 diabetes. *N. Engl J Med*, **345**, 870–878.

Raptis, A.E. and Viberti, G. (2001) Pathogenesis of diabetic nephropathy. *Exp Clin Endocrinol Diabetes*, **109**(Suppl 2), S424–S437.

Ruggenanti, P., Fassi, A., Ilieva, A.P. *et al.* (2004) Preventing microalbuminuria in Type 2 diabetes. *N Engl J Med*, **351**, 1941–51.

UKPDS Study Group (1998) Tight blood pressure control and risk of macrovascular and microvascular complications in Type 2 diabetes (UKPDS 38). *BMJ*, **317**, 703–13.

UKPDS Study Group (1998) Efficacy of atenolol and captopril in reducing the risk of macrovascular complications in Type 2 diabetes (UKPDS 39). *BMJ*, **317**, 713–20.

Viberti, G., Wheeldon,.N.M. (2002) Microalbuminuria Reduction with VALsartan (MARVAL) Study Investigators. Microalbuminuria reduction with valsartan in patients with Type 2 diabetes mellitus: a blood pressure-independent effect. *Circulation*, **106**, 672–78.

Yusuf, S., Sleight, P. *et al.* (2000) Effects of an angiotensin-converting-enzyme inhibitor, ramipril, on cardiovascular events in high-risk patients: The Heart Outcomes Prevention Evaluation Study Investigators. *N Engl J Med.*, **342**, 145–53.

15

Diabetic neuropathy

Nicholas Tentolouris

CASE STUDY 1

A 67 year old woman, with a 15 year history of Type 2 DM, comes to the clinic for a routine visit. She is treated with a mixture of short- and long-acting insulin in the morning and evening and also rapid-acting insulin before lunch. DM control is very good (recent HbA$_{1c}$: 6.9 percent). The patient reports burning pains in the soles for the last year, aggravated at night. Sometimes the discomfort is so intense that she has to get up and walk around or insert her feet in cold water to get some relief. How are her symptoms explained?

Obviously the patient's symptoms are due to peripheral diabetic neuropathy (or chronic sensorimotor peripheral neuropathy). Apart from burning pains, this can present with symptoms of a tingling sensation, 'needles' in the feet and allodynia (i.e., perception of a normal stimulus as painful, for example, pain in the feet when they come in contact with the sheets of the bed or socks, etc.). Some patients report that they feel as if they are walking on marbles, some that their skin 'squeezes' their feet, and others are unable to describe their experience precisely and just report an unpleasant but vague feeling. Peripheral neuropathy symptoms are characteristically aggravated at night. Sometimes they are so intense that they wake the patient up. They get relief by walking, which helps differentiate neuropathic pain from the pain of critical leg ischaemia; the latter pain deteriorates with walking and gets relieved in the sitting position.

It should be emphasized that neuropathic symptoms occur in only 20 percent of patients with peripheral neuropathy, whereas the rest have no obvious symptoms, even in cases where severe sensory deficit can be

Diabetes in Clinical Practice: Questions and Answers from Case Studies.   Nicholas Katsilambros *et al.*
© 2006 John Wiley & Sons, Ltd.

detected at physical examination. Presence of painful symptoms does not mean that the sensation of pain is normal. More often than not, persons with painful symptoms have very severe peripheral neuropathy, with loss of pain sensation. This combination of 'painful-insensitive' feet indicates great risk for development of foot ulcerations, because the presence of symptoms is wrongly considered as a sign of normal sensation.

How do you diagnose peripheral diabetic neuropathy?

The diagnosis is based on physical examination. First of all, inspection can reveal atrophy of intraosseous muscles in the hands and feet, a sign of denervation. When muscle atrophy in the feet is extensive, deformity of the foot architecture can occur, characterized by high foot arch, metatarsal head protrusion, and a shift of the subcutaneous fat normally present under the metatarsal heads towards the bases of the toes, resulting in claw-toe deformity. When autonomic neuropathy coexists, which happens frequently, the foot is reddish, superficial veins are prominent and on palpation it is warm and dry due to lack of sweating. Presence of calluses on pressure sites on the soles is an indication that excessively high pressures are exercised at these sites.

Further examination usually reveals symmetric sensory loss (of touch, pain, temperature and vibration), which starts from the peripheral parts of the extremities and extends centrally (stocking-glove sensory loss distribution). Lower extremity involvement usually precedes the upper extremity involvement. Loss of one type of sensation can be detected at one site (for example, of temperature discrimination), while at the same time another type of sensation (for example, pain) can be normal. Sensory loss can also be segmental, such as complete loss of sensation at one site of the foot and intact sensation at a neighbouring site. Furthermore, the sensory deficient area is not abruptly demarcated from the normal one, but a hypoaesthesia zone usually lies in between. The Achilles tendon reflexes are usually absent and in more advanced disease even knee reflexes can be absent. Deep sensory loss is quite common, with patients reporting imbalance and frequent episodes of falls and trauma.

Special tests (nerve conduction velocity and quantitative examinations of nerve function) are not necessary for the diagnosis in routine clinical practice. A study in the USA found that around 10 percent of diabetics had peripheral neuropathy due to another cause, other than DM.

Table 15.1. Causes of peripheral neuropathy

Metabolic	Diabetes mellitus
	Uraemia
	Amyloidosis
	Hypothyroidism
	Porphyrias
Shortages	Thiamine
	Nicotinic acid
	Vitamin B_{12} or B_6
Medicines	Nitrofurantoin
	Vincristine
	Chrlorambucil
	Isoniazid
	Phenytoin
Toxic substances	Alcohol
Neoplasms	Bronchogenic carcinoma
	Lymphoma
	Paraproteinaemias
Infections	Guillain Barré syndrome
	Leprosy
	Lyme disease
	Chronic inflammatory demyelinating polyneuropathy
Autonomic diseases	Vasculitides (polyarteritis nodosa)
Genetic	Charcot-Marie-Tooth disease

Consequently, before neuropathy can be attributed to DM, other causes need to be ruled out. These causes of peripheral neuropathy are described in Table 15.1.

How frequent is peripheral neuropathy in DM?

Peripheral neuropathy affects 30 percent of diabetic persons. Large epidemiological studies have shown that it is positively associated with DM duration, glycaemic control and body height. Other risk factors are advanced age, hypertension (only for Type 1 DM) dyslipidaemia, smoking and low serum insulin concentrations.

What is the therapy for peripheral neuropathy?

Unfortunately, there are no medicines at present with action on the pathogenetic mechanisms of neuropathy, which could effectively interfere with the natural history of the disease. Ongoing studies examine the effectiveness and safety of newer aldose reductase inhibitors (fidarestate). α-lipoic acid administration (an antioxidant factor) seems, in a series of studies, to be effective in improving the function of small unmyelinated nerve fibres. Small range studies have shown that γ-linolenic acid may be effective in treating peripheral diabetic neuropathy. ACE inhibitor administration resulted in improvement of nerve conduction velocity in patients with mild peripheral neuropathy.

When symptoms of pain are mild, weak analgesics, like paracetamol, are indicated. Non-steroidal anti-inflammatory medicines are also effective, but their potential nephrotoxicity should be taken into consideration in patients with diabetic nephropathy.

Many randomized studies have documented the effectiveness of tricyclic antidepressants in treating neuropathic pain. They act by inhibiting norepinephrine re-uptake from presynaptic neurons. Amitriptyline, imipramine and desipramine have been studied more extensively and are considered medicines of first choice for treating painful symptoms of neuropathy. They are administered at a dose of 25–150 mg once a day, preferably at bedtime, so that side effects are minimized. Since small doses are effective in some patients, it is advised to start with small doses and gradually increase. Most frequent side effects are sleepiness and xerostomia.

Recent publications report a significant improvement of pain after administration of venlafaxine (a serotonin and norepinephrine re-uptake inhibitor) at a dose of 37.5–150 mg/day. Compared to tricyclic antidepressants, venlafaxine has minimal anticholinergic action and no interactions with other medicines. Furthermore, recent studies show that duloxetine, another representative of this class of medicines (serotonin and norepinephrine re-uptake inhibitor), is effective and safe in painful diabetic neuropathy, at a dose of 60 mg/day.

Carbamazepine, essentially an anti-epileptic medicine, at a dose of 200 mg three times a day, was the first of its kind to be used for this condition with fairly good results. Principally, it helps patients with moderate intensity symptoms. It has many side effects as well as many interactions with other medicines. For this reason, carbamazepine is not a first choice medicine for treating neuropathic pain.

Gabapentin is a γ-aminobutyric acid analogue and is used for treating focal convulsions. Administered at a dose of 900–3600 mg/day, it is quite effective in ameliorating neuropathic pain. It has the advantage of lacking side effects and interactions with other medicines and thus it has been extensively used in the symptomatic treatment of painful diabetic neuropathy. Furthermore, it is the only medicine of its class that has been officially approved for administration in this condition. In two recent randomized studies, gabapentin was compared to amitriptyline. The first study showed equal effectiveness in ameliorating pain, whereas the second displayed the superiority of gabapentin. Most frequent side effects are sleepiness and dizziness, with a feeling of tiredness less frequently reported. These side effects usually occur after initiation of therapy, but subside with its continuation.

The usual starting dose of gabapentin is 300–400 mg the first day, and then immediately from the second day a doubling of the dose (300–400 mg twice a day). The dose can subsequently be increased up to 1800 mg/day, depending on the patient's responsiveness. Maximal therapeutic dose is 3600 mg/day. Pharmacokinetic properties are not affected by food intake. An advantage of the medicine is that it does not cause weight gain. Patients with renal insufficiency should receive a smaller dose (creatinine clearance > 60 ml/min: 1200 mg/day; clearance 30–60 ml/min: 600 mg/day; clearance 15–30 ml/min: 300 mg/day; and clearance < 10 ml/min: 300 mg every other day).

The newer antiepileptic medicines topiramate, lamotrigine, oxycarbamazepine and zonisamide have been used in the treatment of painful diabetic neuropathy with variable results. For this reason, none has an official indication for this condition. Potentially these substances have a synergistic action with gabapentin and can be coadministered in resistant cases.

Clonazepam, at doses of 0.5–3 mg/day, is effective in patients with the restless leg syndrome when they do not respond to other medicines. There are no comparative studies of this medicine with others.

Mexiletine is an antiarrhythmic medicine (IB class), analogous to lidocaine. When administered at a relatively small dose (450 mg/day) it is effective in ameliorating pain. This dose does not require frequent electrocardiagraphic evaluation. Nevertheless, experience with long-term use of this medicine is limited and thus its use is recommended only for short periods. As regards lidocaine, although encouraging results have been reported after intravenous infusion, its use is not advocated.

Table 15.2. Therapy of diabetic neuropathy

Symptomatic therapy	Aetiologic therapy
Systemically administered p.o. medicines	Newer aldose reductase inhibitors
Tricyclic antidepressants	α-lipoic acid
Imipramine 25–50 mg/day	γ-linolenic acid
Amitriptyline 25–50 mg/day	Angiotensin converting
Selective serotonin norepinephrine	enzyme inhibitors
re-uptake inhibitors	
Venlafaxine 37.5–150 mg/day	
Duloxetine 60 mg/day	
Antiepileptic	
Carbamazepine up to 800 mg/day	
Gabapentin 900–3600 mg/day	
Topical treatments	
Capsaicin	

There is no consensus concerning the use of opiates in diabetic neuropathy. Many doctors think that they are effective when used at appropriate doses, whereas others that neuropathic pain is quite resistant to them. A recent study showed that the synthetic opioid, tramadole, was quite effective in treating severe neuropathic pain. This medicine has a central analgesic action and is not a member of narcotic analgesics.

Capsaicin is an alkaloid derived from red pepper. Topical application of this substance decreases peptide P concentrations at nerve endings. This peptide is involved in the causation of pain. Capsaicin use causes a temporary burning feeling, which disappears with continued use. It is used for short periods in patients with localized pain.

A concise description of the available medicines for treatment of neuropathic pain is shown in Table 15.2.

How do you manage a patient with findings of severe peripheral diabetic neuropathy but without symptoms?

As mentioned earlier, these cases comprise the vast majority of patients with peripheral neuropathy. For the time being there are no particularly potent medicines for the aetiological treatment of neuropathy. Thus, the patient should be educated so that he or she can avoid the long term complications of neuropathy, such as ulcers and amputations. The best way of substituting sensory loss is by inspecting the feet every single day.

Guidelines for prevention of foot problems are presented in Chapter 17.

CASE STUDY 2

A 37 year old patient with a history of Type 1 DM since the age of 12 comes to the office because of great variations in the blood glucose levels. He reports a 3 month history of frequent vomiting episodes in the morning and after meals as well as early satiety and heaviness in the epigastrium after intake of a small quantity of food. What is the diagnosis?

The most probable diagnosis is gastroparesis. It occurs both in Type 1 and Type 2 diabetic persons and is one of the most severe diabetic complications, because it adversely affects metabolic control and quality of life. It is not, however, associated with other complications or with higher mortality. Gastroparesis can also occur acutely, in cases of diabetic ketoacidosis, but in that case is reversible. It is due to a combination of disturbances (decrease in intensity of gastric muscular contractions, lack of synchronization between gastric and duodenal motility, pyloric spasm) owing to damage of the gastric pacemaker at the fundus of the stomach that regulates motility. Gastroparesis symptoms are morning nausea, burping, flatulence, epigastric pain, early satiety and post-prandial vomiting. The most characteristic symptom of gastroparesis is vomiting of undigested food consumed several hours prior (8–12 hours) or even days before. Symptoms can have exacerbations and remissions or take the form of chronic anorexia and nausea that lasts from a few days to several months, and recurs every so often. A characteristic, albeit not that frequent objective finding, is epigastric splash. Even when symptoms are mild, irregular propulsion of food from the stomach to the intestine is not synchronized with exogenous insulin administration, resulting in great variations of blood glucose levels and unexplained post-prandial hypoglycaemias, mimicking brittle DM.

How do you establish the diagnosis?

Before symptoms can be definitely attributed to gastroparesis, other diseases of the upper gastrointestinal tract must be ruled out. For this reason, an oesophagogastroduodenoscopy (OGD) exam must be performed first. A typical finding of gastroparesis in OGD is undigested food that was consumed 8–12 hours earlier and no pyloric stenosis. The most reliable method for diagnosis of gastroparesis is the study of stomach emptying time after the administration of a certain radiolabeled solid food. When this exam is planned, no prokinetic agents should be given to the patient. Pyloric and duodenal manometry are useful methods for diagnosing pyloric spasm and desynchronization of gastric and duodenal peristaltic waves, but only in selected patients who have relevant symptoms but whose scintigraphy is normal.

How do you treat the patient?

Since hypoglycaemia risk is high, sensible glycaemic control needs to be implemented without exaggerations. Patients with gastroparesis are recommended to have small and frequent meals, with restriction of fat (< 40 g/day) and dietary fibres, to avoid gastric bezoars. Also, the administration of anticholinergic medicines should be stopped. A nasogastric tube for a few days could help in decompressing the stomach.

Drug treatment includes the administration of medicines that increase gastric motility (metoclopramide, domperidone, levosulpiride). Metoclopramide is administered orally or intravenously when symptoms are severe at a dose of 10 mg one hour before meals and at bedtime. Effectiveness of the medicine declines over time and is no longer helpful for the majority of the patients after five months' continuous use. Domperidone is administered at 20–40 mg before meals and at bedtime and contrary to metoclopramide, is effective for long-term use. Levosulpiride is given at 25 mg three times a day before meals. In resistant cases erythromycin at doses of 250 mg 30 minutes before meals p.o. or iv can be useful, as well as clonidine at 0.1 mg 3–4 times a day.

CASE STUDY 3

A 71 year old man with a history of Type 2 DM for 15 years comes to the clinic complaining of diarrhoeal episodes for the last few months, mainly at nights. The episodes last for a few days but are recurrent. Bowel movements are described as bulky and foul smelling. The patient is treated with a mixture of insulin twice a day. What is the diagnosis?

This patient is most likely suffering form diabetic diarrhoea. According to some – but not all – statistics, diabetic diarrhoea is quite frequent. Principally, it occurs in persons with autonomic neuropathy. Factors responsible for its occurrence are stasis of the intestinal content and bacterial overgrowth due to decreased motility, bile acid malabsorption, defective exocrine pancreatic function due to parasympathetic nervous system damage and disturbed water and electrolyte absorption due to sympathetic dysfunction. The typical diabetic diarrhoea is a secretory diarrhoea, occurs more frequently at night, is not associated with food intake, is bulky, lasts for days or even weeks and then subsides without specific therapy, only to recur in a different time. It commonly alternates with periods of constipation. Differential diagnosis should include drug-induced diarrhoea, especially due to metformin and acarbose, lactase deficiency, parasitic infections, various malabsorption syndromes and coeliac disease, which is more common in Type 1 DM.

How do you establish the diagnosis?

There is no pathognomonic test for diagnosing diabetic diarrhoea. Diagnosis is therefore based on the patient's history and exclusion of other diseases that cause chronic diarrhoea.

How do you treat the patient?

As a first step, good glycaemic control and replenishment of water and electrolyte deficits are essential. When bacterial overgrowth is suspected, broad spectrum antibiotics (doxycycline or metronidazole) are administered for at least three weeks. Administration of bile acid sequestrants (cholestyrarmine) can alleviate symptoms. In mild forms, symptomatic treatment with loperamide, diphenoxylate and atropine can be administered. Adrenergic agonists can improve water and electrolyte absorption. Clonidine is especially effective because it improves adrenergic function and thus decreases intestinal motility and increases water and electrolyte absorption. It is initially administered at 0.1 mg twice or three times a day, and the dose can gradually increase up to a total of 0.6 mg/day. In resistant cases, octreotide has been successfully used at 50–75 µg subcutaneously twice a day or even the long-acting synthetic somatostatin analogue once a month.

CASE STUDY 4

A 34 year old patient with Type 1 DM for 30 years reports dizziness and fainting tendency when standing for a few minutes. These symptoms are more intense when standing up from supine or sitting position, after eating and after injecting his insulin. He is suffering from diabetic nephropathy (creatinine 2.5 mg/dl [221 μmol/L]) and bilateral proliferative retinopathy treated with photocoagulation. Apart from insulin, he also receives ACE inhibitors for his nephropathy and coexistent hypertension. What is the diagnosis?

Most likely this patient is suffering from orthostatic hypotension. Orthostatic hypotension is defined as the fall in systolic blood pressure by more than 30 mmHg (or according to some authors by 20 mmHg together with symptoms) or the fall of diastolic blood pressure by more than 10 mmHg, when assuming an erect from supine position. It is characterized by dizziness, weakness, visual disturbances, fainting spells or even loss of consciousness at erection from supine or sitting position and remaining standing for 1–10 minutes. In severe cases it can be very torturous for the patient and symptoms can be wrongly attributed to hypoglycaemia. Orthostatic hypotension can occur or deteriorate 1–3 hours after a meal or administration of various medicines common in DM (vasodilators, diuretics) and tricyclic antidepressants. Furthermore, insulin administration can cause orthostatic hypotension due to its vasodilatory action.

This complication is not very common (frequency of around 5 percent) and is a manifestation of autonomous nervous system dysfunction.

How do you establish the diagnosis?

Diagnosis is based on the patient's history and discovery of blood pressure fall with position change, as mentioned above. The evaluation is performed as follows: the patient is supine for about 15 minutes when the blood pressure is measured. Subsequently, the patient is asked to stand up and stay standing for five minutes. Blood pressure is measured every minute for a total of five minutes and the difference of the lower blood pressure value in the standing position compared to that in the supine is recorded. Variations of blood pressure during this procedure have low reproducibility and can vary from day to day or even at different times of the same day. Thus, the diagnosis can be missed in a patient who is suffering from orthostatic hypotension. For this reason, when clinical suspicion is high but the initial test negative, repeating the procedure on another day is suggested.

How do you treat the patient?

For mild cases, no specific therapy is needed. Advice to avoid sudden changes of body position and gradual erection from supine position are usually sufficient measures for avoiding symptoms. For symptomatic postural hypotension, application of elastic stockings on the lower extremities during the day, mild regular physical activity and raising of the head of the bed by 25–30 degrees are advised. The last measure is necessary to restrict the increase of blood pressure seen in these persons when lying down. When fainting spells are present, manoeuvres that transiently increase blood pressure are recommended, such as bending forward or squatting. Increased intake of NaCl to 4–6 g/day is also recommended, unless contraindications exist. If these measures are not enough, fludrocortisone is administered at a dose of 0.1–0.3 mg/day. Patients with orthostatic hypotension and a decreased erythrocyte mass benefit from small doses of erythropoietin administration (50 IU/kg of body weight) three times a week. Dihydroergotamine, metoclopramide and octreotide have also been used for the treatment of orthostatic hypotension with fairly good results.

CASE STUDY 5

A 45 year old patient with Type 1 DM since the age of 13 reports urinary incontinence and a feeling of incomplete bladder emptying after urination. He also reports that he no longer has the same urge to urinate as in the past. These symptoms first occurred two years ago, and although mild in the beginning, they gradually deteriorated thereafter. What is the diagnosis?

The patient is suffering from neurogenic bladder due to damage of autonomous system nerves from DM. Bladder involvement is not rare in DM and is associated with duration of the disease. In practice, there is no bladder dysfunction in DM of less than 10 years' duration. Its main feature is the asymptomatic gradual onset and progression. In advanced stages, damage of the centripetal sensory fibres of the bladder wall causes a decrease in urination urge. Thus, bladder capacity gradually increases and the detrussor muscle atrophies (neurogenic bladder). The patient may manifest overflow incontinence and urinate once or twice a day. Other clinical symptoms include decrease of the urinary flow rate, a feeling of incomplete emptying of the bladder and need to press the hypogastric area for initiation and continuance of urination.

How do you establish the diagnosis?

For diagnosing neurogenic bladder, urodynamic evaluation is necessary. Findings include an increase in bladder capacity (> 1000 ml), decreased sensation of the wall, increase in urine residual volume after urination (> 200 ml), decreased ability of the bladder wall to contract (pressure at urination < 40 cm H_2O) and decreased urinary flow (< 10 ml/sec).

How do you treat the patient?

The patient is advised to urinate at certain time intervals (every 3–4 hours) with application of pressure on the hypogastric area, so that residual urine volume is decreased. Parasympatheticomimetic medicines, like betanechol, have not proven effective. In advanced cases, intermittent self-catheterization of the bladder is recommended. Transurethral prostatectomy and removal of the bladder neck have also been used with varied results. Decrease of bladder capacity with plastic surgery has only transient results since the bladder resumes its initial size in around one year.

Further reading

Boulton, A.J.M. (1999) Current and emerging treatments for the diabetic neuropathies. *Diabetes Reviews*, **7**, 379–386.

Dyck, J.B. and Dyck, P.J. (1999) Diabetic polyneuropathy, in *Diabetic Neuropathy* 2nd edn, (eds Dyck and Thomas) W.B. Saunders Company, Philadelphia, pp. 255–78.

Young, M.J. and Jones, G.C. (1997) Diabetic neuropathy: symptoms, signs and assessment, in *Diabetic Neuropathy*, (ed. A.J.M. Boulton) Marius Press, Lancashire, pp. 41–61.

Ziegler, D., Hanefeld, M., Ruhnau, K.J. *et al.* (1995) Treatment of symptomatic diabetic peripheral neuropathy with the anti-oxidant alpha-lipoic acid. *Diabetologia*, **38**, 1425–1433.

16

Macroangiopathy in diabetes

Ioannis Ioannidis

CASE STUDY 1

A 50 year old man has an annual laboratory check-up. A plasma glucose level of 153 mg/dl [8.5 mmol/L] is found. Repeat test after five days reveals a plasma glucose level of 138 mg/dl [7.7 mmol/L]. He visits his family physician for advice and is told he is suffering from diabetes mellitus; the doctor stresses the need for good control of his blood sugar. On questioning the reason for such a strict control of blood glucose, the doctor talks about the complications of diabetes, especially for macroangiopathy. Is the doctor's worry legitimate?

The term diabetic macroangiopathy is used interchangeably with the common term atherosclerosis. Unlike other complications, however, macroangiopathy is not specific for DM. Nevertheless, occurrence of various atherosclerotic manifestations tends to be more frequent and earlier and their progression faster in diabetic compared to non-diabetic people. Macroangiopathy manifestations are principally due to involvement of the coronary arteries, the arteries of the lower extremities, as well as the carotid and cerebral arteries.

Morbidity and mortality from macroangiopathy are two to four times higher in diabetic persons. About 75–80 percent of the adult diabetics ultimately die from manifestations attributed to macroangiopathy. The mechanisms of accelerated atherosclerosis in these people are not entirely clear.

The increased risk of macroangiopathy in DM seems to be present very early: even from the stage of impaired glucose tolerance or even earlier at the stage of insulin resistance and hyperinsulinaemia (see Chapter 3). Furthermore, many patients discover they have diabetes simultaneously with the diagnosis of a macrovascular complication.

Diabetes in Clinical Practice: Questions and Answers from Case Studies.   Nicholas Katsilambros *et al.*
© 2006 John Wiley & Sons, Ltd.

The doctor talked to the patient about the need for smoking cessation, baby aspirin intake and strict control of blood pressure and blood lipid levels. Is that necessary? Is control of blood glucose alone insufficient?

Macroangiopathy is a multifactorial phenomenon, which involves the classic atherosclerotic risk factors without any doubt (smoking, hypertension, hypercholesterolaemia), as well as other factors, such as platelet disorders, insulin resistance, central (android-type) body fat distribution, autonomic neuropathy, and possibly hyperglycaemia itself.

Insulin resistance – characteristic of Type 2 DM – seems to play a central role. It is accompanied by a condition of mild, chronic inflammation, triggered and maintained by various cytokines. These are produced by adipose cells as well as by cells that participate in the pathogenesis of the atherosclerotic lesion, such as monocytes, endothelial cells and smooth muscle cells. Furthermore, the presence of oxidative stress, owing to hyperglycaemia and increased free fatty acid levels, contributes to the inflammation, both by promoting the production of various mediators as well as by oxidizing LDL-cholesterol. Oxidized LDL is taken up by macrophages much more easily and leads to the formation of foam cells.

The results of many epidemiological studies (shown in Table 16.1) denote the relative contribution of the risk factors in the appearance of macroangiopathy in diabetic people.

Strict control of all the risk factors, therefore, is necessary together with glycaemic control, for avoidance of macroangiopathy.

Table 16.1. The contribution of risk factors on the occurrence of cardiac episodes, strokes and peripheral vascular disease in persons with diabetes mellitus

Risk factor	Cardiovascular diseases	Strokes	Peripheral Vascular Disease
Hyperglycaemia	+	++	+++
HbA_{1C}	+	++	+++
High total cholesterol	++	+	+
Low HDL cholesterol	+++	++	+
High triglycerides	+++	++	+
Hypertension	+	++	+
Long duration of diabetes	+	+	+++

It should be emphasized here that glycaemic control has been proven sufficient for control of microangiopathy that is associated with it. In fact, the effect of normoglycaemia on macroangiopathy risk is small, as shown in UKPDS study as well.

Our patient is obese (BMI: 32 kg/m^2) and smokes one pack of cigarettes daily. Laboratory results showed the following: HbA$_{1c}$ 7.3 percent, cholesterol 234 mg/dl [6.05 mmol/L]; HDL-cholesterol 31 mg/dl [0.8 mmol/L]; triglycerides 240 mg/dl [2.71 mmol/L]; LDL-cholesterol 155 mg/dl [4.01 mmol/L]. Blood pressure was 145/95 mmHg and reported similar values at other occasions, despite intake of an antihypertensive medicine (ramipril 5 mg/day). Based on these findings, what should the doctor's advice be, so that the patient's cardiovascular risk would be decreased?

Many scientific organizations both in Europe and in the USA have published guidelines for persons with DM. The most recent were published in November 2003 with the cooperation of seven scientific organizations (diabetic, cardiovascular, atherosclerosis). Targets of control in persons with DM are strict:

1. HbA$_{1c}$ < 6.1 percent. (According to the American Association of Clinical Endocrinologists, however, a level of < 6.5 percent is sufficient, and according to the American Diabetes Association a level of < 7 percent is sufficient.)
2. Blood pressure < 130/80 mmHg (usually two to three medicines are necessary to achieve this target).
3. LDL-C < 100 mg/dl (2.59 mmol/L). (When coronary heart disease coexists, a decrease to < 70 mg/dl [1.81 mmol/L] is desirable. In most people with Type 2 DM a statin is necessary, usually in moderate to high doses, to achieve these targets. Furthermore, results of a recent trial (CARDS) showed a decline in cardiovascular events in diabetic persons who received atorvastatin 20 mg daily, even when their initial LDL-cholesterol values were low, < 100 mg/dl [2.59 mmol/L]!)
4. Non-HDL cholesterol (total – HDL cholesterol) < 130 mg/dl [3.36 mmol/L]. (If a statin is not enough for this, increase of the dose or addition of ezetimibe is necessary.)
5. HDL-C > 40 mg/dl (1.03 mmol/L) for men and > 50 mg/dl (1.29 mmol/L) for women.

The administration of antiplatelet agents is also necessary in all diabetics with Type 2 DM older than 35 years, with at least one more cardiovascular disease (CVD) risk factor (acetylsalycic acid 100–325 mg or clopidogrel 75 mg daily).

At the same time, cessation of smoking is necessary. Cigarette smoking is a major risk factor for cardiovascular events, strokes and peripheral angiopathy both in the general population and in diabetics. In the general population, around 21 percent of total mortality from cardiovascular events is due to cigarette smoking.

Weight loss and increase in physical activity are also significant lifestyle changes with dramatic effect on all these CVD risk factors. Diet and exercise guidelines should be simple and comprehensible, and should not be abandoned, even when patients do not totally comply with them.

Physical activity has a beneficial effect on blood cholesterol levels, improves perfusion and vascular elasticity, increases aerobic metabolism, decreases blood glucose variations, prevents or even decreases obesity and improves blood pressure. Furthermore, physical exercise improves insulin resistance.

Finally, it should be emphasized that good control of blood glucose levels, decrease of body weight, increase in physical activity, improvement in insulin resistance by any means and management of dyslipediaemias contribute to the control of blood coagulation disturbances as well. Diabetes is a hypercoagulable state, predisposing to thromboses.

CASE STUDY 2

A 56 year old Type 2 diabetic man is brought to the Emergency Room with intense, pressure-like precordial pain. An ECG and laboratory tests revealed an acute myocardial infarction, and his blood glucose level was especially high (420 mg/dl [23.3 mmol/L]). The patient was transferred to the Intensive Care Unit for treatment and monitoring. What is the proper treatment for his diabetes?

Many studies have shown that diabetic patients have two to three times higher mortality than non-diabetics after an acute myocardial infarction (MI). This is due both to the increased inpatient mortality (congestive heart failure, cardiogenic shock and conduction abnormalities) as well as to the increased outpatient mortality after discharge from the hospital.

Possible explanations are i) painless myocardial infarctions that are more common in diabetic patients and contribute to delayed diagnosis and treatment; ii) the significantly increased frequency of heart failure after an MI, owing to the high degree of atherosclerosis of many vessels but principally to the existence of a special form of cardiomyopathy, irrespective of atherosclerosis, as also seen in patholological specimens; iii) presence of cardiac autonomic neuropathy, leading to increase in myocardial oxygen needs due to acceleration of heart rate, decrease of myocardial perfusion due to increase of vascular tone and decrease in myocardial perfusion during postural hypotension; iv) insulin resistance, even at the level of the heart, which leads to use of free fatty acids from the cardiac muscle. This consumption is less effective energy-wise and does not favour the survival of cardiac muscle territories with borderline perfusion.

Insulin administration in diabetic persons *after an acute MI*, as seen in the DIGAMI-1 study, leads to better metabolic control and is beneficial as regards the progression of the MI and the patients' survival. This finding was not substantiated in the larger DIGAMI-2 trial and the CREATE-ECLA trial. This issue, however, is not considered definitely answered, due to the limitations of these trials.

There are many protocols for insulin administration. Two of the more widely used protocols are mentioned below.

Protocol 1

- Prepare a solution of 250 units of rapid-acting insulin (Regular, Actrapid) in 250 ml 0.9 percent normal saline (1 U = 1 ml).
- Measure blood glucose with a usual portable meter.
- Evaluate the patient's general status.
- Categorize the patient into one of two groups based on the Killip classification. (The Killip classification, published in 1967, categorizes patients with an acute myocardial infarction based upon the presence or absence of simple physical examination findings that suggest left ventricular dysfunction: Class I – no evidence of heart faliure (HF): Class II – finding consistent with mild to modulate HF (S3, lung rates less than one-half way up the posterior lung fields, or jugular venous distension); Class III – pulmonary oedema; class IV – cardiogenic shock.)

  – **Group A:** Patients without heart failure (Killip stage I), patients with mild heart failure (Killip stage II).

  – **Group B:** Patients with severe heart failure (Killip stage III), patients with cardiogenic shock (Killip stage IV).

Table 16.2. Infusion of insulin solution in diabetic persons with acute myocardial infarction (AMI)

Serum glucose	Insulin infusion rate (U/h)	
mg/dl (mmol/L)	Group A	Group B
< 75 (4.2)	0	0
75–120 (4.2–6.7)	1	2
120–200 (6.7–11.1)	2	3
200–240 (11.1–13.3)	3	5
> 240 (13.3)	6	9

Infusion of the solution is done as shown in Table 16.2.

- The infusion rate is increased by 50 percent in obese patients (BMI > 28 kg/m^2).
- Hourly blood glucose monitoring is necessary, until it stabilizes around 75–100 mg/dl (4.1–5.6 mmol/L) in three consecutive measurements. Afterwards, monitoring is done every two hours for four hours and then every four hours for twelve hours.
- Serum K$^+$ levels are measured every twelve hours. Addition of K$^+$ in the solution is done when levels are < 3.6 mmol/L.

We evaluate precision of the portable meter's measurements by comparing them with those of the laboratory every 4–6 hours. This protocol was proposed by Hendra and Yudkin in 1992.

Protocol 2

(This was used in the Swedish DIGAMI-1 study).

- Prepare a solution with 80 units rapid-acting insulin in 500 ml 5 percent dextrose in water (D5W).
- Start an infusion at 30 ml/h.
- Measure blood glucose every 1–2 hours.

We adjust the solution infusion according to Table 16.3.

The intravenous infusion of insulin is continued for 2–3 days. When the patient starts feeding, subcutaneous administration of insulin is initiated. Based on the DIGAMI-1 results, some authors propose insulin

Table 16.3. Insulin infusion rate in diabetic persons with acute myocardial infarction (AMI)

Glucose mg/dl (mmol/L)	Adjustment
> 270 (15.0)	Increase the rate by 6 ml/h and inject 8 units rapid-acting insulin bolus iv.
200–270 (11.1–15.0)	Increase the rate by 3 ml/h
120–200 (6.7–11.1)	Stable infusion rate
70–120 (3.9–6.7)	Decrease the rate by 6 ml/h
< 70 (3.9)	Discontinue infusion rate until blood glucose is > 120 mg/dl (6.7 mmol/L). If symptomatic hypoglycaemia ensues, infuse 20 ml glucose solution 30 percent (about 2 amps Dextrose 35 percent). Readministration of the solution is performed at a lower rate by 6 ml/h.

administration to all diabetic patients after an acute MI, for at least a few months to a year. If receiving insulin prior to the ischaemic event, and as long as he or she was well controlled, the patient returns to the previous regimen. If insulin is to be started for the first time after this event, we follow the same insulin therapy rules that are followed for Type 2 diabetic patients started on insulin, mentioned elsewhere in the book (see Chapter 28).

If the patient is obese (BMI > 30 kg/m^2) or overweight but with a waist circumference > 102 cm (40 in) for men or > 88 cm (34 in) for women, and as long as he or she has a normal renal function (serum creatinine < 1.5 mg/dl [132.6 µmol/L] for men and < 1.4 mg/dl [123.8 µmol/L] for women) and a relatively normal ejection fraction (> 40–45 percent), then metformin administration is necessary as well.

If metformin is not adequate for glycaemic control, a glitazone can also be given provided there is no heart failure or intense diastolic dysfunction (i.e., pioglitazone or rosiglitazone – not yet approved for coadministration with insulin in Europe). There is significant evidence from recent studies that the administration of medicines that potentiate insulin action on the tissues of diabetics is associated with fewer cardiovascular complications in Type 2 diabetic patients with acute MI compared with medicines that potentiate insulin secretion from the pancreas. If an insulin secretagogue is needed, glibenclamide is avoided (it theoretically acts on the myocardium as well and there is fear it might deteriorate ischeamia). Glimepiride 1–6 mg/day or gliclazide 80–240 mg/day are preferred. One of the rapidly acting insulin secretagogues can also be administered, such as nateglinide (60, 120, 180 mg tablets) or repaglinide (0.5, 1, 2 mg tablets) three times a day (immediately before main meals – if a meal is omitted, the medicine is omitted as well).

CASE STUDY 3

A 52 year old man presents to his family physician for a regular follow-up. He is suffering from Type 2 DM and brings in the results of some laboratory tests. His lipid profile is as follows: total cholesterol 218 mg/dl (5.64 mmol/L); HDL-cholesterol 37 mg/dl (0.96 mmol/L); triglycerides 180 mg/dl (2.03 mmol/L); and LDL-cholesterol 145 mg/dl (3.75 mmol/L). The doctor is worried and recommends initiation of hypolipidaemic treatment with a statin. The patient is wondering why a friend of his, with similar lipid profile results, was only given dietary advice and no medications.

The characteristic lipid abnormalities in patients with Type 2 DM are:

1. hypertriglyceridaemia;
2. low HDL-cholesterol;
3. increased concentration of small-dense LDL particles.

Hypertriglyceridaemia is the most common lipid abnormality (see Chapter 23). Nevertheless, the role of hypertriglyceridaemia as a CVD risk factor is partly due to the coexistent low HDL-cholesterol (HDL-C) levels. Most studies have shown a decline in HDL-C levels in diabetic patients. In many studies a reverse association between HDL-C levels and cardiovascular events was observed.

Total- and LDL-cholesterol levels may be normal or mildly increased in diabetic persons compared to non-diabetic ones. It should be noted, however, that the LDL particles have undergone structural changes. The most important is the predominance of 'small and dense particles', which have been associated with increased CVD risk since they are more easily oxidized and are more atherogenic. Thus, for the same LDL-cholesterol levels, diabetic persons have a higher cardiovascular risk.

Presence of qualitative, apart from quantitative, abnormalities is one of the reasons for the differential evaluation of the blood values in a diabetic compared to a non-diabetic person.

Results of large studies, both recent and in the past (such as the Heart Protection Study [HPS] and CARDS), have proven that statin administration aimed at achieving especially low LDL-C levels decreases CVD events in diabetic persons substantially.

CASE STUDY 4

A 47 year old woman has the following blood test results: fasting plasma glucose 117 mg/dl [6.5 mmol/L]; triglycerides 140 mg/dl (1.58 mmol/L); total cholesterol 234 mg/dl (6.05 mmol/L); HDL-C 42 mg/dl (1.09 mmol/L); LDL-C 164 mg/dl (4.24 mmol/L). She is receiving antihypertensive medicines and her blood pressure is 140/90 mmHg. Her weight is 78 kg (172 lb) and her height 164 cm (5 ft, 5 in). Waist circumference is 93 cm (36.6 in). Her doctor tells her she is suffering from 'the metabolic syndrome'. What is the metabolic syndrome and to what is it due?

It is a clinical syndrome, characterized by the clustering/coexistence of a series of metabolic disturbances, associated with insulin resistance and promoting atherosclerosis.

Therefore, diagnosis of the metabolic syndrome identifies persons at high risk of CVD occurrence and should be performed with simple means.

It was described for the first time by Reaven in 1988. He used the term metabolic syndrome X for the congregation of certain abnormal manifestations, the common base of which is insulin resistance and subse-quent hyperinsulinaemia. (Note: insulin resistance is a central point of the metabolic syndrome disturbances and is associated with it aetiologically.)

The following manifestations are included in the classical description of the syndrome:

- impaired glucose tolerance;
- hypertension;
- high triglycerides;
- low HDL.

The presence of the metabolic syndrome has been associated with an increased frequency of coronary heart disease and other forms of macroangiopathy.

During the following years, the concept of the metabolic syndrome was enriched by other metabolic disturbances as well, such as obesity (especially central obesity or android type), microalbuminuria, as well as coagulation and fibrinolysis abnormalities.

Diagnosis of the metabolic syndrome is based on criteria set by international medical organizations. There are mild differences among them. Out of the four groups of diagnostic criteria mentioned below, the first one (NCEP ATP-III) was considered practically more useful, whereas the last one (IDF) was only recently proposed, in April 2005.

NCEP ATP-III (National Cholesterol Education Program, Adult Treatment Panel-III)

Diagnosis of the metabolic syndrome is done when a person fulfils at least three of the following five criteria:

1. fasting plasma glucose $\geq$ 110 mg/dl (6.1 mmol/L);
2. triglycerides $\geq$ 150 mg/dl (1.7 mmol/L);
3. Blood pressure $\geq$ 130/85 mmHg;
4. HDL-C $<$ 50 mg/dl (1.29 mmol/L) for women, $<$ 40 mg/dl (1.03 mmol/L) for men;
5. waist circumference $>$ 88 cm (34 in) for women, $>$ 102 cm (40 in) for men.

WHO (World Health Organization)

Definition of the metabolic syndrome includes diabetes mellitus or impaired glucose tolerance or impaired fasting glucose and/or insulin resistance. It should be noted that it is extremely difficult to determine the presence of insulin resistance at an individual level if the corresponding values of the reference population are not known. Usually we consider that insulin resistance is present when a person has values higher than the upper quintile for the method used (method of choice is the hyperinsulinaemic euglycaemic clamp). The definition of the metabolic syndrome also includes two of the following:

1. triglycerides $\geq$ 150 mg/dl (1.7 mmol/L) and/or HDL-C $<$ 40 mg/dl (1.03 mmol/L) for women, $<$ 35 mg/dl (0.91 mmol/L) for men;
2. blood pressure $\geq$ 140/90 mmHg;
3. waist-to-hip ratio (WHR) $>$ 0.85 (for women), $>$ 0.90 (for men) and/or BMI $>$ 30 kg/m^2;
4. microalbuminuria (albumin excretion rate [AER] $>$ 20 µg/min or albumin-to-creatinine ratio (A/C ratio) $>$ 30mg/g creatinine).

EGIR (European Group for Insulin Resistance)

According to this group, the metabolic syndrome is defined by the presence of hyperinsulinaemia (insulin level higher than the upper quartile of the reference population), together with two of the following:

1. Blood pressure $\geq 140/90$ mmHg;
2. dyslipidaemia (HDL-C < 40 mg/dl [1.03 mmol/L], triglycerides > 180 mg/dl [2.03 mmol/L] or dyslipidaemia under drug treatment);
3. waist circumference > 80 cm (31 in) for women, > 94 cm (37 in) for men;
4. fasting plasma glucose > 110 mg/dl (6.1 mmol/L).

IDF (International Diabetes Federation)

According to these criteria, which were very recently (April 2005) reported, the metabolic syndrome definition includes the presence of central obesity (waist circumference more than 80 cm [31 in] for women and more than 94 cm [37 in] for men), as well as at least two of the following:

1. fasting plasma glucose > 100 mg/dl (5.6 mmol/L);
2. triglycerides ≥ 150 mg/dl (1.7 mmol/L);
3. blood pressure $\geq 130/85$ mmHg;
4. HDL-C < 50 mg/dl (1.29 mmol/L) for women, < 40 mg/dl (1.03 mmol/L) for men.

According to this new definition, central obesity (as defined by high waist circumference values with upper limits lower than those set by NCEP ATP-III) is – as mentioned already – mandatory, and regarding the other coexistent metabolic disturbances, the lower upper limit for fasting plasma glucose at 100 mg/dl (5.6 mmol/L) is noteworthy.

The recognition of a difference between various ethnic groups as regards anthropometric measurements is significant as well. Thus the above mentioned values for the waist circumference of 94 cm (37 in) and 80 cm (31 in) apply only to people of European descent and are different than those of other ethnicities (such as south Asians, African, Japanese, etc.).

The frequency of the metabolic syndrome in the population varies according to different studies (25–40 percent), while in the Type 2 diabetic population it rises to 90 percent.

Insulin resistance seems to be a central disturbance of the syndrome and to be aetiologically associated with it.

Persons with android type obesity have increased intra-abdominal fat (in omentum, mesentery and retroperitoneum) apart from the obvious increase of fat content in the upper half of the body, in the epigastric and the periumbilical area. It should also be noted that intra-abdominal fat is principally channeled through the portal vein system. This fact is extremely important for the metabolic consequences of android obesity, which are also constituents of the metabolic syndrome.

Intra-abdominal adipose tissue shows increased lipolytic activity, derived from its intense sensitivity to adrenergic stimulants that promote lipolysis, i.e., degradation of triglycerides to glycerol and free fatty acids (FFAs) (it shows increased sensitivity to lipolytic action through adrenergic receptors and decreased sensitivity to the antilipolytic activity of insulin).

This particular sensitivity of intra-abdominal adipose tissue regards obese and non-obese men and women with android-type obesity. The role of hormones on accumulation of intra-abdominal fat as well as fat in the upper half of the body is complex and not entirely known, despite a great deal of serious studies (Figure 16.1).

Nevertheless, steroid hormones play an exceptional role. Glucocorticoids, specifically increase intra-abdominal adipose tissue synthesis, whereas female hormones promote fat accumulation on the buttocks and thighs. Generally, in android type obesity, insulin resistance, hyperinsulinaemia, small increase in cortisol and androgen levels is seen, the latest regarding only women. Apart from cortisol levels (which most of the time are within normal limits), a significant role is exerted by the intracellular activity of active cortisol, determined by the concentration of the enzyme 17-HSD1(17-hydroxy-steroid dehydrogenase-1). The activity of this enzyme is increased in the intra-abdominal fat of persons with central obesity and the metabolic syndrome. According, however, to the neuroendocrine theory of obesity (Björntrop, 1992), the central accumulation of adipose tissue and appearance of resistance to the action of insulin are due to an increased activity of the hypothalamus-pituitary-adrenal (HPA) axis. The increased reactivity – due to increased sensitivity – of this axis to various 'central' stimulations (for example, stress) results in a relatively increased corticoid secretion, which promote

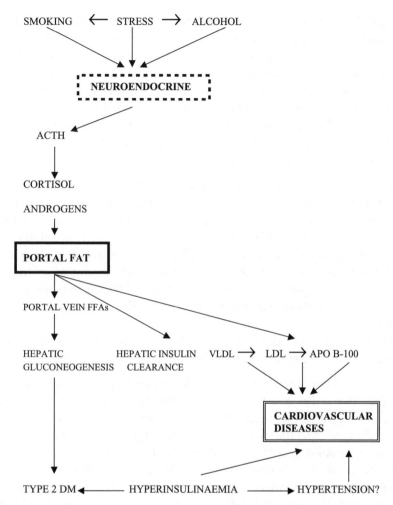

Figure 16.1. Mechanisms involved in intra-abdominal fat deposition (from Björntorp 1992, with modification).

splanchnic fat accumulation. This increased activity of the endocrine HPA axis seems to be potentiated by the defective inhibitory control that is retrogradely exerted through the glucocorticoid receptors.

The hyperactivity of the axis results in an inhibition of growth hormone and the sex hormones' secretion. This also contributes to the development of splanchnic obesity.

Regardless, however, of the hormonal mechanisms contributing to intra-abdominal fat accumulation, an increase of free fatty acids (FFAs) in the portal blood is considered to be a basic underlying cause of a series of 'adverse' events, such as the tendency to hyperglycaemia, hyperinsulinaemia and certain lipid disturbances. Apart from these, FFAs also exert an influence on peripheral tissues, promoting insulin resistance. Resulting hyperinsulinaemia is on its own an independent atherogenic risk factor. Specifically, the described increase in the portal vein of FFAs has the following consequences (see Figure 16.1):

1. An increase in hepatic VLDL synthesis. This leads to an increase in VLDL blood concentration and secondarily in LDL and Apo-B-100.
2. An increase in gluconeogenesis rate, resulting in hyperglycaemia.
3. A partial inhibition of insulin hepatic degradation. This entails hyperinsulinaemia and secondarily insulin resistance and hyperglycaemia. Furthermore, other studies have shown that insulin resistance and subsequent hyperinsulinaemia constitute, through various mechanisms, factors involved aetiopathogenetically in the appearance of hypertension.
4. An increased fat deposition in hepatic parenchyma (hepatic fat infiltration, a characteristic of the metabolic syndrome).

Increased concentration of FFAs decreases muscular glucose uptake (leading to insulin resistance) either through a substrate competition (Randle hypothesis) or, more likely, through products of the intracellular metabolism of FFAs that activate serine/threonine kinase enzymes. These inhibit the insulin receptor and its substrate (insulin receptor substrate, IRS). These actions ultimately result in decreased uptake of glucose from peripheral tissues. Furthermore, it seems that the deposition of fat inside the muscle cells (ectopic fat deposition) contributes to the development of peripheral insulin resistance.

Adipose tissue has been shown in recent years to be an active endocrine tissue and not only simply a storage area that liberates FFAs and glycerol. Thus, adipose tissue produces many substances with autocrine, paracrine or/and endocrine activities, called adipocytokines (cytokines and inflammatory factors). These substances most likely contribute to the development of the metabolic syndrome and its abnormalities, which increase atheromatic and CVD risk.

The most significant adipocytokines (Figure 16.2) are: adiponectin, resistin, tumour necrosis factor-α (TNF-α), interleukin 6, leptin, angio-

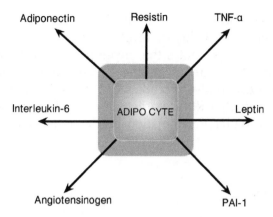

Figure 16.2. Adipocyte as an endocrine tissue.

tensinogen and plasminogen activator inhibitor-1 (PAI-1). The levels of all these substances are increased, depending on adipose tissue size (principally abdominal adipose tissue), with the exception of circulating adiponectin, the levels of which are low in obesity. The substances' actions create an inflammatory environment and also affect the activity of insulin. Thus, as regards to their effect on insulin action, the following points should be noted:

- TNF-α factor inhibits tyrosine phosphorylation of the insulin receptor inhibiting the action of its tyrosine kinase and resulting in insulin resistance.
- Resistin administration decreases glucose uptake from peripheral tissues (the exact mechanism is not known).
- Leptin decreases insulin sensitivity when administered in obese mice.
- Adiponectin, an adipocytokine with particular significance, improves insulin sensitivity and decreases vascular inflammation. Adiponectin levels are low in obese persons (especially in those with central obesity) and increase with weight loss.

As regards to their action on inflammation and atherogenesis:

- TNF-α activates transcription nuclear factor κB (nuclear factor κB), which subsequently orchestrates a series of inflammatory effects on vascular tissues (expression of adhesion molecules on endothelial cells and smooth muscle cells, activation of macrophages and secretion of multiple inflammatory mediators on vascular wall, etc.).

- Leptin promotes fat accumulation in the vascular wall macrophages, especially when blood glucose levels are high.
- Interleukin 6 (IL-6) promotes the inflammatory reactions on its own, and also causes the secretion of other inflammatory cytokines, such as IL-1 and TNF-α. IL-6 also promotes CRP secretion from the liver. hs-CRP (high sensitivity CRP) is particularly useful, because it comprises an index of vascular inflammation and a prognostic atherosclerotic index.

Further reading

Beckman, J., Greagen, M., Libby, P. (2002) Diabetes and Atherosclerosis. *JAMA*, **287**, 2570–81.

Björntrop, P. (1992) Regional obesity, in *Obesity*. (eds P. Bjorntrop and B.N. Brodoff). J.B. Lippincott Co, New York, pp. 576–86.

Colhoun, H.M., Betteridge, D.J., Durrington, P.N., Hitman, G.A., Neil H.A., Livingstone, S.J., Thomason, M.J., Mackness, M.I., Charlton-Menys, V., Fuller, J.H. (2004) Primary prevention of cardiovascular disease with atorvastatin in type 2 diabetes in the Collaborative Atorvastatin Diabetes Study (CARDS): multicentre randomised placebo-controlled trial. *Lancet*, **364**, 685–96.

Gray, R., Yudkin, J. (1997) Cardiovascular disease in diabetes mellitus, in *Textbook of Diabetes*, 2nd edn (eds J. Pickup and G. Williams), Blackwell Science, **57**, pp. 1–22.

Hendra, T.J., Yudkin, J.S. (1992) An algorithm for tight glycaemic control in diabetic infarct survivors. *Diabetes Res Clin Pract.*, **16**, 213–20.

IDF consensus worldwide definition of the metabolic syndrome. www.idf.org April 2005.

Malmberg, K., Ryden, L., Wedel, H., Birkeland, K., Bootsma, A., Dickstein, K., Efendic, S., Fisher, M., Hamsten, A., Herlitz, J., Hildebrandt, P., MacLeod, K., Laakso, M., Torp-Pedersen, C., Waldenstrom, A. (2005) Intense metabolic control by means of insulin in patients with diabetes mellitus and acute myocardial infarction (DIGAMI 2): Effects on mortality and morbidity. *Eur Heart J*, **26**, 650–61.

Malmberg, K. (1997) Prospective randomised study of intensive insulin treatment on long term survival after acute myocardial infarction in patients with diabetes mellitus. DIGAMI (Diabetes Mellitus, Insulin Glucose Infusion in Acute Myocardial Infarction) Study Group. *BMJ*, **314**, 1512–15.

Mehta, S.R., Yusuf, S., Diaz, R., Zhu, J., Pais, P., Xavier, D., Paolasso, E., Ahmed, R., Xie, C., Kazmi, K., Tai, J., Orlandini, A., Pogue, J., Liu, L. (2005) Effect of glucose-insulin-potassium infusion on mortality in patients with acute

ST-segment elevation myocardial infarction: The CREATE-ECLA randomized controlled trial. *JAMA*, **293**, 437–46.

MRC/BHF Heart Protection Study of cholesterol lowering with simvastatin in 20,536 high-risk individuals: a randomised placebo-controlled trial (2002) *Lancet*, **360**, 7–22.

Reaven, G.M. (1988) Role of insulin resistance in human disease. *Diabetes*, **37**, 1595.

Sobel, B.E. (2004) Heart disease and diabetes, in: *Therapy for Diabetes Mellitus and Related Disorders*, 4th edn, American Diabetes Association, (ed. H.E. Lebovitz), pp 465–72.

Third Joint Task Force of European and Other Societies on Cardiovascular Disease Prevention in Clinical Practice. European Guidelines on Cardiovascular Disease Prevention in Clinical Practice. (2003) *Eur Heart J.*, **24**, 1601–10.

17

Diabetic foot

Nicholas Tentolouris

CASE STUDY 1

A 65 year old man with Type 2 DM diagnosed at the age of 52, presents with mild pain on the right sole. He has also recently noticed that his right sock is wet every time he takes off his shoes. He does not recall any trauma. DM control is poor (recent HbA$_{1c}$ 8 percent), treated with oral antidiabetic pills. He lives with his wife and is suffering from hypertension and coronary heart disease. He denies any other symptoms. What is the diagnosis?

It is obvious that the patient has ulceration on the plantar surface of his right foot. The presence of mild symptoms, together with an ulcer, indicates that the patient has a serious degree of sensory loss.

On inspection, there was a purulent ulcer in the area of the 1st metatarsal head. The ulcer was surrounded by a large callus. Peripheral pulses were normal, while the neurologic examination revealed severe peripheral neuropathy with loss of Achilles tendon reflexes and no perception of pain, touch, temperature and vibration sensation up to the middle of the shin. Consequently, it is a neuotrophic ulcer, that is, an ulcer on a foot with neuropathy but normal perfusion (Figure 17.1). An ulcer is termed ischaemic, when there are findings of peripheral arteriopathy, but with normal sensation. Ulcers on the feet of patients with neuropathy and ischaemia are characterized as neuroischaemic (Figures 17.2-17.5).

Neuropathy is the common denominator in up to 85 percent of ulcers in diabetic patients. Neuropathy was present in 87 percent of patients with ulcers in a study (62 percent purely neurotrophic, 25 percent neuroischaemic and 13 percent purely ischaemic). In another study, neuropathy was present in 85 percent of the patients with ulcers (40 percent neurotrophic,

---

Diabetes in Clinical Practice: Questions and Answers from Case Studies. Nicholas Katsilambros *et al.*
© 2006 John Wiley & Sons, Ltd.

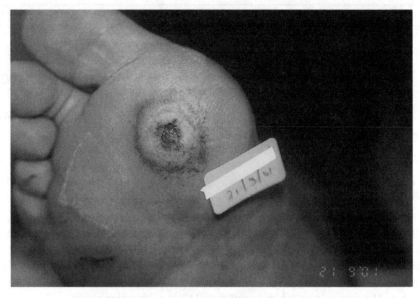

Figure 17.1. Neurotrophic ulcer on the head of the right 1st metatarsal of the patient under discussion. Ample hyperkeratosis around the ulcer is observed, while its base has granulomatous tissue.

45 percent neuroischaemic and 15 percent ischaemic). Differentiation of neurotrophic from ischaemic ulcers is shown in Table 17.1.

As regards the pathogenesis of lower extremities ulcerations, it should be noted that these are the result of a combination of factors. Neuropathy or arteriopathy *per se*, do not cause ulcerations. On the contrary, the principal factor for ulcer occurrence is the combination of neuropathy or arteriopathy together with some trauma, which, due to the presence of neuropathy, goes unnoticed. Trauma can be either endogenous (calluses, anatomical malformations of the feet) or exogenous (inappropriate shoes and soles, foreign bodies inside the shoes, burns). The effects of the various factors that lead to ulcerations are shown in Figure 17.6.

How frequent are the ulcerations of the feet and what is their significance?

The prevalence of feet ulcerations in diabetic persons is in the order of 4–10 percent, whereas their incidence is 2.2–5.9 percent per year. Ulcer frequency is lower in younger persons aged less than 45 years (1.7–

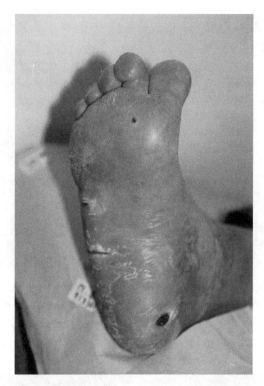

Figure 17.2. Neuroischaemic painful ulcer on the lateral surface of the heel. A second smaller ulcer is observed on the head of the 1st metatarsal. The base of the ulcer is necrotic. The presence of skin cracks is evident due to neuropathy and anhidrosis.

3.3 percent) and higher in persons older than 60 years (5–10 percent), regardless of the type of DM. Many studies have shown that around 5 percent of diabetic people have a history of foot ulceration, while around 15 percent will have an ulceration in their lifetime.

The significance of the ulcers lies in the fact that about 85 percent of leg amputations in diabetic persons have foot ulceration as their underlying cause. These ulcers are difficult to heal. Infections of both soft tissues as well as deeper tissues (abscesses, osteomyelitis) are a frequent complication of chronic ulcerations and are the cause of amputations in 20–50 percent of cases. For this reason, detection of high risk people for development of foot ulceration is of paramount importance as well as their education and the application of measures that decrease the chance of ulcer development. It has been proven that with education and

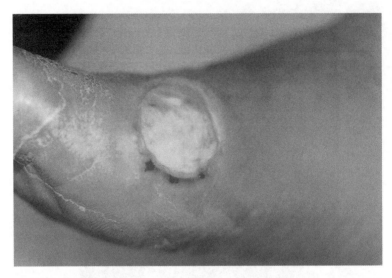

Figure 17.3. Neuroischaemic painful ulcer on the lateral surface of the foot caused by trauma from new shoes. The base of the ulcer is necrotic and the periphery of the lesion is red.

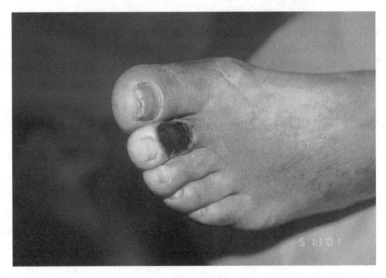

Figure 17.4. Ischaemic ulcer on the dorsum of the second toe in a patient with critical ischaemia. Discoloration of the toe distally to the lesion, the loss of hairs and onychodystrophy of the big toe are also seen.

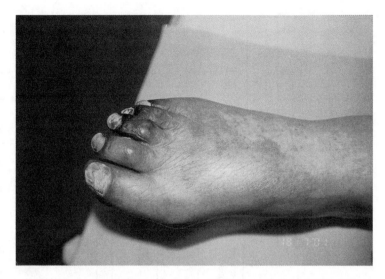

Figure 17.5. Dry gangrene on the periphery of the toes. The precise demarcation of the ischaemic skin necrosis up to the ankle joint is seen.

Table 17.1. The differential diagnosis of ulcers

	Neurotrophic	Ischaemic
Pain	Absent*	Frequent
Localization	In points of increased pressure in the plantar surface (metatarsal heads, heel, plantar surface of big toe)	In the peripheral borders of the foot and in the dorsal surface
Hyperkeratosis	Abundant around the ulcer	Absent
Base	Healthy granulomatous tissue*	Necrotic (yellow or gangrenous tissue)
Periphery of ulcer	Hyperkeratosis	Redness
Findings of peripheral neuropathy	Yes	No
Findings of peripheral arteriopathy	No	Yes

*When neurotrophic ulcers are complicated by infection, pain may be present and their base be dirty.

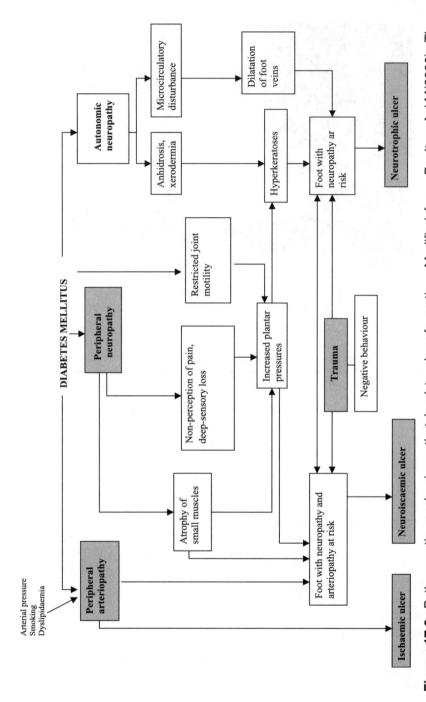

Figure 17.6. Pathogenetic mechanisms that lead to ulcer formation. Modified from: Boulton A.J.M(2000). The pathway to ulceration. Aetiopathogenesis, in A.J.M, Boulton H., Connor P.R. Cavanagh (eds), The foot in diabetes (3rd edn). Wiley, Chichester, p 21.

application of preventive measures, the rate of amputations in diabetic persons can be decreased by at least 50 percent.

Apart from amputations, treatment of ulcerations *per se* implies a great financial burden. The cost of treating an ulcer in the USA in 1997 was $16,850. The psycho-social burden on the patients should be added on this financial cost, since these persons need the continuous care of other people, transiently stop working and significantly restrict their social activities.

Which diabetic patients are at risk of developing an ulcer?

The principal factors for ulcer development are the loss of sensation on the feet and peripheral vascular disease. Peripheral neuropathy, apart from loss of sensation, can also cause anatomic deformities on the feet, since it causes atrophy of the small foot muscles (claw toes, protrusion of the metatarsal heads, shifting of the subcutaneous protective fat pads from the metatarsal heads towards the bases of the toes) and instability when walking. These disturbances, combined with the anatomic deformities, result in an increase of the applied pressure on some areas of the sole (metatarsal heads, plantar surface of the big toe, heel). Peripheral neuropathy of the sympathetic nervous system brings about dryness of the skin in the feet. This, together with the increased pressure on the sole, is responsible for callus formation. The presence of calluses significantly increases the chance of foot ulceration, whereas their frequent removal dramatically decreases the pressure applied on the foot and protects it from ulcer formation.

Other risk factors for ulcer development are long DM duration, the presence of other – microvascular – complications, oedema and non-compliant behaviour of the patients regarding advice given to them for foot care and application of appropriate preventive measures. Also, people living alone or in nursing homes are at increased risk of ulcer development.

How can we detect the diabetic patients at risk of ulcer formation?

As mentioned above, diabetics with loss of sensation or with severe peripheral vascular disease are at risk of developing ulcers.

Specifically, there is an increased chance of ulceration when the following applies:

1. history of ulceration or amputation (increased by five times);
2. callus (increased by eight times);
3. increase of vibration perception threshold (> 25 volts) as measured by a special instrument (biothesiometer) (increased by seven times);
4. inability to feel the Semmes-Weinstein monofilament pressure of 10 g (evaluation of skin pressure) (risk increased of ulceration and amputation by 10 times);
5. inability to feel the Semmes-Weinstein monofilament pressure of 10 g together with anatomic deformities (increased by 32 times);
6. neurologic disability index ≥ 5 (described in the table below) (increased by three times).

Furthermore, the increase of the pressure in various areas of the sole (≥ 6 kg/m^2) and a decrease of conduction motor-nerve velocity have been associated with an increase in the ulcer risk in prospective studies.

The evaluation of the neurologic disability risk is based on the following elements:

Position	Sensation	Right	Left
Big toe	Pain	normal $= 0$ abnormal $= 1$	0/1
Big toe	Vibrations (tuning fork 128 Hz)	normal $= 0$ abnormal $= 1$	0/1
Dorsum of the foot	Temperature (cold-hot sensation)	normal $= 0$ abnormal $= 1$	0/1
Achilles tendon reflexes	–	normal $= 0$ with intensification $= 1$ abnormal $= 2$	0/1/2

Specifically, the sensations tested are: the ability of pain perception with a needle; the ability of vibration perception with a tuning fork of 128 Hz frequency at the base of the big toe; the ability of temperature perception at the dorsum of the foot – using either two sticks or two laboratory tubes with different temperature (difference between cold and hot should be at least 10°C). Sensation is always symmetrically tested in both legs. Normal sensation is graded as zero (0), abnormal with one (1) point.

Furthermore, the Achilles tendon reflexes are evaluated, and normal are graded with zero (0) points, produced with intensification only are graded with one (1) point, and when abolished are graded with two (2) points. The maximum grading for each leg can be up to five (5) points, and for both legs up to ten (10) points.

What will you recommend to people at risk for ulcer development?

These people should take immediate ulcer prevention measures. The measures include proper education (Table 17.2) and provision and use of special shoes and soles (preventive shoes). These shoes are made of soft leather or other synthetic material that takes the shape of the foot; they do not have interior seams and have a proper depth so that special soles can be applied if needed.

How will you treat the patient?

It is necessary to surgically debride the ulcer, remove the callus and cover its surface with a bandage. Callus removal decreases the applied pressure on the ulcer area. A foot X-ray, focused on the ulcer area, is also necessary for ruling out obvious osteomyelitis. If there is foul odour, accompanying cellulitis or a dirty ulcer base, it is indicated to get a culture from the ulcer base, after surgical debridement, for identification of infection-causing bacteria and administration of the proper antibiotics.

As mentioned above, the corner-stone of ulcer treatment is the decrease of the applied pressure in the ulcer area, until complete healing is achieved.

How will decompression in the ulcer area be performed?

Bed confinement and use of a special wheelchair for moving around are very effective measures, but patient compliance can be difficult. For this reason, measures that permit some restricted mobility are applicable. The use of a cane, and support of the foot on the heel when there is no ulceration, are also effective.

Table 17.2. Guidelines for the individuals that are in danger of developing ulcers in their feet

---

Individuals that are at increased risk of developing ulcers should:
1. Look at their feet daily (dorsum, sole, regions between the toes). Inspection of the soles can be performed by another person or with the use of a mirror. When sight is poor, inspection should be performed by another individual.
2. Avoid walking barefoot (without shoes or slippers), even inside the house.
3. Never wear shoes without socks, even for small intervals.
4. Buy the right size of shoes. Iindividuals with neuropathy get used to buying footwear of smaller size, so that they press their feet a lot.
5. Not wear new shoes for more than one hour per day. After taking off the shoes, they should inspect their feet carefully.
6. Change their shoes once a day (in midday) and if possible in the afternoon as well. With the change of shoes, unloading of certain regions of the foot is achieved.
7. Feel inside their shoes for presence of foreign bodies before they wear them.
8. Wash their feet daily and dry them carefully. Particular care (cleanness and dryness) is required for the regions between the toes.
9. Not put their feet on or very close to thermal bodies.
10. Check the temperature of water in the bathroom with the elbow of their arm.
11. Not try to remove hyperkeratosis of the feet on their own, using sharp tools or various chemical dressings. Removal should be performed by a physician or trained podiatrist.
12. Cut the nails straight (not in the sides of nails).
13. Wear the socks with the seams outside or better wear socks with no seams.
14. Not use footwear in which the interior is worn out.
15. Use special ointments for hydration of the skin (these are applied only in the plantar and dorsal surface of the foot, never between the toes, because the risk of infections and superficial ulcerations is increased with the increase of humidity).
16. Check their feet carefully for presence of minute trauma after walking for a long time.
17. Ask for medical help immediately when there is pain, trauma, even shallow, oedema, redness or black regions in the feet.

There are special therapeutic shoes available for decompression of the front or hind part of the foot (half shoes). These are worn until complete healing of the ulcer. Furthermore, specially-designed shoes and soles that reallocate the pressures in the sole, decompressing the ulcer area, are also helpful. Existing studies have shown, however, that people with ulcers very frequently prefer their usual shoes and not the special shoes in daily activity. Sometimes the duration of usual shoe use is almost double that of the therapeutic ones, despite the fact that the patients report using the therapeutic shoes during most of their activities.

The most effective way to decompress the ulcer area is the application of a total contact cast with a proper base so that restricted walking is permitted (method of choice). It has the disadvantage, however, that it is not appropriate for infected ulcers, when frequent inspection and bandage change is needed, or for heel ulcers or when peripheral vascular disease exists. The cast should be changed every 1–2 weeks. A hole under the surface of the ulcer permits its frequent inspection and bandage changes. Another effective decompression method (maybe equally effective as the application of a cast) is the application of a removable cast (instant total-contact-cast). To increase patient compliance, a band of plaster or a strong adhesive band is wrapped around the cast at the height of the calf, so that its removal is difficult. Other decompression methods include special boots (Scotchcast and aircast boots) that are removable and suitable for infected ulcers or with lots of exudates, although their effectiveness is not proven.

How are ulcers classified?

Apart from their classification to plain neurotrophic, plain ischaemic and neuroischaemic ulcers, as mentioned earlier, there are two classification systems for the severity of the ulcers. Traditionally, classification by Meggitt-Wagner was considered as the 'classification of choice'. Relatively recently, however, a new classification system was proposed by the University of Texas in the USA, which is considered to be superior. Its main advantage is that it takes into consideration the presence of infection and ischaemia in the more superficial ulcers, two factors that are related to outcome and survival. Furthermore, this newer classification scheme was evaluated in a prospective study and was found to predict outcome (Tables 17.3 and 17.4).

Table 17.3. The Meggitt-Wagner ulcer classification system

Degree	Description of ulcer
0	Completely healed ulcer
1	Superficial ulcer in the epidermis that is not extended in the chorion
2	Ulcer that extends in the subcutaneous tissue or even beyond it (tendons, fascia, synovium) without, however, abscesses or osteomyelitis
3	Deep ulcer with osteomyelitis or formation of abscess
4	Gangrene localized in the toes or the forefoot
5	Extensive gangrene

CASE STUDY 2

A 68 year old woman with a chronic neurotrophic ulcer in the 3rd metatarsal head for six months, comes to the diabetic foot clinic for re-evaluation. She has an ulcer 2 × 3 cm in diameter and 1 cm in depth. It is foul smelling and the surface is dirty, with accompanying cellulitis extending 3 cm around it. She denies any pain and receives no antibiotics. Her temperature is normal and she

Table 17.4. The University of Texas ulcer classification system

Stage	0	1	2	3
A	Ulcer completely healed	Superficial ulcer, without involvement of tendons, synovial membranes or bone	Ulcer with involvement of tendons or synovial membranes	Ulcer with involvement of joints or bone
B	With infection	With infection	With infection	With infection
C	With ischaemia	With ischaemia	With ischaemia	With ischaemia
D	With infection and ischaemia	With infection and ischaemia	With infection and ischaemia	With infection and ischaemia

wears special therapeutic shoes for decompression of the ulcer area. How should this patient be managed?

It is obvious that the ulcer has been complicated by an infection. In this case, thorough debridement and curettage of the ulcer base is indicated, followed by culture of the deep tissues inside it (this is preferable to obtaining culture by swabbing the ulcer surface) with fast dispatch of the specimens to the laboratory for identification of the inciting aerobic and/or anaerobic pathogens. When clinical signs of infection are present, empirical initiation of antibiotic treatment is indicated, while awaiting the results of the culture. However, when the ulcer shows no signs of infection, no culture should be sent and, most importantly, no antibiotics should be prescribed.

Which antimicrobial(s) will you empirically prescribe for ulcers with infection?

The decision concerning the prescribed antimicrobials is derived from an interrelation of the severity of infection and the presumed presence of resistant microbial strains. Infections of the diabetic foot are categorized as follows:

- *Mild:* Localized cellulitis without ulcer is observed, or cellulitis (redness, pain, increased temperature, sensitivity to touch) around the ulcer, or purulent exudate (Figure 17.7). The patient does not have systemic symptoms and is metabolically and haemodynamically stable. The majority of these infections are due to aerobic Gram positive pathogens (with most frequent *Staphylococcus aureus*) and often these are the only pathogens.
- *Moderate severity:* There is cellulitis of > 2 cm in diameter or deep tissue infection (abscess, septic arthritis, osteomyelitis, septic tenosynovitis). Systemic symptoms are absent or mild and the patient is metabolically and haemodynamically stable. The principal pathogens are – as in mild infections – aerobic Gram positive microbes. When chronic ulcers are involved, or patients that have recently received antimicrobial agents, more than one pathogen is usually isolated.
- *Severe:* There are signs of systemic toxicity threatening the extremity or even the life of the patient (fever, rigours, confusion, hypotension) and metabolic instability (excessive hyperglycaemia, metabolic acidosis, azotaemia). Moreover, the involvement of deep tissues,

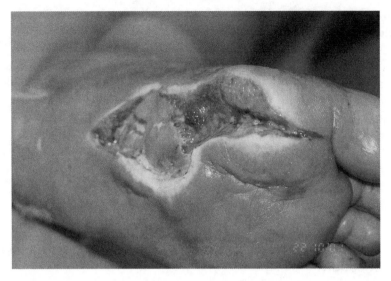

Figure 17.7. Deep neurotrophic ulcer on the plantar surface with dirty base and adjacent cellulitis. The ulcer was caused by a mild trauma 2 years prior when the patient walked barefoot in her house.

wet gangrene, extensive tissue necrosis and the fast extension of infection constitute (each one separately) signs of serious infection. When critical ischaemia of the lower extremities is present, a mild infection can very rapidly progress into a serious one. Other manifestations of a serious infection are the existence of vesicles, ecchymoses, undetermined pain, muscular weakness and sensory loss. Severe infections are polymicrobial with involvement of Gram (+), Gram (−) and anaerobic microbes.

The antimicrobial medicines that are prescribed, depending on the severity of the infection, are presented in Table 17.5 and the doses of the frequently used antimicrobials in Table 17.6.

When is hospitalization of a patient with foot problems indicated?

Hospitalization is indicated in any case where intravenous administration of treatment is required, when signs of systemic infection, metabolic instability or critical ischaemia of the lower extremities are present, when

Table 17.5. Proposed empiric antimicrobial treatment of infections of the diabetic foot

Severity of infection	Usual pathogen	Antimicrobial
Mild or moderate (the required treatment can be given p.o.)		
Without recent use of anti-microbials and without necrosis	Gram +	Semisynthetic penicillins **or** first generation cephalosporins
Recent use of antimicrobials	Gram + **with or without** Gram −	Fluoroquinolones **or** b-lactame antimicrobials with inhibitors of b-lactamases
Allergy to penicillins/cephalosporins		Clindamycin **or** fluoroquinolones **or** TMP/SMX
Severe infection * (the iv administration of antibiotics is recommended until the patient is stabilized)		
Without recent use of anti-microbials and without necrosis	Gram + **with or without** Gram −	b-lactam antimicrobials with inhibitors of b-laktamases **or** 2nd **or** 3rd generation cephalosporins
Recent use of antimicrobials / signs of necrosis	Gram+ **and** Gram − /anaerobes	Cephalosporins 3rd or 4th generation **or** fluoroquinolones + clindamycin
Life-threatening infection (prolonged administration of antimicrobials iv)		
Small probability for MRSA	Gram+ **and** Gram− **and** anaerobes	Carbapenemes **or** amino-glycoside + clindamycin
High probability for MRSA		Cephalosporin 3rd or 4th generation + glycopeptide or linezolid **or** fluoroquinolone + metronidazole

In cases where a high probability for MRSA exists (methicillin-resistant *Staphylococcus aureus*) the addition of linezolide or glycopeptide is indicated.

Hemisynthetic penicillins: oxacillin, dicloxacillin. First generation cephalosporins: Cephalexin, cephazolin, cephapirin. Cephalosporins of 2nd/3rd/4th generation: cephaclor, cefuroxime, ceforanid, cefoxitin/cefotaxime, ceftriaxone, ceftazidime/cefipime. B-lactame antimicrobials with inhibitors of b-lactamases: amoxycillin/clavulanate, ampicillin/sulbactam, ticarcillin/clavulanate, piperacillin/tazobactam. Glycopeptides: teicoplanin, vancomycin. Fluoroquinolones: ciprofloxacin, levofloxacin. TMP/SMX: trimethoprim/sulfomethoxazole. Aminoglycosides: gentamycin, amikacin, tobramycin, netilmicin. Carbapenems: imipenem/cilastatin, meropenem, ertapenem. Other medicines active against MRSA are also expected in the market (e.g. pristinamycin).

Table 17.6. The doses of certain antimicrobial factors that are often used in the treatment of infections of the diabetic foot

Antimicrobial	Dose
Oxacilin	100 mg/Kg/day in 3 doses. Not suitable for p.o administration
Cefalexin	100 mg/Kg/day p.o
Fusidic acid	500 mg q8 hours p.o or iv
Rifampicin	600 mg/day p.o or iv
TMP/SMX	160/800 mg twice a day
Amoxycillin/clavulanate	625 mg q8 hours or 1 g q12 hours p.o or 1.2 g q6 hours iv
Imipenem/silastatin	50 mg/kg/day in 2 doses. The highest daily dose is < 4 g
Pristinamycin	1 g q8 hours p.o.
Clindamycin	600–900 mg q8 hours p.o or iv
Levofloxacin	750 mg/day p.o or iv
Ciprofloxacin	750 mg q12 hours p.o or iv
Vancomycin	1 g q12 hours
Teicoplanin	600 mg/day iv or im
Linezolid	600 mg q12 hours p.o or iv. No dose adjustment is needed in renal insufficiency or hepatic disease. Should not be given for more than 28 days.

TMP/SMX: trimethoprim-sulfomethoxazole

extensive surgical procedures are needed and when social reasons dictate (in individuals that are unable to take care of their feet or to receive the recommended treatment on their own).

How can you rule out or confirm the diagnosis of osteomyelitis?

All chronic ulcers, particularly when their dimensions are more than 2 cm, can be complicated by osteomyelitis. Acute osteomyelitis manifests radiological findings two weeks after involvement of the bone. These consist of osteolysis or even a significant degree of bone absorption, with or without periosteal reaction (Figure 17.8). It is recommended

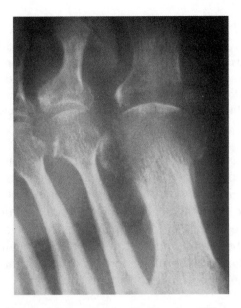

Figure 17.8. The X-ray of the patient with the ulcer (Figure 17.7). Osteolysis of the head of the 1st metatarsal and the proximal part of the last phalanx, with periosteal reaction due to osteomyelitis is seen.

that an X-ray is performed on all chronic ulcers (sensitivity in diagnosing osteomyelitis is in the order of 55 percent but increases more when the radiograph is repeated at a two weekly interval). In cases when the radiograph is negative and the clinical suspicion high, it is recommended to treat the infection as osteomyelitis and repeat the X-ray in two weeks. A complete blood count (CBC) may show anaemia of chronic disease. Erythrocyte sedimentation rate (ESR) and C-reactive protein (CRP) levels are usually slightly elevated and are useful for disease monitoring and follow-up. Probing of bone with a metal object through the ulcer (probe-to-bone test) has a sensitivity of more than 90 percent for diagnosing acute osteomyelitis. Three-phase technetium bone scan scintigraphy is indicated when the radiograph is negative. Computed tomography (CT) can reveal more subtle damage than the simple radiograph (periosteal reaction, small cortex erosions) as well as damage of soft tissues. Magnetic resonance imaging (MRI) tomography can also help in cases where the other tests are non-diagnostic, because it has higher sensitivity and specificity for the diagnosis of osteomyelitis.

CASE STUDY 3

A patient with a relapsing neurotrophic ulcer at the head of his right 5th metatarsal presents for a follow-up visit. On examination, he has an ulcer 2 × 1.5 cm in diameter and 0.8 cm in depth, surrounded by a callus. The gauzes that the patient uses to cover the ulcer are impregnated with serosanguinous fluid, but there are no clinical signs of infection. How will you manage the patient?

As mentioned above, surgical debridement of the ulcer border for removal of the hyperkeratotic rim is necessary. Adequate tissue should be removed, up to the point of mild bleeding from the ulcer rim. The surface of the ulceration is cleansed initially with ample NaCl 0.9 percent or 15 percent solution and then debrided with a scalpel, aimed at removing microbes and macrophage products (proteases), which act by suspending the action of fibroblasts and locally produced healing factors. The surgical debridement of the ulcer borders times to transform a chronic ulcer into an acute one that heals faster.

Apart from surgical debridement, are there other ways of debriding an ulcer?

The enzymatic and chemical debridement methods are available. In the first case, autolytic, proteolytic enzymes (papain, collagenase and streptokinase) are applied on the ulcer surface daily. This type the debridement is recommended when there is extensive necrosis or when surgical debridement is not possible due to pain. Disadvantages of enzymatic debridement are its high cost and the irritation it can cause when applied on healthy skin. Use of sterile maggots (larvae) is included in the enzymatic debridement as well. Maggotts are the larvae of the green fly (gender Lucilia sericata). The larvae are received and developed in a special sterile environment. When they are applied on ulcers with necroses or infection, they have the attribute to 'only eat' the abnormal tissue while leaving the healthy tissue intact, thus cleansing the surface of the ulceration. This treatment is painless, safe, relatively cheap and effective.

Chemical debridement is performed by applying hydrogels (Table 17.7). Hydrogels help in the cleansing of the ulcer surface when this cannot be performed surgically. They are, however, inferior to the surgical debridement, because, on the one hand, onset of their action is delayed and on the other hand, their effectiveness is lower.

Table 17.7. Characteristics and indications of various dressings

	Advantages	Disadvantages
Gauze impregnated with NaCl solution	Cheap and available everywhere Suitable for ulcers with dry gangrene as well	It is attached on the surface of the ulcer and may cause bleeding at removal
Membranes	Hemi-transparent, low cost, form a barrier for the microbes, should be changed every 4–5 days	Suitable only for superficial ulcers
Foamy dressings	Suitable for ulcers with abundant exudate, easily applied	Absorbance ability of the various foamy dressings varies
Hydrogels	Effective, easily applied, not irritant for the healty skin, decrease the risk of infection, remove exudates, suitable for ulcers with crpts	Surgical debridement is superior, unsuitable for ischaemic/ neuroischaemic ulcers, frequent inspection of ulcer is required for timely diagnosis of possible infection
Hydrocolloids	Suitable for necrotic ulcers with moderate quantity of exudates. They do not require daily removal	They predispose to superinfections, especially from anaerobes
Alginate	Very useful when there is abundant exudate, suitable for superinfected ulcers as well, some also have haemostatic properties	Unsuitable for neuroischaemic ulcers with small exudate. They predispose to superinfections. They dryout the ulcer surface and may cause bleeding at removal

Which dressing will you apply?

The dressing that is considered to be the 'dressing of choice' at present is the sterile gauze impregnated in NaCl 0.9 percent or even better 15 percent solution. Ulcers heal better when their surface is humid and for this reason dressings that dry out the ulcer surface should not be used. An exception to this rule is the existence of dry gangrene, when it is desirable to maintain the affected area dry, to avoid wet gangrene. There are various different dressings available with varied characteristics and certain small studies support their effectiveness. These dressings, their characteristics and their indications are presented in Table 17.7. The cost of the dressings is quite large and no comparative studies exist that suggest the supremacy of one against the other. This is also the reason that the impregnated with NaCl 0.9 or 15 percent solution gauze constitutes at present the 'method of choice'. Special dressings can be used in resistant ulcers.

In ulcers that are not infected or necrotic, the use of povidone solution is not advisable, because it is toxic for the fibroblasts. Dressings should be changed by the patient in his or her environment on a daily basis (or even more often, if the quantity of exudate is large). The frequency of outpatient visits in the diabetic foot clinic should be once a week provided the ulcer does not manifest any complications. The patient should be informed that the appearance of signs of infection should indicate the search for urgent medical help and no postponement until the next programmed visit in the diabetic foot clinic.

Are there any other factors, apart from dressings, that can accelerate healing?

Apart from the dressings mentioned previously, biotechnology has developed substitutes of human skin and growth factors. Cultivated human chorion (Dermagraft) is produced from human fibroblasts that are multiplied in a biodegradable matrix. After culture for two weeks a live substitute of chorion is produced, which can later support the production of epidermis. Dermagraft produces, as does the physiologic skin, all growth factors that promote healing. This biologic substitute of skin is particularly effective for ulcers of long duration.

Another substitute of skin is the biotechnologically manufactured substitute of skin of two layers (Apligraf, Gaftskin). This is comprised of a layer of epidermis from human keratinocytes and a layer of chorion that consists of human fibroblasts in a matrix of bovine collagen type I. Apligraf seems to heal more ulcers, in a shorter period of time, compared to the classic dressings.

Apart from skin substitutes, the local application of growth factors derived from platelets (platelet-derived growth factor-BB [becaplermin] and platelet releasate), accelerates the healing time. Local application of the recombinant epidermal growth factor and the transforming growth factor-beta (TGF-β) has good results as well.

The administration of ketanserin (systematically or locally), the local application of phenytoin, lyophilized collagen and gel that contains low-molecular-weight heparin have given satisfactory results in small studies, but sufficient documentation of their effectiveness does not exist.

Local and systemic treatment with hyperbaric oxygen is indicated mainly for ulcers with signs of ischaemia and infection. The intravenous administration of the synthetic prostacyclin analogue (Illoprost) is indicated and is effective for ischaemic or neuroischaemic ulcers. The application of negative pressure in the foot with ulceration, using a special appliance, is also effective and is indicated principally for ulcers with abundant exudate. The negative pressure also helps in the reduction of oedema and results in a better perfusion of the ulceration.

CASE STUDY 4

A 58 year old man, with Type 1 DM that was diagnosed at the age of 24 years, presents with discomfort in his right foot for the previous 15 days. He also observed oedema and redness in the middle of the foot. He denies any trauma. He had initially visited an orthopaedic surgeon, who had diagnosed ligamentous damage. Non-steroidal anti-inflammatory pain-killers were prescribed together with advice for rest. A small improvement of symptoms was noticed with this treatment. What is the most likely diagnosis?

For every patient with more than 10 years' duration of DM, who presents with oedema, redness and feeling of heaviness or mild pain in the foot or ankle joint (with or without history of recent ligamentous damage [sprain]), the diagnosis is acute Charcot arthropathy (or acute neuro-osteo-arthropathy), until proven otherwise.

How does acute Charcot arthropathy manifest itself?

The typical picture consists of the sudden installation of heaviness or even pain, as a rule, mild, in the foot. Sometimes acute Charcot arthropathy can present itself after an infection of the foot, intervention for any reason in the ipsilateral or contralateral foot, and a few cases have been reported after interventions of lower extremity revascularization. Physical examination reveals the presence of serious degree of peripheral neuropathy, with normal peripheral pulses. The majority of patients have increased temperature, redness and oedema in the involved region. An invariable finding is the existence of at least 2°C temperature difference between the affected and the healthy foot. Moreover, this temperature difference constitutes a criterion of response to the therapeutic regimen. Erythrocyte sedimentation rate and CRP may be slightly elevated. The number of white blood cells is normal.

How can the diagnosis be confirmed?

The diagnosis will be confirmed by confirming compatible radiological findings. In the acute phase (phase of installation), oedema of the soft tissues, subluxations of the affected joints, erosions of cartilages and the subchondrial bone, stenosis or abolition of the intra-articular spaces, diffuse osteopenia and fragmentation of one or more bones are manifested. In the second phase (phase of coalescence), there are signs of efforts to repair the damage. The affected joints are stabilized, the broken bony pieces are attached to the adjacent bones and periosteal reaction and the formation of new bone appear. The last phase (phase of reconstruction) is characterized by osteosclerosis of subchondrial bone, formation of osteophytes between adjacent bones and ossification of ligaments and tendons. For this reason, the mobility of the affected joint is limited.

It should be noted, however, that in the very early stages, the radiological findings may be non-diagnostic. Therefore, it is imperative to repeat the radiological examinations when the clinical suspicion is high.

Radionucleotide scan (three-phase technetium scintigraphy bone scan), magnetic resonance tomography and computed tomography may help in difficult cases, but they cannot differentiate acute Charcot arthropathy from osteomyelitis.

How frequent is Charcot arthropathy and which persons are at risk of developing this complication?

Charcot neuroarthropathy is an infrequent but important condition, which is recognized more often if the physician is sensitive to the complication. It equally affects men and women, both with Type 1 and Type 2 DM. The mean age of appearance is 60 years and the known duration of DM is at least 10–15 years. In order for Charcot arthropathy to manifest itself, severe peripheral neuropathy, neuropathy of the autonomous (sympathetic) nervous system and sufficient blood perfusion of the foot should be present. In the literature it is stressed that this complication does not present in individuals with an important degree of peripheral vascular disease.

What is the pathogenesis of the disease?

The pathogenesis is not precisely known. It is speculated that a small trauma, that often goes unnoticed because of the sensory loss, can initiate the process of joint and bone destruction. The inability to perceive pain, due to loss of sensation, allows the continued utilization of the foot, resulting in deterioration of the damage. Simultaneously, increased perfusion in the affected region (most likely and intraosseously) is observed, through an abnormal – due to the neuropathy of the peripheral sympathetic nervous system – opening of arteriovenous anastomoses, that results in increased absorption of bone. The body tries to restore the damage, but this is done without organization, due to the continuous pressure-loading of the foot. The final result can be big deformities of the foot (Figures 17.9 and 17.10), especially when the offence concerns the middle and the rear department of the foot as well as the ankle joint.

What is the treatment?

Treatment consists in immobilization of the foot with the application of a plaster that includes the whole foot, except for the toes, up to the knee. The plaster should be changed every 2–3 weeks. There are no explicit guidelines for the time interval of immobilization, but a

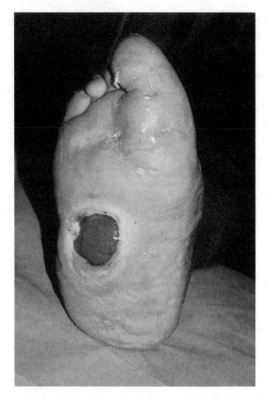

Figure 17.9. Chronic recurrent neurotrophic ulcer on a foot with Charcot athropathy. The ulcer develops under an area with abnormal osseous protrusion in the middle of the foot. The foot arch has been destroyed.

criterion of successful treatment is the return of the temperature of the foot to a normal level. There are recent studies in small numbers of patients that show that the intravenous administration of bisphosphonates has very good results in the treatment of acute Charcot arthropathy. One dose of pamidronate 60 mg (or even another bisphosphonate in equivalent dose) intravenously causes a decrease of pain or the feeling of heaviness, amelioration of inflammation signs, and more rapid return of the temperature to the normal range. Moreover, the indicators of increased bone metabolism (bony fraction of alkaline phosphatase, urine dihydroxypyridoline) more quickly return to normal levels.

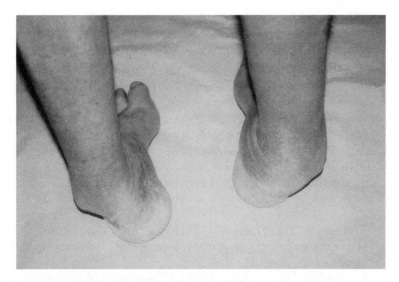

Figure 17.10. Significant deformity of the foot joints bilaterally due to bilateral Cahrcot arthropathy.

What are the consequences of Charcot arthropathy?

Timely diagnosis and treatment are of paramount importance for the leg of the patient. Otherwise, foot anatomy, especially when the middle or the rear foot has been affected, is deformed to such a degree that walking and balance are difficult (Figures 17.4–17.5). Frequently, because of foot collapse and suppression of the foot arch, ulcerations under bony protrusions develop that heal with difficulty and often relapse. In many cases the only therapeutic choice is amputation.

Further reading

Assal, J.P., Mehnert, H., Tritschler, H.S., Sidorenko, A., Keen, H. (2002) 'On your feet' workshop on the diabetic foot. *J Diabet Comp*, **16**, 183–91.

Boulton, A.J.M. (2004) The diabetic foot: from art to science. The 18th Camillo Golgi lecture. *Diabetologia*, **47**, 1343–53.

Boulton, A.J.M. (2000) The pathway to ulceration. Aetiopathogenesis, in *The Foot in Diabetes* 3rd edn (eds A.J.M. Boulton, H. Connor P.R. Cavanagh), Wiley, Chichester, 19–31.

Eldor, R., Raz, I., Yehuda, A.B., Boulton, A.J.M. (2004) New and experimental approaches to treatment of diabetic foot ulcers: a comprehensive review of emerging treatment strategies. *Diabet Med*, **21**, 1161–73.

International Working Group on the Diabetic Foot (1999) in *International consensus on the diabetic foot*. International Working Group on the Diabetic Foot eds, Netherlands.

Katsilambros, N., Tentolouris, N., Tsapogas, P., Dounis, E. (2003) Atlas of the Diabetic Foot, in *Atlas of the Diabetic Foot* (eds N. Katsilambros, N. Tentolouris, P.Tsapogas, E. Dounis), Wiley, Chichester, pp. 3–21, 25–40, 187–212.

Lipsky, B.A. (2004) A report from the international consensus on diagnosing and treating the infected diabetic foot. *Diabetes Metab Res Rev*, **20**(Suppl 1), S68–S77.

Pham, H., Armstrong, D.G., Harney, C., Harkless, L.B., Giurini, J.M., Veves, A. (2000) Screening techniques to identify people at high risk for diabetic foot ulceration. *Diabetes Care*, **23**, 606–11.

Reiber, G.E., Ledoux, W.R. (2002) Epidemiology of diabetic foot ulcers and amputations: evidence for prevention, in *The Evidence-base for Diabetes Care* (eds B. Williams., W. Herman., A.L. Kinmonth., N.J. Warehan) Wiley., Chichester, 641–65.

Tentolouris, N., Al-Sabbach, S., Walker, M., Boulton, A.J.M., Jude, E.B. (1990) Mortality in diabetic and nondiabetic patients after amputations performed from 1990 to 1995: a 5-year follow-up study. *Diabetes Care*, **27**, 1598–1604.

Tentolouris, N., Jude, E.B., Smirnof, I., Knowles, E.A., Boulton, A.J.M. (1999) Methicillin-resistant *Staphylococcus aureus*: an increasing problem in a diabetic foot clinic. *Diabet Med*, **16**, 767–71.

18

Skin disorders in diabetes

Konstantinos Makrilakis

What are the main skin manifestations in DM?

Certain cutaneous disorders appear to be specific for DM (for example, diabetic thick skin), whereas others are present in the general population but are more frequent in diabetic individuals.

Diabetic dermopathy is the most common skin disorder associated with DM. It is quite frequent and presents at a rate, according to various authors, ranging up to 50 percent in diabetic patients, but only 3 percent in the general population. It is more prevalent in men older than 50 years of age, with long-standing DM. It is characterized by well circumscribed, brownish, atrophic, round or oval macules and scars, 0.5 to 2 cm in diameter (Figure 18.1). Usually these are located on the extensor surfaces of the shin bilaterally (hence the use of the term *shin spots* in this situation). They are asymptomatic and usually resolve in 1–2 years, but often relapse in other regions of the shins. There is no special treatment. The cause of the disorder is attributed to microangiopathic changes of the skin vessels.

Necrobiosis lipoidica diabeticorum is a rare dermatosis, with prevalence roughly around 0.3 percent among diabetic patients. Its name emanates from the characteristic necrobiosis, that is the degeneration of collagen in the dermis, the yellow colour of most lesions (due to carotene and lipid deposition) and its association with DM. It is characterized by asymptomatic, red, red-brown or violet plaques on the skin that often enlarge and become yellow centrally. Furthermore, there is atrophy of the epidermis that leads to shiny, transparent skin and visualization of the underlying dermal and subcutaneous vessels (Figure 18.2). The most

Diabetes in Clinical Practice: Questions and Answers from Case Studies.   Nicholas Katsilambros *et al.*
© 2006 John Wiley & Sons, Ltd.

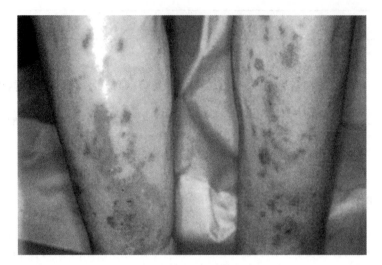

Figure 18.1. Diabetic dermopathy or shin spots.

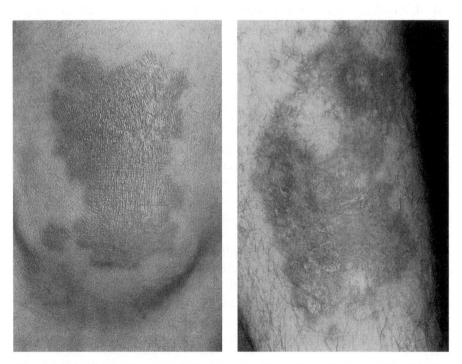

Figure 18.2. Necrobiosis lipoidica diabeticorum. (Reprinted from Textbook of Diabetes, 3rd edn., J. Pickup & G. Williams, Copyright 2003, with permission from Blackwell Science Ltd.)

frequent location is the shins (90 percent), but it can also present on the scalp, face or hands. The plaques may eventually ulcerate, become painful and predispose to infection. There is no satisfactory treatment. Improvement of hyperglycaemia does not result in corresponding improvement of the dermal lesions. Topical corticosteroids have been tried (either applied locally or by intralesional injection), as well as anticoagulants and antiplatelet agents (heparin, aspirin, dipyridamole) and immunosuppressants (cyclosporin, mycophenolate mofetil), without particular success. In a relatively small study, positive results were reported with the use of ultraviolet radiation (PUVA) and topical application of methoxypsoralen. In more infrequent cases, excision and grafting of the skin may even be needed.

The *diabetic bullae* (*bullosis diabeticorum*) are an uncommon dermal manifestation of DM. They occur more frequently in men as tense blisters containing clear liquid, more often on the dorsal and lateral surfaces of the hands and feet, on a normal, non-inflammatory base. They are usually asymptomatic and disappear within a few weeks. They do not usually require particular treatment (except perhaps for drainage when they are big in size [Figure 18.3] and local application of antibiotics if there is suspicion of superinfection). Their aetiology is unknown.

Periungual telangiectasia, that is the dilatation of capillaries and venules in the nail folds, is more frequent in DM (up to 50 percent in diabetics compared to 10 percent in the non-diabetics). The nail-fold capillary loops are examined easily through a magnifying lens and have

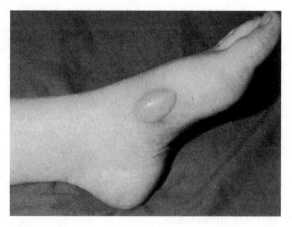

Figure 18.3. Bulla on the dorsum of the foot in a diabetic patient.

been used for functional studies of diabetic microangiopathy, because they are thought to represent the general status of the microcirculation in DM.

The skin of diabetic individuals is often thicker than in non-diabetics, and less elastic. In certain cases this thickness of the skin is pronounced and can potentially lead to *scleroedema of the skin*, with more frequent localization at the posterior surface of the neck and upper back. Seldom does it extend to the face, arms and abdomen. Scleroedema affects roughly 2.5 percent of Type 2 diabetic patients and is related to obesity and poor diabetes control. In certain cases the combination of skin thickness together with involvement of the small and large joints of the hands leads to *cheiroarthropathy*, with the inability to approximate the palmar surfaces of the hands (see also Chapter 20: 'Musculoskeletal system and diabetes', and Figure 20.1).

Carpal tunnel syndrome and *Dupuytren contracture* are also more common in DM.

Which cutaneous manifestations are associated with chronic complications of DM?

Skin infections

The view that cutaneous infections are more frequent in diabetic individuals has recently been disputed. Perhaps the better control of DM with oral medicines and insulin has contributed to a reduction of severe dermal infections. *Furuncles, carbuncles, styes* and *erythrasma* were in the past (before the introduction of insulin and antibiotics) much more common in diabetic individuals, but now their frequency has definitely decreased. Furuncles and carbuncles are due to *Staphylococcus*, and erythrasma are due to *Corynebacterion (C. minutissimum)*. *Malignant otitis externa* due to *Pseudomonas* infection is also infrequent today, but potentially lethal. *Fungal dermal infections* are also common in diabetic individuals, mainly from *Candida albicans*. This yeast can cause *vulvovaginitis* in women, *balanoposthitis* in men, *intertrigo* and *chronic paronychia*. Intertrigo is an infection occurring on opposing skin surfaces (under the breasts, in the axillae, the groins, the skin of the abdomen, etc.). Proper antibiotic and antifungal treatment (local or systemic) will usually help in the confrontation of these infections.

Ulcers and relevant damage of the lower extremities

These are related to the development of neuropathy and ischaemia and are described in Chapters 15 ('Diabetic Neuropathy') and 17 ('Diabetic foot').

Which cutaneous manifestations occur in other endocrine and metabolic disorders that are related to DM?

Acanthosis nigricans is characterized by hyperpigmentation of the skin in regions where this forms folds, as in the axillae, the neck and the groins (Figure 18.4). Generalized acanthosis nigricans is usually related to development of neoplasia, mainly of the gastrointestinal tract, whereas the more limited form is related to conditions of insulin resistance, such as obesity, Type 2 DM, the polycystic ovary syndrome and acromegaly.

Eruptive xanthomata are due to deposits of triglycerides in the skin and are more frequent in diabetic men with hypetriglyceridaemia and poor metabolic control of DM. They present as small, red or yellow nodules, up to 0.5 cm in diameter, on the extensor surfaces of the extremities and the buttocks (Figure 18.5). Their occurrence is usually abrupt and they disappear slowly with the improvement of hypetriglyceridaemia.

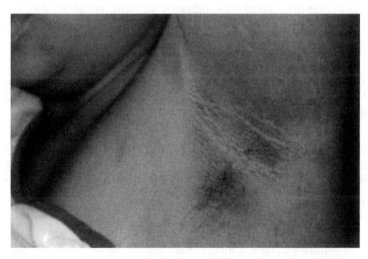

Figure 18.4. Acanthosis nigricans of the axilla.

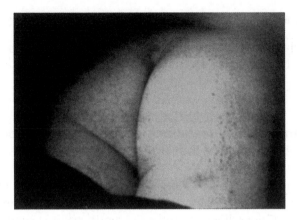

Figure 18.5. Xanthomata on the buttocks. (Reprinted from Textbook of Diabetes, 3rd edn., J. Pickup & G. Williams, Copyright 2003, with permission from Blackwell Science Ltd.)

Vitiligo is also more frequent in diabetic individuals (mainly with Type 1 DM). It is due to an autoimmune destruction of the skin melanocytes and presents as symmetrical, usually, white (because of discoloration), patches of skin.

Other endocrine conditions that cause cutaneous manifestations and are related to the appearance of DM are glucagonoma (causes the characteristic migratory necrolytic erythema), haemochromatosis (dark pigmentation of the skin), Cushing syndrome (atrophy of skin, striae in the abdomen, hirsutism), acromegaly (thickness of skin), the polycystic ovary syndrome (hirsutism, acanthosis nigricans) and the lipodystrophy syndromes.

Which cutaneous manifestations are associated with complications of DM treatment?

Treatment with insulin can cause local or systemic allergic reactions (itching, urticaria, seldom angioneurotic oedema, etc.); however, these are now extremely rare due to the use of the purified human insulins that are available. Lipoatrophy (localized loss of subcutaneous tissue) or lipohypertrophy (increase/thickening of subcutaneous tissue) at sites of insulin injection are also relatively rare today with the new insulins.

Oral antidiabetic medicines, and mainly sulfonylureas, may also cause allergic reactions from the skin, within 6–8 weeks from onset of

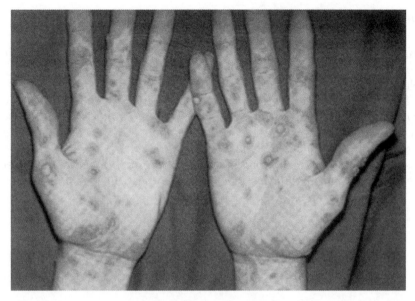

Figure 18.6. Erythema multiforme with the typical target lesions (Reprinted from Color Atlas of Dermatology, G.M. Levene, Copyright 1974, with permission from Elsevier).

treatment. These range from the simple urticaria to erythema multiforme (Figure 18.6) and its severe form (Stevens Johnson syndrome, see Figure 18.7), as well as eczema, blisters in the skin, photosensitivity, purpura and erythema nodosum.

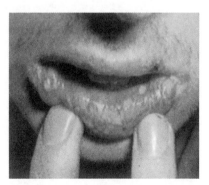

Figure 18.7. Mouth ulcerations in Stevens-Johnson syndrome, the severe form of erythema multiforme (Reprinted from Color Atlas of Dermatology, G.M. Levene, Copyright 1974, with permission from Elsevier).

Further reading

Almeyda, J. and Baker, H. (1970) Drug reactions. X. Adverse cutaneous reactions to hypoglycemic agents. *Br J Dermatol*, **82**, 634–7.

Bolognia, J.L. and Braverman, I.M. (2004) Skin and subcuataneous tissues, in *Therapy for Diabetes Mellitus and Related Disorders*, 4th edn, American Diabetes Association, (ed. H.E. Lebovitz), pp 318–330.

Katsambas, A., Lotti, T. (2004) *European Handbook of Dermatological Treatments*. Springer-Verlag, 2nd edn, Heidelberg.

Sharpe, G.R. (2003) Skin disorders in diabetes, in *Textbook of Diabetes*, 3rd edn, (eds J. Pickup and G. Williams) Blackwell Science Ltd, Oxford, pp 60.1–60.13.

19

Sexual function and diabetes

Ioannis Ioannidis

CASE STUDY 1

A 32 year old married man visits his family doctor with complaints of progressive loss of erectile ability. He has been suffering from Type 1 DM for 15 years, with relatively satisfactory control. Over the previous three years he has also experienced neuropathic type pains (coexistence of peripheral neuropathy signs) in the lower extremities. In the past he had observed larger fluctuations in his blood sugar levels.

Initially his main problem was the inability to maintain erections so that he could achieve a satisfactory sexual contact. During the last six months, however, he also observed reduction in the quantity of sperm, despite preservation of orgasm. Very recently, he noticed the complete inability to achieve satisfactory erections.

His family doctor recommends that he speaks to a urologist.

Answers with regard to the reasons for this condition and its management are given below.

Repercussions of DM in sexual life

Erectile dysfunction is defined as the inability of a man to achieve and/or maintain sufficient erection for sexual activity.

This complication (less often called 'impotence' these days) often occurs in middle-aged men. In a large study performed in Massachusetts, 52 percent of healthy middle-aged men manifested some degree of erectile dysfunction. The same study showed that the frequency increases with age, while it is three times more frequent in diabetics compared to non-diabetics of a similar age.

Diabetes in Clinical Practice: Questions and Answers from Case Studies.   Nicholas Katsilambros *et al.*
© 2006 John Wiley & Sons, Ltd.

Table 19.1. Erectile dysfunction evaluation scale (International scale of erectile function, IIEF)

During the last 4 weeks:	
1. How often did you have an erection during any sexual activity?	0–5
2. During sexual activity, how often did you have an erection that allowed penetration?	0–5
3. Out of all the times you sought sexual contact, how many times did you succeed?	0–5
4. How often did you maintain the erection after penetration?	0–5
5. How difficult was it for you to maintain the erection up to the completion of the contact?	0–5
6. How do you grade the confidence in yourself with regard to your ability to succeed and maintain a satisfactory erection?	0–5
Total score: 25–30: normal, 17–25: mild dysfunction, 11–16: moderate dysfunction, < 10: severe dysfunction.	

In various studies, diabetic individuals manifest disturbances of erectile function at a rate from 33 to 75 percent.

The problem of erectile dysfunction considerably influences the patient's quality of life because it decreases self-esteem while at the same time creates problems in their personal life. Often the patient does not report his problem, but is willing to discuss it when asked by his treating physician. It is consequently essential, because of its frequency, that this sensitive problem is discussed discreetly, with the initiative of healthcare professionals in the diabetic clinics. Erectile dysfunction is basically diagnosed with a detailed medical history (Table 19.1) and is much less dependent on physical examination and special tests. Recently specific questionnaires with detailed questions concerning sexual activity have been developed, and if answered sincerely, they usually reveal the problem.

In order to exclude psychological causes, the confirmation or absence of automatic morning erections is (details of the first morning hours are reported at history taking and are recorded with a special instrument).

Erectile dysfunction is associated, in most cases, with diseases that affect the blood vessels, causing atherosclerosis. Thus, hypertension, hypercholesterolaemia, DM and smoking increase the risk of the problem. At the same time, it can be also due to psychological or emotional factors. Finally, the use of medicines (diuretics, beta-blockers) but also psychotropic substances (alcohol, marijuana, cocaine, etc.) can cause erectile dysfunction.

Erection involves the blood vessels and the nervous system of the body. The penis consists of two parallel structures, the *corpus caverno-sum* and the *corpus spongiosum penis*, which originate from inside the pelvis and end up at the tip of the penis. These structures consist of spongy tissue that contains many blood vessels. Usually the walls of the vessels are constricted and impede any additional blood to flow into the penis. Thus, the penis is relaxed most of the time. When a man is sexually aroused these blood vessels begin to dilate and blood flow is increased. Simultaneously, the veins that remove the blood from the penis constrict and prevent the fast and quantitative removal of blood. The combination of a big surge of blood with its decreased removal leads to the inflation and hardening of the penis and causes erection.

It should be noted that DM can cause hardening and stenosis of the arteries that impede the smooth and sufficient flow of blood into the penis. At the same time, DM can cause damage in the nerves that connect the nervous system with the penis, thus leading, through this additional mechanism, to erectile dysfunction. The presence of other factors, from those already mentioned, can also aggravate the problem (mainly smoking, hypertension, alcoholic abuse and certain categories of medicines). In rare cases the existence of hypogonadism is also a contributory factor. Overweight or obese diabetic individuals very frequently suffer from this metabolic syndrome and are characterized, among other things, by low levels of sex hormone binding globulin (SHBG). This globulin is connected in plasma with the sex hormones. Decreased levels, although affecting the total levels of testosterone, do not influence the levels of free testosterone, which are the active levels. Thus, the determination only of levels of total testosterone in these individuals can create a false picture of hypogonadism.

In the context of investigating erectile dysfunction, apart from the classical routine tests, serum testosterone is often also ordered. If total testosterone is < 300 ng/dl, a second sample should be drawn between 7 and 10 a.m. in order to determine total testosterone, LH (luteinizing hormone) and prolactin levels. Measurement of free testosterone is performed when the levels of total testosterone are marginal and when there is indication for decreased levels of SHBG. If LH levels are low or normal with levels of testosterone < 200 ng/dl, or if hyperprolactinaemia or abnormal thyroid function are present, the patient should be referred to a specialist.

Erectile dysfunction in DM can be transient and reversible when diabetes is not controlled well. Good DM control is essential, although there are no large studies showing that the improvement of glycaemic control ameliorates erectile dysfunction. In certain cases, however, especially when a man has had DM for a long time, the disturbance may not be completely reversible.

The problem can occur in both types of DM. Men with Type 1 DM suffer from the illness for a long time and usually from a young age. They consequently stand a higher chance of manifesting erectile problems at a younger age. Patients with Type 2 DM are adults, frequently smoke and consume alcohol, and also have hypertension. Thus, they too frequently manifest erectile problems.

The problem of erectile dysfunction should be discussed with the doctor, becames nowadays pharmacological management of the problem may be possible.

Can we cure erectile dysfunction?

The treatment of erectile disturbances requires initially an excellent control of blood sugar and arterial pressure, with a parallel cessation of smoking and alcohol. These measures are necessary, but are often not enough.

Today, a lot of pharmaceutical and other means are available to confront the problem. Decisions on the most suitable and safest treatment should be taken in collaboration between patient and doctor.

The wide and large availability of medicines for treatment of erectile dysfunction is the 'good' news. The basic category of medicines used since 1998 is the Type 5 phosphodiesterase inhibitors, including the medicines *sildenafil*, *vardenafil* and *tadalafil*. The use of these medicines over the past few years has created new data and naturally a large amount of optimism. Their administration requires the existence of arousing stimuli, since they do not produce automatic erections nor do they act as aphrodisiacs.

So, how do they act anyway? These medicines are inhibitors of Type 5 phosphodiesterase (PDE5) and thus inhibit the action of this enzyme.

Sexual excitation is produced through a complex chain of events that begins with signals from the central nervous system and the release of chemical messengers in the tissues of the penis. The sexual excitation fires the release of nitrogen oxide (NO), which in turn releases guanylate cyclase, causing an increase of intracellular concentration of cyclic guanosyne monophosphate (cGMP), reduction of intracellular calcium and in consequence relaxation of the smooth muscles of the vessel walls in corpora spongiosum facilitating the surge of blood in the penis. This results in its hardening and inflexibility. Cyclic GMP is degraded in smooth muscles of the penile vessel walls by Type 5 phosphodiesterase. These medicines, with the inhibition of the action of this enzyme, improve the maintainance of the dilation, thus improving the flow of blood in the penis and maintaining the erection. Through them the action of the chemical messengers responsible for the beginning and maintenance of excitation and erection is augmented. This means that the sexual stimulus *is required* in order to cause and maintain the erection.

The inhibitors differ with regard to their pharmacokinetic character- istics as well as their selectivity of inhibiting the various PDE isoenzymes. However, they share the same levels of effectiveness and safety of use.

The most frequent undesirable effects of these medicines are related to their mild vasodilatory action and include headaches, flushing, optical disturbances, indigestion and nasal congestion or rhinitis, present at a rate of 10–15 percent.

The undesirable effects are reversible and are usually decreased with the continuation of treatment. Sildenafil and vardenafil have a shorter duration of action (roughly four hours) compared to tadalafil, the action of which lasts up to 36 hours (it was characterized as 'the pill of the weekend').

However, consumption of a fat-rich meal slows down the absorption of sildenafil and vardenafil, although the absorption of tadalafil is not influenced by the intake of a fatty meal.

The effectiveness of these medicines in diabetic individuals reaches 60–70 percent of cases, and it appears that these patients require larger doses (50 to 100 mg sildenafil and 20 mg vardenafil and tadalafil) componed to non-diabetics. In any case, the initial doses of the medicine are often unsuccessful and patience is required (frequently successful erection is achieved with time, after seven or eight doses).

Special attention is needed for patients with coronary heart disease who are treated with nitrates. The simultaneous use of nitrates and PDE inhibitors can produce a big fall in blood pressure (even shock), tachycardia, stroke, myocardial infarction and even death. Attention is also needed when a-blockers, like doxazosin, are used (medications that are often prescribed for treatment of prostate hypertrophy).

Very few deaths have globally been reported in connection with the use of these substances. These that have been reported involved patients above 60 years of age, who used nitrates or had a history of one or more risk factors for coronary heart disease (diabetes, hypertension, smoking, hypercholesterolaemia). Many diabetic individuals, particularly those with erectile dysfunction, have underlying coronary heart disease which is often silent (without symptoms). Thus, in individuals to be prescribed this treatment, it would be prudent to first exclude the presence of coronary illness by any means (electrocardiogram, exercise stress test and if needed scintigraphy with thallium or even coronary angiography).

These medicines should not be prescribed for individuals with normal erectile function or in women.

Another medicine that is also available for this problem is apomorphine. Apomorphine stimulates the paraventricular nucleus in the brain. When used sublingually (2 and 3 mg) it acts after 20 minutes. The results in diabetic individuals are not encouraging. The main undesirable effects are nausea, headaches and dizziness.

Another potent medicine that is used for erectile dysfunction is the prostaglandin E1 (PGE1, alprostadil). This is used as a medicine of second choice. Alprostadil stimulates adenylate cyclase increasing the levels of cyclic AMP (cAMP) in the corpora cavernosum penis. This results in the reduction of intracellular calcium and muscular relaxation.

The medicine can be administered either through an intrapenile injection in the corpora cavernosum or intraurethrally. Intraurethral administration was successful in 65 percent of the patients. The intracavernous injection is even more effective (94 percent success rate). The side-effects of the medicine include pain (10 percent) and less often priapism.

Finally, many diabetic individuals use either vacuum appliances (they increase penile blood flow by creating vacuum conditions and negative pressure) or special rings (they press on the base of the penis, preventing the venous removal of blood). In other cases, the placement of an intrapenile prosthesis can be preferred.

What other sexual disturbances, apart from erectile dysfunction, can occur?

Apart from erectile dysfunction, one out of three men with DM can manifest ejaculation disturbances. The most frequent disturbance is retrograde ejaculation, during which some sperm, instead of exiting through the urethra, regresses into the urinary bladder. This condition is due to damage of the nervous system and can (and should) be managed with certain medicines, since it can cause sterility problems as well.

CASE STUDY 2

A 55 year old man has suffered from Type 2 DM for 5 years, and is treated with oral antidiabetic medicines. He does not regularly monitor his blood sugar levels (he is rather negligent). He has smoked since the age of 37 years (1–2 packs/day), and has high blood pressure and cholesterol levels. He was recently prescribed an ACE inhibitor with diuretic combination and a statin for this reason. Recently, he also complained of pains in his calves when walking. He visited his family doctor, who detected decreased peripheral pulses in the lower extremities bilaterally. When asked by the doctor, the patient admitted to recent, significant problems with achieving and maintaining an erection, which he attributes to the blood pressure medicines, and which he contemplated stopping. What is the proper management of the patient?

The patient has many vascular disease risk factors which he is not managing well. It appears that he has already developed serious peripheral vascular complications, as evidenced by the symptomatology of intermittent claudication and the decreased pulsations of the lower extremities.

The doctor ought to discuss with the patient the need for smoking cessation and the need for aggressive control of the metabolic disturbances. He ought to reassure the patient regarding the unfavourable effect of blood pressure medicines 'on his problem'. He should add an antiplatelet agent (aspirin or clopidogrel) to the patients regimen.

He should also check, in collaboration with a vascular surgeon, the patency of the lower extremity vessels with triplex ultrasonography and if the possibility for surgical intervention arises, with digital angiography as well.

Finally, if he decides to prescribe a medicine for erectile dysfunction, it would be prudent to have a cardiac evaluation beforehand (the patient is at high risk of coronary heart disease and a cardiologic evaluation would be useful any way, either through an exercise stress test or even better in association with thallium scintigraphy or a dobutamine stress echocardiogram).

CASE STUDY 3

A 46 year old woman has been suffering from Type 2 DM for the last five years. Her blood sugar is under good control. She has been married for 20 years and has three children. For most of her life, sexual activity has been normal.

Recently, however, she is trying to avoid sexual contact. Even when emotion- ally aroused, a long time had to pass before she can feel physically ready for sexual contact. Her doctor recommended a lubricant ointment for the vagina and discussion of the problem with her husband.

Do such sexual problems often occur in diabetic women?

The presence of sexual function disturbances in women is revealed with more difficulty than men. The physiological sequence of events comprises the following: wish, excitation, orgasm, satisfaction. The wish is borne in the brain, caused by external and internal stimuli, and then produces secretion of hormones and the stimulation of corresponding nervous paths.

The excitation is the emotional and physical response to the erotic wish and is mainly characterized by concentration of blood in the region of the genital organs. In this phase, the vagina is moistened. The orgasm, which is controlled by the nervous system, is characterized by a series of repeated, rhythmical twitches of the perineal and genital organs muscles.

The most frequent problem of women, regardless of whether they are diabetics or not, is the decreased sexual wish.

Chronically high blood sugar levels can cause disturbances in the physiologic sexual maturation, and can also lead to disturbances of menstruation.

Another problem that diabetic women manifest is insufficient moisten- ing of the vagina. Together with the dryness of the vaginal mucosa, the insufficient accumulation of blood in the genital organs during intercourse causes irritation and pain at sexual contact (dyspareunia). This symptom most likely also adds to the problem of the woman in this case study.

Furthermore, high blood sugar levels increase the chance of vaginal infections (vaginitis) due to common bacteria and yeasts. These infec- tions, with the local disturbance that they cause, obviously intervene with the physiologic sexual function and worsen the dyspareunia.

Finally, damage of the nervous system related to DM, can be incrimi- nated for orgasmic disturbances.

Can women with DM receive oral contraceptive pills?

The use of oral contraceptive pills requires particular attention and advice from experts. These pills can increase the tendency for thromboses and consequently the tendency for thrombophlebitis, pulmonary embolism and other undesirable complications.

Their use is decided in collaboration with the treating physician, who also selects the specific compound, after taking into consideration all parameters of risk and benefit.

Further reading

Alexander, W. (1997) Sexual function in diabetic men in *Textbook of Diabetes*, 2nd edn, (eds J. Pickup and G. Williams), Oxford, **59**, pp. 1–12.

American Diabetes Association (1998) Men's Sexual Health in *The Uncomplicated Guide to Diabetes Complications* (eds. M. Levin and M. Pfeiffer), pp. 304–17.

Hijazi, R., Betancourt-Albrecht, M., Cunningham, G. (2004) Gonadal and erectile dysfunction in diabetics. *Med Clin N Am*, **88**, 933–45.

Jackson, G. (2004) Treatment of Erectile Dysfunction in Patients with Cardiovascular Disease Guide to Drug Selection. *Drugs*, **64**(14), 1533–45.

Jackson, G. (2004) Sexual dysfunction and diabetes. *Int J Clin Pract*, **58**, 358–62.

Steel, J. (1997) Sexual function and contraception in diabetic women in *Textbook of Diabetes*, 2nd edn, (eds J. Pickup and G. Williams) Oxford, **60**, 1–9.

20

Musculoskeletal system and diabetes

Ioannis Ioannidis

Which disturbances of the musculoskeletal system occur characteristically or with higher frequency in the diabetic individuals?

Cheiroarthropathy

Many patients with Type 1 DM (up to 30 percent), especially those with long duration of the disease, manifest waxy skin and stiffness of the small and large joints. This damage is correlated with the presence of microvascular complications.

The involvement of the small hand joints leads to the characteristic inability of palmar surfaces approximation (Figure 20.1, the prayer sign) and the inability of complete extension of the palm.

The skin on the dorsal surfaces of the hands is hard, waxy and cannot be easily tented (see Chapter 18).

These disturbances are partially improved with glycaemic control but do not require any special treatment.

Dupuytren syndrome and carpal tunnel syndrome

People with DM manifest carpal tunnel syndrome as well as Dupuytren syndrome more often (contracture of the palmar fascia, Figure 20.2). This contracture is indeed present in up to 63 percent of diabetics. The third and fourth fingers are involved more frequently (the small finger is not involved as in classic types of the disease). Furthermore, there are often sclerotic nodules on the heels and on the dorsal surfaces of the central interphalangeal joints (Garrod's nodules).

Diabetes in Clinical Practice: Questions and Answers from Case Studies. Nicholas Katsilambros *et al.*
© 2006 John Wiley & Sons, Ltd.

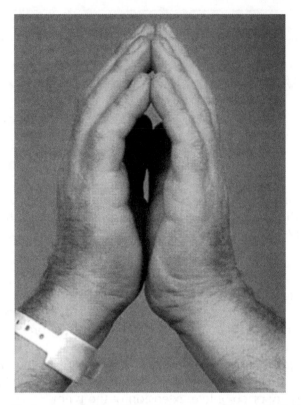

Figure 20.1. Cheiroarthropathy . (Reprinted from Textbook of Diabetes, 3rd edn., J. Pickup & G. Williams, Copyright 2003, with permission from Blackwell Science Ltd.)

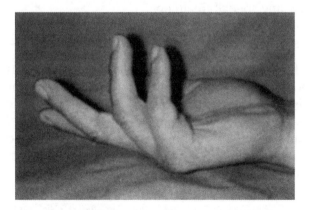

Figure 20.2. Dupuytren contracture.

Shoulder periarthritis

This condition occurs more frequently in diabetics as well as at younger ages. Periarthritis leads to a significant reduction in joint mobility and is rather resistant to treatment. Radiologically, calcifications in ligaments around the shoulder joint are visible, and often these calcifications are asymptomatic.

Osteoarthritis

The relatively increased occurrence of osteoarthritis in individuals with Type 2 DM is probably due to the coexisting obesity.

Charcot neuroarthropathy

Charcot neuroarthropathy is a rare disease (1–2 cases in every 1000 patients) in persons with DM. It usually affects (monoarthritis) the foot (tarsal and metatarsophalangeal joints). The characteristics of the person with DM who develops the disease are:

1. long duration of the illness (> 10 years);
2. poor glycaemic control;
3. usually insulin-dependent DM;
4. peripheral neuropathy and absence of pain (causative factor);
5. coexistence of other complications.

This condition is due to invisible small trauma and microfractures that are favoured both by the diabetic osteopenia and by the severe neuropathy. It leads to destruction and complete disorganization of the joint. The foot is deformed and oedematous and predisposed to the appearance of neuropathic ulcers (see detailed description in Chapter 17 and Figure 17.3 and 17.4).

Diabetic osteopathy

In this lesion, progressive osseous absorption and alterations that almost exclusively concern the leg are observed, initially with circumscribed or diffuse osteoporosis and subcartilagenous osseous cysts. Later on, peripheral erosions, osteolyses and characteristic softening-absorption of the peripheral metatarsal and the central phalangeal edges, sublaxations, fractures and osseous segmentation, appear gradually.

Ankylosing hyperostosis

This condition is characterized by osseous overproduction in the vertebral column, pelvis and peripheral bones. It equally affects both sexes and is more frequent in diabetic individuals. Mild backache and lumbago are characteristic and, radiologically, the lower thoracic spine is more frequently involved. The lesions are mainly found in the anterior segments of the vertebrae and the radiological pictures are 'like half-melt wax in the candlestick' (meloreostosis).

Vertebral hyperostoses (syndesmophyta) present in the anterior and lateral segments of the vertebral bodies. The diagnostic criteria of the disease are:

1. age > 40 of years;
2. explicit involvement of the thoracic spine with hyperostoses in at least four vertebrae with or without osseous conjunction, and only or more in the right side of the vertebral bodies;
3. normal intervertebral spaces;
4. absence of perceptible osteoporosis; normal form-outline of vertebral bodies (apart from hyperostoses);
5. normal sacroiliac joints; absence of osseous ankylosis of the posterior joints;
6. mild backache or lumbago with normal mobility of the spine;
7. absence of symptoms of severe degenerative spondyloarthropathy.

Osteomyelitis and infectious arthritis (see also Chapter 17)

Osteomyelitis and infectious arthritis are more common in persons with DM and often develop in Charcot neuroarthropathy.

Stenotic tenosynovitis de Quervain; other stenotic tenosynovitides

Fibrous hyperplasia and thickening of the tendon sheaths without explicit points of inflammation are often observed in diabetics. This usually involves flexor muscles of the fingers leading to 'trigger finger'.

Is osteoporosis more frequent in diabetic individuals?

According to several studies, the frequency of osteoporosis is higher in individuals with long duration of Type 1 DM. These individuals manifest a reduction of the osseous trabecular mass and significant demineraliza-tion. Both the increased bone absorption and the decreased formation of bone contribute to the pathogenesis of osteoporosis.

Osteoporosis is related to the long-lasting poor control of the disease.

Insufficient insulin availability contributes to the decreased composi-tion of proteoglycans in the bones and in the ligaments.

In Type 2 diabetics, bone mass density is increased compared to that of individuals with Type 1 DM. Moreover, it is not clear if there is increased frequency of osteoporosis compared to the non-diabetic individuals. The usual confounding factor is obesity.

Further reading

Katsilambros, N., Tentolouris, N., Tsapogas, P., Dounis, E. (2003) *Atlas of the Diabetic Foot*. Ed: Wiley.

Katsilambros, N., Verykokkidou, H., Sfikakis, P., Tzanou, A., Daikos, G.K. (1984) *Dupuytren's contracture in diabetes*. European Diabetes Epidemiology Study Group.

Pal, B. (2003) Rheumatic disorders and bone problems in DM. In *Textbook of Diabetes*, (eds J. Pickup and G.Williams) 3rd edn, Blackwell Science Ltd, Oxford, **61**, 1–13.

21

Infections in diabetes

Stavros Liatis

Do diabetic individuals have a higher susceptibility towards infections compared to non-diabetics?

Sufficient data do not exist to substantiate the opinion that diabetics, as a whole, have a higher susceptibility towards infections. However, some infections are more common in diabetic patients, and others present nearly exclusively in these people. Moreover, some infections have a more severe clinical course and manifest a higher frequency of complications in diabetics.

The increased susceptibility of diabetics to certain infections is due to many factors. The polymorphonuclear neutrophils of diabetics have been found to have decreased chemotactic and phagocytic abilities. Furthermore, it seems that the ability of leukocytes to counter the microorganisms after the process of phagocytosis is diminished.

What are the specific characteristics of the common infections in persons with diabetes?

Respiratory tract infections

It has not been proven that DM is an independent risk factor for the development of common upper and lower respiratory tract infections. However, infections from certain micro-organisms are definitely more common in individuals with diabetes. Such micro-organisms are *Staphylococcus aureus*, Gram (−) bacteria and mycobacterium tuberculosis.

Diabetes in Clinical Practice: Questions and Answers from Case Studies. Nicholas Katsilambros *et al.*
© 2006 John Wiley & Sons, Ltd.

Diabetes is a risk factor for bacteraemia in patients with pneumococcal pneumonia and is associated with increased mortality in these individuals. Increased mortality is also seen in patients with DM in whom a respiratory tract infection occurs from streptococcus, *Legionella* and the influenza virus.

It should also be noted that diabetics have a normal immunologic reaction to vaccines. The American Diabetes Association, in their annual guidelines, recommend the vaccination of all individuals with DM against the influenza virus and pneumococcus.

Urinary tract infections

Most studies agree that women with DM have a 2–4 times higher incidence of bacteriuria compared to those without diabetes. Asymptomatic bacteriuria is also definitely more frequent in diabetic women. Nevertheless, the clinical and microbiological characteristics of urinary tract infections do not appear to differ compared to the general population. DM constitutes a predisposing risk factor for the development of serious infections of the upper urinary tract. Thus, diabetic individuals manifest bilateral infections of the upper urinary tract more often, and emphysematous pyelonephritides are also more frequent in these individuals. Finally, DM constitutes a risk factor for the development of urinary tract infections from fungi.

Infections of soft tissues

The infections of the foot are the most frequent infections of soft tissues in individuals with DM and are described in detail in Chapter 17.

Which infections are observed with particularly increased frequency in individuals with DM?

Certain fungal infections

The most frequent fungal infections that present in diabetics are oral candidiasis and candidiasis of the external genital organs. Occasionally, the initial diagnosis of DM is done after measurement of a blood glucose level due to the appearance of similar infections (balanoposthitis or fungal vaginitis).

Malignant otitis externa

This a rare (on absolute frequency) but potentially lethal infection of the outer acoustic canal. The responsible micro-organism, in the majority of cases, is *Pseudomonas aeruginosa*. It presents with pain, otorrhoea and reduction of the acoustic acuity, without fever. If the diagnosis is delayed, the infection can spread, resulting in osteomyelitis of the skull and/or intracranial infection. Ciprofloxacin is usually prescribed, although in neglected cases surgical treatment may also be needed.

Necrotizing fasciitis and myonecrosis

This is a very serious infection of the soft tissues, accompanied by clinical signs of sepsis and constitutes an emergency condition. The infection begins from the subcutaneous tissues and spreads deeper. It is distinguished as either monomicrobial (streptococci are the responsible micro-organisms) or polymicrobial (caused by enterobacteria and anaerobic bacteria – mainly clostridia). The most common sites of infection include the upper and lower extremities and abdominal wall. Mortality reaches 40 percent. Immediate surgical debridement and administration of the proper antibiotics are required, because the patient can very rapidly manifest signs of multiple organ failure.

Fournier's gangrene is a form of necrotizing fasciitis that affects the male genital organs.

Rhinocerebral mucormycosis

Around 50 percent of cases are observed in individuals with DM. The usual predisposing factor is diabetic ketoacidosis. Initially, this condition presents with local symptoms (pain, nasal congestion, rhinorrhoea), whereas later intense headache, fever, visual disturbances and symptoms due to a cranial nerve palsy can occur. Thrombosis of the internal jugular vein or carotid artery can also be evident. The treatment consists in surgical debridement and administration of amphotericin B.

Emphysematous cholecystitis

This is an uncommon infection of the gallbladder, during which there is production of air. Around 35 percent of cases are observed in individuals with diabetes. The clinical picture is initially similar to the usual form of acute cholocystitis, however, there is a male preponderance and gangrene and perforation of the gallbladder are more often observed, resulting in a much higher mortality rate (15 versus 4 percent of patients with the common form of acute cholocystitis). The infection is usually polymicrobial with Gram (−) and anaerobic micro-organisms. A plain abdominal radiograph can reveal the presence of air in the right upper quadrant. The definitive diagnosis is done with the revelation of air in the gallbladder wall on a computed tomographic scan of the abdomen.

Should asymptomatic bacteriuria be treated in diabetic individuals?

Asymptomatic bacteriuria (ASB) is defined as the recovery of the same microbe in at least two consecutive urine cultures in quantity of $< 10^5$ CFU/ml (colony forming units) with a simultaneous absence of clinical symptoms of urinary tract infection. It is seen more frequently in diabetic individuals and especially in diabetic women. In a recent European epidemiological study it was found that 26 percent of diabetic women had ASB versus 6 percent of control subjects.

Factors that have been incriminated in the increased incidence of ASB in diabetic women are hyperglycaemia (and the resultant disturbance of leukocytes' function), poor glycaemic control, more frequent use of urinary bladder catheters (as is observed in diabetics), presence of autonomous nervous system neuropathy and relapsing vaginal infections, as well as the more frequent presence of anatomic abnormalities (also observed in diabetics) such as cystocoele, cystourethrocoele and rectocoele. It appears that the presence of diabetic neuropathy has particular importance. Decreased sensation of the urinary bladder leads to its distention, urinary retention and increased residual urine volume, resulting in an increased sensitivity towards infections as well as the appearance of infections with a smaller initial number of pathogenic micro-organisms.

According to all large studies, there is no difference between the responsible pathogenic microbes in diabetics and non-diabetics.

The importance of ASB lies in the probability of it causing complications and more specifically in the production of upper urinary tract infections and decrease in renal function. It has indeed been observed that upper urinary tract infections are more frequent and more serious in women with Type 2 DM and ASB. This has not, however, been proven for women with Type 1 DM. As regards the effect of ASB on renal function, there are no sufficient data. Only one prospective study (of 18 months' duration) showed that women with Type 1 DM and ASB had a tendency for deterioration of renal function compared to Type 1 diabetic women without ASB; however, the amounts did not reach statistical significance. It should also be noted that the follow-up interval was relatively small. For the resolution of this question, larger and longer-lasting prospective studies are required.

Therefore, returning to the initial question of whether ASB in diabetic women requires treatment or not, it has to be stressed that this question cannot be answered definitively. There are certainly selected cases in which the treatment of ASB is absolutely indicated. Thus, ASB should, without any doubt, be treated in pregnant women with DM, in whom treatment of ASB has been proven to decrease the probability of pyelonephritis as well as the probability of premature birth and low birth-weight infants. The treatment of ASB is also absolutely indicated in individuals who are to undergo urological operations as well as those who have had kidney transplantation.

In the general diabetic population, several experts, mainly Americans, believe that ASB should be treated, aiming at the reduction of upper urinary tract infections, but also – probably – at the protection of the kidneys. European specialists, however, do not on the whole conform to this opinion. The scepticism of many researchers is based on the absence of a large study that proves the benefit of treatment. Recently, a well-planned study in 105 diabetic women with ASB (half of whom received at the beginning of the study antimicrobial treatment for 14 days, while the others received a placebo) showed no difference in the probability of urinary tract infection in the following 27 months between the two groups. In other words, women who received the initial antimicrobial treatment had no benefit at all.

Nevertheless, in order to answer with certainty the question of treatment of ASB in diabetic women, large prospective studies, for longer duration and probably with other treatment strategies are required.

Based on the above evidence, it is not surprising that there is a lack of a generally accepted position concerning the necessity of screening all diabetic women for detection of ASB. The supporters of treatment are in favour of regular screening while the sceptics do not support the regular screening of all diabetic women but only of those at high risk for upper urinary tract infection, such as individuals with neuropathy and/or with urogenital system anatomic abnormalities.

CASE STUDY 1

A 62 year old woman was brought to the hospital because of fever and pain in the left lower extremity. The symptoms had begun two days prior and had shown a constant deterioration. The patient had had known Type 2 DM for 10 years, under treatment with insulin, with poor metabolic control. She also had known diabetic background retinopathy and diabetic neuropathy. Physical examination revealed fever 38.8° C (101.8° F), a pulse rate of 125 beats/min, respiratory rate of 24 breaths/min and arterial pressure of 90/60 mmHg. The entire left lower extremity was oedematous, dark red, hot and sensitive. There were a few haemorrhagic blisters on the anterior surface of the thigh and shin. There was coexistent pain, redness, warmth and sensitivity in the ipsilateral groin, the left lower quadrant and the lower part of the left lateral abdomen. Palpation of the whole left lower extremity, but also the left lateral abdominal wall, revealed crepitus. There was ulceration in the big toe of the left foot with a necrotic eschar. Routine laboratory examinations revealed a haemoglobin level of 13.7 g/dl, white cell count of 13.6 k/mm^3 and plasma glucose level of 358 mg/dl (19.9 mmol/L).

What is the diagnosis? How should the patient be managed? What is the responsible micro-organism? Was there a predisposing factor that led her to this condition?

A plain radiograph of the left lower extremity, and subsequently a computed tomographic scan of the same extremity and the abdomen, were performed. Both exams revealed the presence of a large quantity of air in the soft tissues along the fasciae of the affected lower extremity and the left lateral abdomen. A small quantity of air was also observed in the gastrocnemius muscles. Based on the clinical picture and the above mentioned findings, the diagnosis of necrotizing fasciitis and myonecrosis was considered.

This necrotizing infection is an emergency medical condition. It manifests itself with signs of sepsis, has a fulminant course and a mortality rate of 30–60 percent. The most frequent localizations are the upper and lower extremities as well as the abdominal wall. The prognosis depends on prompt diagnosis and treatment. The revelation of air in the soft tissues, which can be demonstrated on a plain radiograph, ultrasound, computed or magnetic tomography, is very important for the diagnosis. Computed tomography has the advantage of offering information on the extent of necroses as well as on the possible coexistence of intra-abdominal or pelvic abscesses, and it is usually more easily available and cheaper than the magnetic tomography. Computed tomography findings include asymmetrical thickening of fasciae in combination with the presence of air along them. In advanced cases, air is observed in contiguous muscles, and the diagnosis of myonecrosis is complete.

Based on the above diagnosis, the patient was immediately led to the operating room for debridement of necroses. Simultaneously, parenteral administration of liquids, insulin and antibiotics was begun. Specifically, crystalline penicillin G at a dose of 6×10^6 units every 6 hours, clindamycin 900 mg every 8 hours and piperacillin-tazobactam, 4.5 g every 8 hours were administered. The prognosis was poor due to the large extent of affected tissues.

During surgery, extensive necroses of the soft tissues in the muscular aponeuroses of the whole left lower extremity and the abdominal wall were detected, and these extended to the subcutaneous tissue and partly to the gastrocnemius muscles. There was a copious quantity of malodorous purulent fluid with brown colour. Gram stain showed a polymicrobial colonization with Gram (+) cocci and Gram (−) bacteria. Later on, the cultures of necrotic tissues certified the presence of the following microbes: *Staphylococcus epidermidis, Bacteroides ureolyticus, Bacteroides fragilis, Pseudomonas aeruginosa* and *Enterococcus faecalis.*

Necrotic fasciitis is categorized as Type I (infection from at least one anaerobic micro-organism and one or more aerobic) and Type II (caused by group A streptococci, with or without staphylococci). Port of entry of the micro-organism(s) can be some small or large trauma, although often it cannot be found and remains unknown. In the case of this particular patient, the port of entry was very probably the ulcer in the big toe.

In 50 percent of cases of necrotizing fasciitis, DM is the underlying disease (mainly in patients with poor metabolic control). Other predisposing factors for the appearance of this severe infection are alcoholism and morbid obesity.

The cornerstone of treatment is surgical debridement. At the same time antibiotics should be administered. The combination of penicillin with clindamycin and additionally an aminoglycoside or second generation cephalosporin or piperacillin/tazobactam or co-trimoxazole is recommended.

The patient underwent a surgical intervention, during which multiple incisions of the affected soft tissues were performed, with extensive debridement of the necrotic tissues. Afterwards, she was transferred to the intensive care unit, where despite the administration of large doses of antibiotics (as mentioned before), she developed septic shock and died 24 hours later.

Note: It is stressed that necrotizing fasciitis/myonecrosis is more frequent in persons with DM but, in the diabetic population as a whole, it is an infrequent disease. However, the gravity of the illness and the need for immediate medical intervention to save the patient's life necessitated the inclusion of the present case.

In DM, lower extremity gangrene (dry or wet) is much more frequent. Analogous patient cases are reported in Chapter 17.

CASE STUDY 2

A 57 year old woman presented to the hospital because of continuous, blunt pain in the left side of the abdomen, extending to the back, high fevers and vomiting for the previous four days. She also reported mild dysuric symptoms for the last week. She had a history of Type 2 DM for seven years, under treatment with oral antidiabetic medicines. Her glycaemic control was not satisfactory. Physical examination revealed fever (39.2° C [102.6° F]), tachycardia (110 per min), tachypnoea (26 per min) and mild confusion. Arterial blood pressure was normal (130/80 mmHg). Chest and heart examinations were normal. Palpation of the abdomen and percussion of the left flank area revealed tenderness over the left upper quadrant and left lateral abdomen.

The initial haematologic/biochemical tests showed increased white blood cell count (16.6×10^9/L) with 94 percent neutrophils, normal number of platelets (247×10^9/L), ESR 130 mm/hour, plasma glucose 315 mg/dl (17.5 mmol/L), urea 85 mg/dl (14.1 mmol/L), creatinine 1.5 mg/dl (132.6 µmol/L), alkaline phosphatase 623 U/L (normal < 260 U/L), and γGT 83 U/L (normal < 32 U/L). Serum bilirubin levels were within normal limits and transaminase levels slightly elevated (1.5 × above upper limits of normal). Blood pH was 7.33 and HCO_3^- 16 mEq/L. Urinalysis showed 25–30 WBCs per high power field with no ketones. Plasma ketone concentration was normal as well.

A plain abdominal radiograph showed the suspicion of air in the parenchyma of the left kidney, and an abdominal ultrasound revealed a small subcapsular collection of fluid ipsilaterally. A computed tomographic scan of the abdomen showed an increase in the size of the left kidney and intraparenchymal collection of air, and also confirmed the small subcapsular collection of fluid.

A diagnosis of sepsis due to emphysematous pyelonephritis was considered. The patient was hospitalized and hydration and immediate intravenous administration of antibiotics was started. Immediately after blood and urine cultures were taken, she was started on intravenous piperacillin/tazobactam treatment. A urologist was consulted because of the possible need for nephrectomy. It was initially decided to insert a transutaneous (under ultrasound guidance) drainage catheter in the subcapsular fluid collection, through which a small quantity of haemorrhagic fluid was drained. The patient was placed under very close monitoring with a low threshold for nephrectomy in case her condition deteriorated.

Blood and urine cultures isolated *Klebsiella pneumoniae*, which was sensitive to the already administered antibiotics.

Hyperglycemia was controlled within the first 24 hours. After 72 hours the patient's fever had subsided and the acidosis had recently been reversed. The transutaneous catheter was removed because fluid drainage had ceased. The patient was afebrile 15 days later. A computed tomography of the abdomen was repeated, which showed disappearance of both the air from the renal parenchyma as well as of the subcapsular fluid collection. The patient was discharged from the hospital and continued treatment with oral antimicrobials for another 15 days with co-trimoxazole, based on the culture's sensitivities.

Emphysematous pyelonephritis is a rare but serious infection of the kidney, characterized by the production of air, either intrarenally or perirenally. More than 90 percent of cases are observed in diabetic patients. The main microbes that cause the disease are those involved in the usual infections of the upper urinary tract. In most cases *E. coli* is isolated. Less frequently *Klebsiella pneumoniae*, *Proteus mirabilis*, *Pseudomonas aeruginosa*, *Aerobacter aerogenes* and *Citrobacter* are isolated. In 20 percent of cases more than one microbe is isolated. Very occasionally, even fungi can be involved. The typical anaerobic bacteria that produce air are extremely seldomly reported as causes of emphysematous pyelonephritis.

There are no specific symptoms of the disease. Pneumaturia can be present, but this is also observed in fistulas between the intestine and the urinary tract. Only in one third of cases does the plain radiograph detect the presence of air in the parenchyma or perirenally. However, according to other studies, this percentage can be much larger. Ultrasound, although useful for the diagnosis of possible obstructions of the urinary tract, is not sensitive for the localization of air in the kidney. The preferred examination method is the computed tomography of the abdomen, which determines the extent of the disease both intra- as well as perirenally.

There are various classifications of emphysematous pyelonephritis, mainly regarding the localization, extent and form of the presence of air. According to the simplest of these, Type I emphysematous pyelonephritis is characterized by complete absence of fluid collection in the computed tomography as well as by the scattered presence of air. In the Type II form of the disease, collection of fluid intrarenally or perirenally is observed as well as presence of air under the form of small or bigger bubbles in the parenchyma or inside the urinary drainage tract. The latter form has a better prognosis. Other unfavourable prognostic factors are acute renal insufficiency, thrombocytopenia (implying diffuse intravascular coagulation), a disturbed level of conscience and shock.

Together with the proper antimicrobial treatment, the substitution of the usually existing fluid deficit and the correction of hyperglycaemia and electrolyte disturbances are of paramount importance. Traditionally, emergency nephrectomy was the treatment of choice for all cases. Today, this treatment is indicated when the disease is extensive and/or has a fulminant course as well as when there is no response to the initial conservative treatment. Drainage with placement of a transutaneous catheter (under computed tomography or ultrasound) is often used in cases of localized disease and fluid collection.

Further reading

Brook, I. and Frazier, E. (1995) Clinical and microbiological features of necrotizing fasciitis. *J Clin Microbiol*, **33**, 2382–7.

Geerlings, S.E., Stolk, R.P., Camps, M.J., *et al*. (2000) Asymptomatic bacteriuria may be considered a complication in women with diabetes. Diabetes Care, **23**, 744–49.

Geerlings, S., Stolk, R., Camps, M., Netten, P., Collet, J.T., Schneeberger, P., Hoepelman, A. (2001) Consequences of asymptomatic bacteriuria in patients with DM. *Arch Intern Med*, **161**, 1421–7.

Harding, G., Zhanel, G., Nicolle, L., Cheang, M. (2002) (for the Manitoba urinary tract infection study group). Antimicrobial treatment in diabetic women with asymptomatic bacteriuria. *N Engl J Med* **347**, 1576–83.

Hoepelman, A., Meiland, R., Geerlings, E. (2003) Pathogenesis and management of bacterial urinary tract infections in adult patients with DM. *Intern J Antimicrob agents*, **22**, S35–S43.

Huang, J. and Tseng, C. (2000) Emphysematous pyelonephritis. *Arch Intern Med*, **160**, 797–805.

Joshi, N., Caputo, G., Weitekamp, M., Karchmer, A.W. (1999) Infections in patients with DM. *N Engl J Med*, **341**, 1908–12.

Joshi, N., Mahajan, M. (2003) Infection and diabetes in *Textbook of Diabetes*, 3rd edn (eds J. Pickup and G. Williams) Blackwell Science Ltd, Oxford, **40**, pp. 1–16.

Mallet, M., Knockaert, D.C., Oyen, R.H., Van Poppel, H.P. (2002) Emphysematous pyelonephritis: no longer a surgical disease? *Eur J Emerg Med*, **9**, 266–9

Stapleton, A. (2002) Urinary tract infections in patients with diabetes. *Am J Med*, **113**, 80S–84S.

22

Hypertension and diabetes

Konstantinos Makrilakis

How is hypertension defined in DM and what are the targets of therapeutic intervention?

Hypertension in the general (non-diabetic) population is defined as the presence of arterial blood pressure (BP) levels above 140/90 mmHg. These limits were set based on large epidemiological studies (e.g. Framingham Study, Multiple Risk Factor Intervention Trial, etc), which revealed that the risk of cardiovascular complications is considerably increased above these levels, while the risk for lower BP levels, although existent, is not significant enough to justify therapeutic interventions, apart from lifestyle advice. For DM, however, the data from large, controlled, randomized, clinical studies showed that the reduction of BP should be more aggressive in order to decrease the risk of cardiovascular complications. Thus, the UKPDS 36 study (Adler, *et al.* 2000) showed that the reduction of BP levels from 154/87 mmHg (for the control group) to 144/82 mmHg (for the treatment group) decreased considerably the chance of micro- and macro-vascular complications. The HOT (Hypertension Optimal Treatment) Study (Hansson, *et al.*, 1998) showed the benefit of a target diastolic BP reduction to under 80 mmHg for diabetic patients. A later analysis of the data from the UKPDS 38 study examined the risk of cardiovascular complications in relation exclusively to systolic BP and led to the conclusion that the risk in diabetics is smallest for arterial pressures near 120 mmHg for the systolic BP.

Diabetes in Clinical Practice: Questions and Answers from Case Studies.   Nicholas Katsilambros *et al.*
© 2006 John Wiley & Sons, Ltd.

Thus, based on the above studies the guidelines of the Hypertension and Diabetes Executive Working Group of the National Kidney Foundation of the USA include a reduction of BP < 130/80 mmHg. These guidelines were also adopted by the American Diabetes Association. BP levels > 130/80 mmHg in a diabetic individual are considered as hypertension and treatment is recommended. Moreover, in the event of diabetic nephropathy coexistence, with proteinuria of > 1 g 24 hours, more aggressive control of BP for the protection of the diabetic kidney is recommended, with target BP levels of < 120/75 mmHg.

What is the frequency of hypertension in DM?

Hypertension constitutes a frequent problem among diabetic patients. Its frequency differs, however, between Type 1 and Type 2 DM.

Specifically, in Type 1 DM the frequency of hypertension increases with the duration of the disease and has a direct relationship to the appearance of nephropathy in these patients. Hypertension is relatively unknown in patients without nephropathy, and the coexistence of nephropathy and hypertension appears to worsen both conditions. Thus, the incidence of hypertension increases from 5 percent for duration of DM of 10 years, to 33 percent for duration of 20 years and 70 percent for duration of 40 years. Blood pressure begins to increase in these patients (even within the considered normal limits) within three years of the appearance of microalbuminuria (which constitutes the first clinical indication of diabetic nephropathy). Finally, the incidence of hypertension as a whole is roughly 15–25 percent for patients with microalbuminuria and 75–85 percent for those with clinically evident diabetic nephropathy.

For Type 2 DM, however, the relationship of hypertension and DM is more complex. Hypertension often coexists from the beginning of DM diagnosis, together with the other parameters of the metabolic syndrome (obesity, dyslipidaemia, insulin resistance, increased thrombogenesis, endothelial dysfunction). Thus, roughly 40 percent of Type 2 diabetics have hypertension at the time of DM diagnosis. As a whole, roughly up to 75 percent of patients with Type 2 DM develop hypertension during their lifetime.

What is the pathogenetic mechanism for the development of hypertension in DM?

In Type 1 DM, as was already mentioned, hypertension is usually due to the development of nephropathy.

For Type 2 DM, things are not that simple. Both Type 2 DM and hypertension are frequent abnormalities in the general population and it could be considered that their coexistence is subject to chance. In certain cases, however, it appears that there is likely to be common cause for their development. Insulin resistance (see Chapter 3) has been incriminated as the common pathogenetic factor for the development of both Type 2 DM and hypertension. This is due to the fact that certain insulin actions are intensified in situations of insulin resistance, when it appears that there is in reality increased insulin sensitivity for certain actions of insulin. Thus, the hyperinsulinaemia that insulin resistance causes (as regards its action in the entry of glucose into the cells), results as a consequence in an intensification of other insulin actions, for which its sensitivity is preserved. Such actions include increased sodium and water retention from the distal convoluted tubules of the kidney (which leads to an increase in the total sodium load and total blood volume of the body) and the increased activity of Na-K-ATPase activity in the vascular smooth muscle fibres, resulting in increased intracellular concentration of sodium and subsequently of calcium, leading to vasoconstriction and increase of peripheral vascular resistances. In addition, insulin, through actions in the central nervous system, increases the excitation of the sympathetic nervous system, which can contribute to an increase of BP. Also, abnormal activity of insulin on the vascular endothelium in situations of insulin resistance, resulting in decreased production of nitrogen monoxide (NO), has been incriminated in increased vasoconstriction and final development of hypertension. Finally, as is the case in Type 1 DM, in Type 2 the development of nephropathy can also lead to the development and deterioration of hypertension.

It should not be overlooked, however, that certain medicines used in the treatment of idiopathic hypertension (especifically the thiazide diuretics and beta-blockers) most likely have a diabetogenic action, especially when given at high doses, which sometimes complicates the relationship between hypertension and DM. But, on the other hand, certain secondary forms of DM – especially due to endocrine disorders (such as pheochromocytoma, acromegaly, Cushing syndrome, etc.) or due to administration of medicines (such as glucocorticoids, oral contraceptive pills, etc.) – may be associated with development of both DM and hypertension.

What is the effect of hypertension in diabetic patients?

Both hypertension and DM constitute extremely important risk factors for the development of cardiovascular events (coronary artery disease, strokes, peripheral obstructive arteriopathy). However, the coexistence of these two abnormalities has a multiplicative effect on the risk, rather than a simple additive effect. The effects of hypertension on the risk of coronary heart disease mortality in diabetic individuals are increased two to five times, compared to non-diabetics. The frequency of strokes, the appearance of cardiac failure and the probability of peripheral obstructive arteriopathy are also significantly increased in hypertensive diabetic individuals.

Furthermore, the probability of microvascular diabetic complications, mainly nephropathy and retinopathy, are considerably increased by the presence of hypertension. This has also been proven by the beneficial effects that the treatment of hypertension has on the reduction of microvascular complications progress in Type 2 diabetics, as shown in the UKPDS (1998) study.

How often should BP be measured in diabetic patients? What is the recommended method of follow-up?

BP should be measured at diagnosis of DM and then at each doctor's visit. Due to the variability of its measurement, proper conditions and the right technique are of utmost importance for correct recording. The dimensions of the sphygmomanometer cuff should properly fit the size of the patient's arm – the length of the cuff should cover at least 80 percent of the circumference of the arm (bigger than needed cuffs will show false lower blood pressure values, whereas smaller cuffs will show false higher values. The systolic and diastolic blood pressures should also be measured in both arms the first time (and then the arm with the higher pressure should be used). The measurement should be performed both in a sitting and standing position (after at least 1 minute of standing) in order to exclude potential orthostatic hypotension – i.e., fall of systolic BP by 20 mmHg and/or of diastolic by 10 mmHg – which is not that infrequent in diabetic patients (the coexistence of supine hypertension with orthostatic hypotension is a difficult therapeutic problem that can require modification of the pharmaceutical regimen). The patient should rest quietly for at least 10 minutes before the measurement, should not have consumed alcohol, caffeine or nicotine for the previous half an hour and the room temperature should be normal. The BP should ideally be measured at least three times (with intervals of 1–2 min) and the mean of the last two measure- ments used for its recording. It is essential that the cuff deflation be performed slowly, at a rate of 2 mmHg per second during BP measurement.

Sometimes it is useful to record 24-hour ambulatory BP with the use of special equipment for automatic recording, in order to exclude the possibility of 'white-coat hypertension' as well as to diagnose the likely existence of 'not-falling' of BP during the night (non-dippers). This phenomenon increases the cardiovascular risk, even if the BP during the day is normal (it is more frequent in diabetic patients with nephropathy).

Are other examinations needed for patient follow-up?

The diabetic patient should be thoroughly followed up from the standpoint of cardiovascular risk. The interest of the treating physician should not only be focused on the control of arterial pressure and DM, but also on the reduction of the cardiovascular risk as a whole. This requires additional examinations of the cardiac and renal function, the peripheral vessels (mainly of the lower extremities and the carotid arteries) and a lipid profile, as well as intervention in the event of abnormal findings. Routine examinations, such as a 12-lead electrocardiogram and probably an echocardiogram, are usually essential for the detection of possible ischaemic abnormalities, arrhythmias and left ventricular dysfunction-hypertrophy. In the event of symptoms compatible with myocardial ischaemia, an exercise stress test should be performed. Routine tests should also include presence of urine microalbuminuria, blood urea and creatinine measurement, as well as serum electrolytes and lipid levels. Special examinations (for example, scintigraphy of the kidneys, Doppler ultrasound of renal arteries, endocrine examinations for secondary hypertension hyperaldosteronism, pheochromocytoma, etc.) will be ordered depending on the findings of the physical examination and the initial routine tests.

When should the treatment of hypertension in diabetic patients begin and in what way? How long will the treatment last?

Since hypertension in the diabetic individual is defined as the presence of BP levels > 130/80 mmHg, it is obvious that the therapeutic approach should begin when its values exceed these limits. Initially, for blood pressure levels of 130–139/80–89 mmHg, it is advisable for the first approach to be non-pharmaceutical, and to try to reduce the BP with lifestyle modification measures. These include an effort of body weight reduction in obese patients (with diet and exercise), reduction of salt and alcohol consumption, and smoking cessation. Weight loss is the most efficient of these measures, as regards the success of BP reduction (a loss of 10 kg body weight usually produces a BP fall by 5–20 mmHg). A reduction of dietary caloric consumption is very important, with fat restriction, mainly saturated animal fat, being the basic factor. Salt should be limited to less than 6 g per day. Alcoholic beverages should also not exceed 2–3 glasses of wine (or equivalent alcohol quantity in other drinks) for men and 1–2 glasses of wine (or equivalent) for women. Regular physical activity (30–45 min brisk walking per day, for 5–7 days a week, is recommended) will also contribute to the stabilization of weight loss and also has beneficial effects on BP independent from the weight loss. Smoking contributes to vasoconstriction and to an increase of atherogenesis risk, and thus its cessation has multiple beneficial effects.

The effects of the application of these lifestyle modification measures should be monitored by the treating physician. If after three months the BP has not fallen to the target levels (< 130/80 mmHg) or if from the beginning BP was > 140/90 mmHg, it is recommended that antihypertensive pharmaceutical treatment be started. The continuation of treatment (always in combination with lifestyle modification measures) should probably be continued for life, since hypertension is a chronic disease that is almost never cured (unless secondary curable causes are found in the initial physical and laboratory examinations).

Which medicines can be used in the treatment of hypertension in DM and what is the medicine of first choice?

In the event that hypertension is present in a diabetic individual without complications (nephropathy, heart disease, etc.), all categories of anti-hypertensive medicines can be used (Table 22.1). It has not been proven that any category is superior to another with regard to the antihypertensive effect *per se*. The five main categories of antihypertensives (diuretics, beta-blockers, angiotensin converting enzyme inhibitors [ACEIs], angiotensin receptor blockers [ARBs], calcium channel blockers) are usually preferred initially, whereas the remaining categories (a-adrenergic blockers, centrally acting antiadrenergic agents, direct vasodilators) are used when the medicines of first line do not suffice or are not well tolerated. Thus, it is rational to prefer initially cheap and time-honoured medicines, such as diuretics and beta-blockers. Nevertheless, there are adequate data (experimental and clinical) that support the view that ACEIs and/or ARBs exert a particular renoprotective action on diabetic individuals (see also Chapter 14). For this reason many consider these medicines to be the first choice in antihypertensive treatment. It is emphasized, however, that in moderate to severe degree hypertension, it is very frequent that the addition of small doses of a thiazide diuretic is required (see below). Moreover, based on the results of the HOPE study (Heart Outcome and Prevention Evaluation) and MICRO-HOPE (sub-study of HOPE in 3577 diabetic patients), the administration of an ACEI (in this particular study, ramipril) in diabetic patients with history of a cardiovascular event or at least one cardiovascular risk factor, resulted in a significant reduction of cardiovascular risk and cardiovascular mortality. Based on these results the FDA (Food and Drug Administration) in the USA has approved the administration of ramipril in high risk individuals, as defined in this study (including diabetic patients), even if there is no hypertension. It should be emphasized, however, that the very strict goals that have been set for the treatment of hypertension in diabetic patients ($< 130/80$ mmHg) are very difficult to achieve with only one antihypertensive medicine and *most diabetics will need two (or often even three or four) different antihypertensive medications in order to control their blood pressure*. Thus, which medicine to use first is usually of secondary importance, since ultimately more than one will soon be needed. It should be also noticed that thiazide diuretics are preferred against loop diuretics, because they are more effective antihypertensives when the renal function is normal;

Table 22.1. Categories of antihypertensive medicines

Category of medicines	Drastic substance	Dosage (mg/day)	Doses/day
Thiazide diuretics	Indapamide	1.25–2.5	1
	Hydrochlorothiazide	12.5–25	1
	Chlorthalidone	12.5–25	1
Loop diuretics	Furosemide	20–80	2
Thiazide + potassium sparing diuretics	Hydrochlorothiazide + amiloride	12.5–25/ 1.25–2.5	1
Loop diuretics + potassium diuretics	Furosemide + amiloride	20–80/ 2.5–10	1
beta-blockers (without intrinsic sympatho-mimetic activity)	Atenolol	25–100	1
	Betaxolol	5–20	1
	Bisoprolol	2.5–10	1
	Metoprolol	50–200	1–2
	Nebivolol	2.5–10	1
	Propranolol	40–180	1–2
beta-blockers (with intrinsic sympatho-mimetic activity)	Oxprenolol	80–320	2–3
	Pindolol	10–60	2
	Celiprolol	200–400	1
alpha- and beta-blockers	Carvedilol	12.5–50	1–2
Angiotensin converting enzyme inhibitors (ACEIs)	Benazepril	10–40	1–2
	Enalapril	5–40	1–2
	Zofenopril	30–60	1–2
	Imidapril	5–20	1
	Captopril	25–100	2–3
	Quinapril	10–40	1
	Lisinopril	10–40	1
	Perindopril	2–8	1
	Ramipril	2.5–20	1
	Cilazapril	2.5–5	1
	Trandolapril	1–4	1
	Fosinopril	10–40	1
Angiotensin receptor blockers (ARBs)	Valsartan	80–320	1
	Eprosartan	400–800	1–2
	Irbesartan	150–300	1
	Candesartan	8–32	1
	Losartan	25–100	1–2
	Olmesartan	20–40	1
	Telmisartan	40–80	1

(continued)

Table 22.1. (*Continued*)

Category of medicines	Drastic substance	Dosage (mg/day)	Doses/day
Calcium channel	Amlodipine	5–10	1
blockers	Varnidipine	10–20	1
(diydro-pyridines)	Isradipine	5–20	2
	Lasidipine	4–8	1
	Lercanidipine	10–20	1
	Manidipine	10–20	1
	Nisoldipine	10–40	1
	Nitrendipine	10–40	1–2
	Nifedipine	30–60	1
	Felodipine	5–20	1
	Fendiline	50–150	1
Calcium channel	Verapamil	80–360	1–3
blockers (non-diydropyridines)	Diltiazem	120–540	1–2
a-1 blockers	Doxazosin	1–16	1
	Prazosin	2–20	2–3
	Terazosin	1–20	1–2
Antiadrenergics with	Clonidine	0.15–0.8	2
central action	Methyldopa	250–1000	2
Direct vasodilators	Minoxidil	2.5–80	1–2
	Hydralazine	25–100	2

when the serum creatinine is > 2–2.5 mg/dl (176.8–$221.0\,\mu$mol/L), however, their action is deficient and in this case furosemide is preferred.

Certain antihypertensives, however, may in fact have some unfavourable metabolic effects in DM, for example the thiazide diuretics and b-adrenergic blockers – and mainly their combination: they cause a deterioration of glycaemia through induction of insulin resistance and decreased insulin secretion from the pancreas. As a rule, however, this happens with the administration of large doses (as used to happen in the past) and not with the small doses (e.g., hydrochlorothiazide 12.5–25 mg/day) that are usual today. Hypokalaemia and hyperuricaemia from the administration of thiazide diuretics is a characteristic of large doses. Besides, their beneficial effect in the reduction of cardiovascular events in diabetic patients has been shown in many studies, and generally speaking they are considered safe medicines in DM. Characteristically, in the recent ALL-HAT (2000) study, the biggest study ever conducted in hypertension (and with the participation of thousands of diabetic patients), the thiazide diuretic, chlorthalidone, was found to be equally effective in the reduction of hypertension and cardiovascular events as the calcium channel blocker (amlodipine) and the ACEI (lisinopril). The small disturbance that the administration of chlorthalidone caused in the metabolism of blood glucose was without clinical importance.

Based on the above, the practicing physician should be able to use a wide spectrum of antihypertensive medicines and to know their appropriate combinations. Such combinations are the ones that use medicines with a synergistic action as regards to the antihypertensive result and decrease the risk of undesirable effects (since smaller doses from each medicine are used). Examples of such combinations are thiazide diuretics with ACEIs, thiazide diuretics with ARBs, ACEIs with the calcium channel blockers, the a-adrenergic blockers with the b-adrenergic blockers and recently the combinations of ACEIs with ARBs (although larger further studies of this combination are expected). The combination of non-dihydropyridine calcium channel blockers (diltiazem or verapamil) with b-adrenergic blockers should be avoided because of the common negative action of these medicines on cardiac conductivity.

It should also be stressed that in diabetics with particular complications or coexistent diseases, there is an indication for specific medicines in priority (unless certain contraindications exist). Thus, for example, in the event of history of myocardial infarction, the b-adrenergic blockers and ACEIs are indicated, since they have been shown to increase survival. In the event of cardiac insufficiency the ACEIs, the beta-blockers, the ARBs and the loop-diuretics are indicated. In the event of diabetic nephropathy, the ACEIs and ARBs are specifically indicated (see Chapter 14). At the initial administration of these medicines, a usually small increase of serum creatinine is expected (up to 30 percent) that does not constitute a reason for interrupting treatment. Loop-diuretics also help in the event of renal insufficiency with volume overload. In the event of prostate hypertrophy, the a-adrenergic blockers will have a beneficial effect on both conditions. It should be noticed here that in the previously mentioned ALL-HAT study, the a-blocker doxazosin caused an increase in the frequency of cardiac insufficiency and was prematurely withdrawn from the study, but this finding has not been completely evaluated yet as regards its significance (it is likely that the increase in the frequency of new cases of cardiac insufficiency could be due to the interruption of other medicines [ACEIs, beta-blockers] in patients with pre-existing, latent cardiac insufficiency).

CASE STUDY 1

A 63 year old man with a history of Type 2 DM for 10 years, myocardial infarction for five years, hypertension for 10 years and bronchial asthma from a young age, presents to the diabetes clinic for a follow-up visit. His pharmaceutical regimen includes an insulin mixture (slow-rapid acting) 70–30 percent morning-evening and a rapid-acting insulin injection before lunch, together with metformin for his DM, as well as metoprolol 50 mg bid and indapamide 2.5 mg once a day for his hypertension. His DM is under satisfactory control (HbA$_{1c}$: 6.9 percent), without severe or unaware hypoglycaemias. His arterial blood pressure is also under good control (usually 120–130/70–80 mmHg) and his renal function is normal, without microalbuminuria. His primary physician has recommended a change of metoprolol, telling him that there is a risk of it causing hypoglycaemias, that it is contraindicated because of the asthma and that because of his diabetes it would be scientifically more correct to use an antihypertensive medicine of another category, called an angiotensin receptor blocker (ARB), because 'it has been found that it is better in Type 2 diabetics'. The patient asks the opinion of the diabetes centre about this statement. Is the primary physician of the patient right?

Although there are well-founded fears that the use of beta-blockers can cover the symptoms of hypoglycaemia, especially in insulin-treated diabetic patients, this disadvantage should 'be balanced' against the advantages of the use of these medicines. Beta-blockers *do not cause hypoglycaemias on their own,* but can in fact cover the hypoglycaemic adrenergic symptoms (tachycardia, palpitations, perspiration, tremor, nervousness, etc.). Also they can worsen the glycaemic control and perhaps, to some degree, they can even cause the development of DM in predisposed individuals, as was shown in the ARIC (Gress, *et al.*, 2000) study (Atherosclerosis Risk in Communities Study – 28 percent increase in the risk of DM development with the use of beta-blockers). However, their use has been proven to be beneficial in countless studies of hypertensive diabetic patients. In the UKPDS (1998) study for example, atenolol was equally effective as captopril regarding hypertension control and regarding the reduction of microvascular and macrovascular complications as well as the reduction in DM related mortality (by 32 percent). Also, it is proven that in post-myocardial infarction patients, beta-blockers increase survival. The presence of asthma (as well as chronic obstructive pulmonary disease) is only a relative contraindication for the use of these medicines, and depends on the gravity and the frequency of the lung disease exacerbations. Equally relative is the contraindication in the event of peripheral obstructive vascular disease.

Consequently, in this particular patient, there is no particular reason at the moment to the beta-blocker with another medicine. His arterial pressure, as well as his DM, are under good control with the current pharmaceutical regimen. The presence of a history of myocardial infarction makes the use of a beta-blocker imperative (not only should its use not be interrupted, but on the contrary, even if the patient was not using a beta-blocker, a significant reason would exist to start using it, irrespective of blood pressure control, simply because of the increase of post-infarction survival). The history of bronchial asthma in childhood no longer constitutes a problem. The patient also does not report serious or unaware hypoglycaemias. Moreover, the notion that ARBs have a special indication in *all* Type 2 diabetic patients, is not correct. The medicines that inhibit the rennin-angiotensin system (such as the ACEIs and the ARBs) are indicated with priority against other antihypertensives in the event of DM with nephropathy (micro- or macro-albuminuria or renal dysfunction [increase in serum creatinine]). It was already mentioned that antihypertensive treatment can be initiated with medicines of any category, although there are data suggesting that the ACEIs are advantageous in high cardiovascular risk patients (which includes indeed our patient). When there is no nephropathy, any antihypertensive medicine can be used. Since, therefore, BP is under good control ($<130/80\,mmHg$), the medicines (metoprolol and indapamide) are well tolerated, the DM is under satisfactory control and there is no nephropathy, there exists no reason whatsoever for replacement of the antihypertensive medicines at the moment. If the BP were not well controlled, then definitely, given the patient's history of coronary heart disease, another medicine should be added. In this case, a medicine of the ACEI category would be a good choice, given the fact that these medicines also increase the survival in post-infarction patients or generally in patients of high cardiovascular risk, as diabetics are (MICRO-HOPE Study). In any case, the addition (not the replacement of metoprolol) of an ACEI already at this point, should not be considered a mistake, on condition that the patient tolerates it well.

Besides, a small dose of aspirin (80–325 mg/day) should be recommended to the patient for secondary prevention of myocardial infarction.

CASE STUDY 2

A 76 year old woman with a 15-year history of Type 2 DM, and a 20-year history of hypertension and dyslipidaemia, is treated with a sulfonylurea and metformin for her DM and a statin for her dyslipidaemia. Her HbA_{1c} is 8.2 percent. Her antihypertensive regimen includes an inhibitor of angiotensin II receptors (e.g., irbesartan 150 mg) in combination with a thiazide diuretic (e.g., hydrochlorothiazide 12.5 mg) daily. The BP is 150–170/70–80 mmHg in repeated measurements at home and in the doctor's office. Other medicines include aspirin 100 mg daily and a benzodiazepine (e.g., bromazepam 1.5 mg) in the evening before bedtime. Recently the patient complains of frequent episodes of dizziness, weakness, blurred vision and tendency to faint, especially in the morning after rising. This has influenced her quality of life significantly and has created some depression. Her relatives express fears that the patient may suffer a stroke.

It is obvious that the patient is a very high risk individual for cardiovascular diseases, given the multiple risk factors (DM, hypertension, dyslipidaemia, old age). It is also obvious that her DM is under poor control (increased HbA_{1c}), as is her BP. The patient exhibits isolated systolic hypertension (systolic BP > 140 mmHg and diastolic BP < 90 mmHg) with increased pulse pressure (difference of systolic and diastolic pressure). This phenomenon is quite frequent in elderly individuals (> 65 years of age) and also increases their cardiovascular risk. However, this particular patient also presents symptoms compatible with orthostatic hypotension (dizziness, weakness, blurred vision and tendency to faint, especially in the morning after rising) that influence her quality of life.

Orthostatic hypotension is defined as the fall of systolic BP by at least 20 mmHg and/or of diastolic BP by at least 10 mmHg (with or without compatible symptoms) after rising from supine position for 1–5 minutes. It is by no means unusual in elderly individuals (roughly 18 percent in individuals > 65 years), but it is not always symptomatic. Its causes are many, among which DM and the autonomous nervous system (ANS) insufficiency caused by DM are among the most frequent. Dehydration and the use of antihypertensive medications (mainly diuretics and sympatholytics) and antidepressant medicines often also contribute.

The ANS insufficiency (see also Chapter 15: 'Neuropathy') can influence the cardiovascular ANS, with the common appearance of resting tachycardia at early stages and orthostatic hypotension. The mortality increases (roughly 25 percent in 5 years), mainly because of an increase in the sudden death rate. Unfortunately there is no specific therapy for ANS neuropathy, apart from the best possible metabolic control of DM.

Orthostatic hypotension can be treated with various non-pharmacological or even pharmacological interventions. The patient should be educated to rise slowly and gradually from the supine position (first sitting and then standing), especially in the morning when the sensitivity towards orthostasis is more pronounced. Walking under extremely warm conditions should be avoided, because this decreases the venous return and increases the probability of orthostatic phenomena. The reduction of night-time diuresis with the elevation of the head of the bed during sleep by 20 to 30° (it decreases renal perfusion during sleep and increases the activity of the renin-angiotensin-aldosterone system, thus increasing the extracellular fluid volume) is very subsidiary. The patient should be guided not to stand upright without reason and told that crossing the legs periodically when standing (if it is necessary to stand) creates muscle tension and increases BP, with alleviation of orthostatic symptoms. The recommendation for elastic stockings of gradually increasing pressure (from the feet up to the waist) is not well tolerated by most patients. A lot of patients also manifest orthostatic phenomena after a meal (within 60–75 minutes) and the recommendation to eat small meals, with lots of liquids and to avoid work immediately afterwards, is often beneficial. The cessation of medicines that are probably involved in the manifestation of orthostatic hypotension (in the present case diuretics) and the addition of larger salt quantities in the diet can also help in the disappearance of the symptoms. If these lifestyle change interventions have no success, a pharmaceutical approach can be tried. The mineralocorticoid fludrocortisone (Florinef) at doses of 0.1–0.4 mg per day (in combination with increased salt consumption) is the medicine of choice and often helps in the disappearance of symptoms. Side effects can include an increase of supine BP, hypokalaemia, appearance of lower extremity oedema and, rarely, of pulmonary oedema. Furthermore, in patients with anaemia it has been shown that the addition of erythropoietin (25–50 IU/kg subcutaneously, three times a week) ameliorates the orthostatic phenomena.

The coexistence of supine hypertension with postural hypotension when rising (as in this particular patient) constitutes a difficult therapeutic problem. The cessation of the antihypertensive medicines and the addition of salt in the diet or even fludrocortisone for the management of the orthostatic problems may worsen the supine BP. The best solution is an individualized approach of various interventional methods, and mainly the non-pharmaceutical ones that were mentioned above. The recommendation to these patients not to lay down during the day (if they are tired they should rest sitting) and manage the night-time elevated BP with a nitroglycerine patch (only for the evening – remove it in morning before rising) has been proven effective in some studies, but the effectiveness of this approach needs to be confirmed in more studies.

In this particular patient, first of all the existence of the problem should of course be ascertained, with measurement of the BP and pulse in the supine and then in the standing position, after 1–5 minutes of orthostasis. The fall of BP (by at least 20/10 mmHg) with/or without the appearance of symptoms will confirm the diagnosis. The simultaneous failure of an increase in the pulse rate (by more than 20 beats/minute as is the normal physiologic response) will create the suspicion of autonomous nervous system insufficiency. The complete range of the Ewing tests and other more sophisticated and complicated ones are only performed in specialized centres for a more detailed study of the autonomous cardiac nervous system. If an orthostatic disturbance is confirmed, the therapeutic approach could first include the behavioural changes that were previously mentioned, replacement of the diuretic with another antihypertensive medicine (e.g., a calcium channel blocker), recommendation for ample fluid consumption, and perhaps a trial of fludrocortisone. More intensive control of DM should also be attempted. A possible addition of small doses of insulin should be done with caution, because patients with autonomous nervous system insufficiency often manifest a deterioration of their orthostatic hypotension with insulin.

Further reading

Adler, A.I., Stratton, I.M., Neil, H.A., Yudkin, J.S., Matthews, D.R., Cull, C.A., Wright, A.D., Turner, R.C., Holman, R.R. (2000) Association of systolic blood pressure with macrovascular and microvascular complications of Type 2 diabetes (UKPDS 36): prospective observational study. *BMJ*, **321**, 412–9.

ALL-HAT (2002) Major outcomes in high-risk hypertensive patients randomized to angiotensin converting enzyme inhibitor or calcium channel blocker vs diuretic: The Antihypertensive and Lipid-Lowering Treatment to Prevent Heart Attack Trial (ALL-HAT) *JAMA*, **288**, 2981–97.

Biaggioni, I. (2004) Postural hypotension, in *Therapy for Diabetes Mellitus and Related Disorders*, 4th edn, American Diabetes Association, (ed H.E. Lebovitz), pp 458–64.

Gress, T.W., Nieto, F.J., Shahar, E., Wofford, M.R., Brancati, F.L. (2000) Hypertension and antihypertensive therapy as risk factors for Type 2 DM. Atherosclerosis Risk in Communities Study. *N Engl J Med*, **342**, 905–12.

Hansson, L., Zanchetti, A., Carruthers, S.G., Dahlof, B., Elmfeldt, D., Julius, S., Menard, J., Rahn, K.H., Wedel, H., Westerling, S. (1998) Effects of intensive blood pressure lowering and low-dose aspirin in patients with hypertension: principal results of the Hypertension Optimal Treatment (HOT) randomized trial. HOT Study Group. *Lancet*, **351**, 1755–62.

Heart Outcomes Prevention Evaluation Study Investigators. (2000) Effects of ramipril on cardiovascular and microvascular outcomes in people with diabetes mellitus: Results of the HOPE study and MICRO-HOPE substudy. *Lancet*, **355**, 253–9.

Nilsson, P.M. (2003) Hypertension in diabetes mellitus in *Textbook of Diabetes*, 3rd edn (eds J. Pickup and G. Williams), Blackwell Science Ltd, Oxford, **55**, pp. 1–16.

UKPDS Study Group (1998) Tight blood pressure control and risk of macrovascular and microvascular complications in Type 2 diabetes (UKPDS 38) *BMJ*, **317**, 703–13.

23

Lipids and diabetes

Konstantinos Makrilakis

What are the lipids and what is their physiologic function in the body?

The lipids constitute a heterogeneous group of substances, their main characteristic being that they are insoluble in water. They are split into two types: the simple lipids (cholesterol, fatty acids) and the complex ones (triglycerides [glycerin with three fatty acid molecules], cholesterol esters [cholesterol with fatty acids], phospholipids [glycerin with fatty acids and phosphorus] and sphingolipids [ceramides, sphingomyelins]). Depending on the number of double bonds that is contained in the molecules of their fatty acids, the lipids are distinguished by being saturated, mono-unsaturated or poly-unsaturated (with none, one or more double bonds, respectively). The poly-unsaturated fatty acids with their first double bond in the third carbon atom from the end of their carbonic skeleton (this is called 'ω' [omega] carbon atom), are called ω-3 (or n-3), whereas when the first double bond is found in the sixth from the end of the carbonic atom, they are called ω-6 (or n-6) fatty acids.

The lipids play a very important role in the physiologic functions of the body. They are used for storage but also for production of energy when needed (triglycerides and fatty acids in the adipose tissue), for heat insulation, for steroid hormone and vitamin D production (cholesterol), for the production of bile salts (cholesterol), for the structure of cell membranes (cholesterol and phospholipids) and for the co-ordination of various cellular activities (prostaglandins).

Diabetes in Clinical Practice: Questions and Answers from Case Studies.   Nicholas Katsilambros *et al.*
© 2006 John Wiley & Sons, Ltd.

What are the lipoproteins and what are they used for in the body?

Because lipids are insoluble in water, they cannot circulate freely in the blood. For this reason, they are linked with special proteins (the apolipo- proteins or apoproteins) and form complex substances (the lipoproteins) that are soluble in water and can be transported through the blood circulation all over the body. More specifically, the lipoproteins contain a lipid core (from free cholesterol, cholesterol esters, triglycerides and phospholipids) and a protein cover, the apolipoproteins. Lipoproteins are distinguished into five main categories (Table 23.1), depending on their density: chylomicrons, very low density (VLDL), intermediate density (IDL), low density (LDL) and high density lipoproteins (HDL). There are many apolipoproteins (A-I, A-II, A-IV, B-48, B-100, C-I, C-II, C-III, D, E, apo(a)), which not only participate as structural components in the molecule of the various lipoproteins, but also have very important biologic participation in their metabolism. The lipoprotein Lp(a) is a special form of low-density-lipoprotein (LDL), which is surrounded by a special apolipo- protein, the apo(a). It should also be noticed that the fatty acids can circulate in the serum as free fatty acids (FFAs), bound to albumin.

Table 23.1. Classification of lipoproteins

Lipoproteins	Chylomicrons	VLDL	IDL	LDL	HDL
Subclasses				1, 2, 3	2, 3
Diameter (nm)	500	43	27	27, 26.6, 26	9.5, 6.5
Composition (%)					
Proteins	2	10	18	25	55
Triglycerides	85	50	26	10	4
Cholesterol	1	7	12	8	2
Cholesterol esters	3	13	22	37	15
Phospholipids	9	20	22	20	24
Apolipoproteins	B-48, A-I, A-II, C-I, C-II, C-III, E	B-100, A-I, A-II, C-I, C-II, C-III, E	B-100, B-48, E	B-100	A-I, A-II, C-I, C-III, D, E

VLDL: Very low density lipoproteins; IDL: Intermediate density lipoproteins; LDL: Low density lipoproteins; HDL: High density lipoproteins

Epidemiological studies have shown that an increase in the level of total cholesterol (TC) and of low-density-lipoprotein cholesterol (LDL-C) is associated with an increased risk for cardiovascular events. The level of high-density-lipoprotein cholesterol (HDL-C), however, is associated with low risk, both in the general population and in diabetic patients. The lipoprotein Lp(a) level has also been associated with elevated risk for such events.

How are the lipids and lipoproteins metabolized in the body?

The metabolism of lipids and lipoproteins can generally be divided into two overlapping metabolic pathways, the exogenous and the endogenous (Figure 23.1).

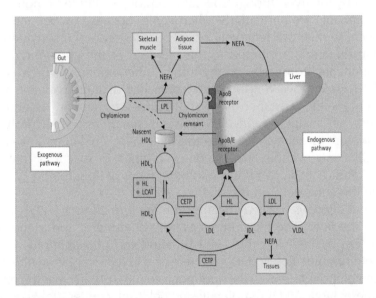

Figure 23.1. Endogenous and exogenous lipid metabolism pathway. LPL = Lipoprotein Lipase, HL = Hepatic Lipase, CETP = Cholesterol Ester Transfer Protein, LCAT = Lecithin Cholesterol Acyltransferase, VLDL = Very low density lipoproteins, IDL = Intermediate density lipoproteins, LDL = Low density lipoproteins, HDI = High density lipoproteins, FFA = Free fatty acids, apoB = apolipoprotein B (Reprinted from Textbook of Diabetes, 3rd edn., J. Pickup & G. Williams, Copyright 2003, with permission from Blackwell Science Ltd.).

In the *exogenous pathway*, the dietary lipids (mainly triglycerides and less so cholesterol), but also the cholesterol emanating from the bile, are absorbed by the intestine in the form of chylomicrons (the main protein component of which is the apolipoprotein B-48). These enter the systemic circulation via the lymphatics and undergo the hydrolytic effect of lipoprotein lipase (LPL), an enzyme found in capillary endothelium (the activity of LPL is increased by insulin and is decreased by apolipoprotein C-III). The FFAs that are released from the chylomicrons are transported in the tissues for storage (as triglycerides in the adipose tissue) or for energy production in the muscles, depending on the needs of the body at that point in time. During the chylomicron hydrolysis, many of their surface components (mainly apolipoproteins) are extracted and transported for the formation of HDL lipoproteins. The residual chylomicron remnants that remain after the hydrolysis of triglycerides are removed by the liver through special receptors. It should be noticed that these remnants are particularly atherogenic, because of their small size and because they are relatively rich in cholesterol. The so-called postprandial lipaemia, attributed to the increase of the chylomicrons and their remnants, constitutes a physiologic phenomenon, which is particularly evident, however, in poorly controlled diabetic patients, as well as when insulin resistance is present (since LPL activity is under the influence of insulin, in insulin resistant situations the hydrolysis of chylomicrons is deficient). Inside the liver cells, chylomicron remnants (that still contain cholesterol) undergo a chain of reactions that 'reassemble' their constitutive lipids into other types of lipoproteins (VLDL) or excrete the cholesterol in the bile.

The *endogenous pathway* begins with the formation of VLDL lipoproteins in the liver. The liver produces both cholesterol and triglycerides, which 'are packed' together with proteins and phospholipids in large lipoprotein-molecules ($VLDL_1$) and released in the circulation (their main protein component is now the apolipoprotein B-100). Due to the effect of LPL, these large $VLDL_1$ molecules expel triglycerides, take on other apolipoproteins and convert into smaller molecules ($VLDL_2$). Then, with the effect of hepatic lipase [HL], they are converted into still smaller molecules, the IDL-lipoproteins, from which finally the LDL-lipoproteins are formed. These are removed from the circulation via special hepatic LDL-receptors (apo B/E receptors). The cholesterol of these LDL molecules is ultimately removed through the intestine (as free cholesterol in the bile or with the bile acids) or is used by the liver cells for their needs.

LDL receptors exist also on all body cells, serving the purpose of taking up cholesterol from the blood and using it for their needs (steroidogenesis, cell membrane synthesis, etc.). In the event that the clearance of LDL by the liver is deficient for various reasons (lack or reduced number of receptors, disturbance in binding with the receptor, etc.), the LDL molecules remain for a long time in the blood, undergo oxidative modification and become atherogenic (they are taken up by macrophages of the vessel wall, which are converted into foam cells – the precocious cells of the atheromatous plaque). During the process of food-derived chylomicron catabolism and the liver-derived VLDL catabolism (i.e., catabolism of the triglycerides containing lipoproteins), many of their surface components are degraded and are transported into small 'nascent' HDL particles, which are initially deprived from cholesterol and cholesterol esters (they contain apolipoproteins A-I and A-II and phospholipids) and can take up cholesterol from the tissues (HDL_3). This cholesterol is subsequently esterified under the effect of a special enzyme (LCAT – Lecithin Cholesterol Acyl Transferase). These mature, larger molecules (HDL_2) can then transfer cholesterol outside of the body (either through special scavenger receptors [$SR-B_1$ receptors] in the liver and the kidneys, or through an exchange of cholesterol esters with triglycerides between the HDL and the apo-B containing lipoproteins [VLDL, IDL, LDL], with the effect of the enzyme CETP [Cholesterol Ester Transfer Protein]). The HDL lipoprotein is therefore useful for the *'reverse cholesterol transport'* from the tissues to the liver and then outside the body. The more efficient the catabolism of the triglycerides' enriched lipoproteins (for example, due to increased activity of the LPL), the higher the concentration of HDL-cholesterol will be.

How is diabetic dyslipidaemia defined and what is its cause?

Blood lipid disturbances differ somewhat between Type 1 and Type 2 diabetic patients.

The lipid profile in Type 1 DM depends, for the most part, on glycaemic control. Poor glycaemic control is associated with hypertriglyceridaemia and, in certain cases, with increased LDL-cholesterol and reduced HDL-cholesterol concentrations. Hypertriglyceridaemia in poorly controlled Type 1 DM is due to two consequences of insulin shortage: to increased VLDL production from the liver and to decreased clearance of these lipoproteins (as well as of chylomicrons) from the circulation, because of decreased activity of the LPL (the action of which is under the influence of insulin). The serum triglycerides levels can be extremely high (> 1600 mg/dl [18.08 mmol/L]), resulting in the likely appearance of skin xanthomata (see Chapter 18, Figure 18.5) from triglyceride deposition. This also increases the risk of acute pancreatitis. Improvement of DM control with the administration of insulin results in normalization of blood lipids.

The typical dyslipidaemia in Type 2 DM includes a slight increase of triglycerides, low levels of HDL-C and normal to slightly elevated levels of total (TC) and LDL-cholesterol (LDL-C). The main problem, however, is that the molecules of low density lipoproteins (LDL) are 'small and dense' and consequently more atherogenic. Thus, focusing only on the measurement of LDL-C concentration can underestimate the risk related to the concentration of the atherogenic lipoprotein molecules in DM. The diabetic hypertriglyceridaemia also emanates (the same as in Type 1 DM) from the overproduction of VLDLs in the liver and the decreased clearance of the triglyceride rich lipoproteins (VLDLs and chylomicrons) from the circulation. This is due to the insulin resistance that accompanies Type 2 DM, resulting in increased lipolysis, with increased supply of FFAs to the liver, as well as to the decreased activity of the LPL. One of the main actions of the latter is to convert the large $VLDL_1$ molecules into smaller $VLDL_2$ ones.

The extended stay of the triglycerides' rich lipoproteins in the circulation leads to the increased exchange of their triglycerides with cholesterol esters in the HDL (as well as in the LDL) through the effect of the enzyme CETP. These exchanges lead to a reduction of the contained cholesterol in the HDL and LDL molecules, that thus become smaller and denser (also due to the hydrolysis of their triglycerides by the hepatic lipase). These small LDL molecules have a decreased affinity for the LDL receptor on the cell surface, remain more in the circulation, undergo oxidation more easily and penetrate the vascular wall more easily, resulting potentially in more vascular damage. They consequently are more atherogenic. This so-called 'type B dyslipidaemia', with the elevated triglycerides concentration (mainly the large $VLDL_1$ molecules), the low HDL-cholesterol concentration (with increase mainly of the small-dense HDL_3) and the increase of the small dense LDL molecules, is not detected during the routine lipid examinations, because the size and the composition of LDL is not measured in everyday practice (these can be measured with special techniques of nuclear magnetic spectro-scopy [NMR spectroscopy]).

An indication of the presence of this kind of dyslipidaemia is the elevated concentration of triglycerides and apolipoprotein B (or the ratio of TC/HDL-C). Indeed, various studies have shown that an increase in the concentration of apo-B can predict cardiovascular events better than the LDL-C level (apo-B reflects the total concentration of the atherogenic molecules VLDL, IDL and LDL, with the LDL containing 95 percent of the circulating apo-B). Furthermore, glycosylation of apo-B (i.e., the non-enzymatic binding of glucose to an aminogroup in apo-B) is considered to be increased in diabetic individuals, which can contribute to the development of atherosclerosis. The glycosylation causes a reduction of the ability to recognize LDLs from the hepatocyte receptors (apoB together with apoE participate in this recognition) and consequently the time of LDL stay in the circulation is increased. The glycosylated LDL is then taken up by macrophages preferentially (via another special receptor). This leads to the formation of the well-known foam-cells, the precursors of the atherosclerotic plaque.

What is the proper treatment of dyslipidaemia in DM?

In poorly controlled Type 1 DM with coexistent hypertriglyceridaemia, as already mentioned, good metabolic control of the blood sugar with insulin therapy usually also restores the triglycerides level to normal.

In Type 2 DM – where obesity and insulin resistance usually coexist – weight loss with diet and physical activity constitute the cornerstone of treatment. It is remarkable, however, that although weight loss and better metabolic control of DM with antidiabetic pills or insulin usually improve the dyslipidaemia, they do not completely restore it to normal levels. The reduction of the particularly elevated cardiovascular risk of these diabetic individuals requires the multifactorial and simultaneous confrontation of all risk factors that are related to the metabolic syndrome (glycaemia, hypertension, obesity and dyslipidaemia) and also the cessation of smoking. Although blood sugar control *per se*, when the other elements of the metabolic syndrome coexist, does not appear to decrease – at least to the expected degree – the risk for cardiovascular complications, reduction of the levels of the individual components of this syndrome (including dyslipidaemia) has been proven to decrease considerably the rate of cardiovascular events, both primary as well as secondary.

What are the targets for reduction of blood lipid levels in the diabetic patient?

The current guidelines from the USA National Cholesterol Education Program – Adult Treatment Panel III (NCEP-ATP III, 2002) determine that initially the concentration of LDL-C (a level of LDL-C < 100 mg/dl, and not the level of other lipids such as HDL-C, triglycerides, etc.) should be taken into consideration before therapy is initiated, since abundant data exist from analyses of diabetic subgroups of large clinical studies (and recently from studies exclusively in diabetic patients as well), that the reduction of LDL-C improves these patients' survival. The treatment target for LDL-C in diabetic individuals is the same as for non-diabetics with a history of coronary heart disease (CHD), since DM is considered equivalent to CHD. Thus, the objective is to achieve an LDL-C level < 100 mg/dl (2.59 mmol/L), while an LDL-C level > 130 mg/dl (3.36 mmol/L) is considered to be an indication to start pharmaceutical hypolipidaemic treatment. For LDL-C levels 100–129 mg/dl (2.59–3.34 mmol/L), a lifestyle change with diet and exercise for 3–6 months is recommended, and if this does not result in the fall of LDL-C to < 100 mg/dl (2.59 mmol/L), the beginning of pharmaceutical treatment is recommended. Furthermore, based on the results of the recently published Heart Protection Study (Collins, *et al.* 2003), the administration of a statin is even considered in diabetic patients > 40 years old with total cholesterol levels > 135 mg/dl (3.49 mmol/L). The aim is to reduce the LDL-C level by roughly 30 percent, independent of the initial LDL-C levels (even for LDL-C levels < 100 mg/dl [2.59 mmol/L]). Afterwards the levels of HDL-C and triglycerides will also be taken into consideration for treatment, aiming at HDL-C of > 40 mg/dl (1.03 mmol/L) for males (> 50 mg/dl [1.29 mmol/L] for females), and at triglycerides of < 150 mg/dl (1.7 mmol/L).

Which medicines are used in the treatment of diabetic dyslipidaemia?

There are currently many medicines in the physician's arsenal for the treatment of diabetic dyslipidaemia (Table 23.2).

Table 23.2. Effect of various hypolipidaemic medicines on serum lipids in the general population

Medicine	LDL-cholesterol	HDL-cholesterol	Triglycerides
Statins*	−20 to −60%	+5 to +10%	−10 to −33%
Bile acid sequestrants (cholestyramine)	−15 to −30%	0 to slight increase	−
Statin + Bile acid sequestrants	−50%	+11 to +18%	−10 to −20%
Gemfibrozil	−10 to −15%	+15 to +25%	−35 to −50%
Micronized Fenofibrate	−6 to −20%	+18 to +33%	−41 to −53%
Nicotinic acid	−10 to −25%	+15 to +35%	−25 to −30%
Inhibitors of cholesterol absorption (ezetimibe)	−18%	−	−

*Atorvastatin and rosuvastatin are more powerful than the other statins and decrease LDL-C by 60% at high doses.

For Type 2 diabetic patients with LDL-C levels > 100 mg/dl (2.59 mmol/L), the statins are recommended as medicines of first choice, since it is proven that not only do they decrease the LDL-C levels with safety and more effectively than any other category of hypolipidaemic medicine, but moreover they decrease the mortality of these patients (both in primary as well as secondary prevention studies). There are nowadays six different statins on the market (Table 23.3), with very good tolerance and effectiveness, although there are differences among them regarding the effective dosage (the most effective statins are rosuvastatin, atorvastatin and simvastatin). These medicines act by inhibiting the hepatic enzyme hydroxyl-methyl-glutaryl-coenzyme A (HMG-CoA) reductase, therefore preventing the production of cholesterol by the liver. In this way the intrahepatic concentration of cholesterol is decreased initially, leading to a compensatory increase in the number of LDL receptors on the hepatocyte surface, aiming at LDL uptake from the blood in order to substitute for the low intrahepatic cholesterol levels. Thus, the concentration of LDL-C in the blood is decreased. The triglycerides levels are also decreased in a dose dependent way and the levels of HDL-C slightly increase.

The most serious side effect of statins is myositis, which is manifested with diffuse myalgias, muscular weakness and increased serum creatine phosphokinase (CPK) concentrations (more than 10 times above the

Table 23.3. Characteristics of statins

Statin	Dose range (mg/day)	Maximum LDL-C reduction (%)	Reduction of serum LDL-C (%)[*]	Reduction of serum triglycerides (%)[*]	Increase of serum HDL-C (%)[*]
Lovastatin	20–80	40	34	16	8,6
Pravastatin	10–80	39	34	24	12
Fluvastatin	20–80	30	24	10	8
Fluvastatin XL	80	35		19	12
Simvastatin	5–80	47	41	18	12
Atorvastatin	10–80	60	50	29	6
Rosuvastatin	5–40	58	58	26	12

[*]The reduction of LDL-C or triglycerides and the increase of HDL-C concern in doses of 40 mg of the various statins. (Modified from: Knopp, R.H., 'Drug treatment of lipid disorders'. *N Engl J Med* 1999; 341: 498 and Schneck, D.W., *et al.* 'Comparative effects of rosuvastatin and atorvastatin across their dose ranges in patients with hypercholesterolemia and without active arterial disease'. *Am J Cardiol* 2003; 91: 33–41)

upper limits of normal). In rare cases it can even lead to rhabdomyolysis and renal damage. The frequency of myositis is exceptionally small (roughly 0.05–0.1 percent), but increases mainly in diabetics with nephropathy (proteinuria), hypothyroidism and liver disease. The appearance of myalgias without myositis presents, in the various studies, at a rate of 2–11 percent. The preventive measurement of serum CPK is not recommended, because it does not predict the future appearance of myositis (a measurement at the beginning of treatment, however, is nonetheless recommended for potential future comparison). The patient should be informed about the symptoms of myositis and be told to stop the medicine in the event of compatible symptoms, to drink lots of fluids and contact their treating physician for measurement of CPK. The incidence of clinically important myopathy is increased in the event of coadministration of a statin with other medicines that inhibit the cytochrome P450-3A4, mainly gemfibrozil, cyclosporin and macrolide antibiotics. The incidence of myositis appears in any case to be smaller with pravastatin, perhaps because of its water solubility. A small percentage of patients (1–2 percent) can also manifest a clinically insignificant, reversible increase of the transaminase levels. It is recommended that their levels should be monitored at the beginning of treatment, after three months and then periodically (especially after each increase of the dose).

After achievement of the LDL-C targets, attention is focused on the triglycerides and HDL-C levels. *Fibrates* – gemfibrozil (at a dose of 600 mg twice a day) and fenofibrate (in the form of micronized capsules 200 mg/day) – are agonists of the nuclear receptors PPAR-α (peroxisome proliferator activated receptors-a) and act mainly in the liver, decreasing serum triglycerides, up to 53 percent (Table 23.2). They also cause a small reduction of the LDL-C (up to 20 percent) and increase the HDL-C quite satisfactorily (up to 33 percent). For this reason they are considered the medicines of first choice for diabetic patients with hypertriglyceridaemia. Fibrates decrease the triglyceride-rich lipoproteins by stimulating (via the activation of PPAR-α receptors) the expression of the LPL gene and by inhibiting the expression of the apoC-III (a powerful inhibitor of LPL). The increased catabolism of the triglycerides-rich lipoproteins leads to the transfer of their surface components for the formation of new HDL molecules. Furthermore, the synthesis of apoA-I and apoA-II is stimulated, which further increases the HDL synthesis. Fibrates also have the advantage of increasing the concentration of the large LDL molecules, which favours the removal of these molecules from the circulation via the special apoB/E receptor in the liver, thus decreasing the diabetic patients' type B dyslipidaemia. These substances can be co-administered with statins (in the event of a combined increase of LDL-C and of triglycerides), but it should be taken into consideration that the risk of myositis increases (to 1–5 percent), most likely because fibrates increase the levels of statins. In as far as it is described, the safest combination of a statin with a fibrate is pravastatin or fluvastatin with fenofibrate (unlike gemfibrozil, it does not interact with statins). Studies utilizing either gemfibrozil (VA-HIT [Veterans Affairs High-Density Lipoprotein Cholesterol Intervention Trial] Study) or fenofibrate (DAIS study [Diabetes and Atherosclerosis Intervention Study]) have shown a reduction of cardiovascular events and mortality in diabetic patients with low HDL-C levels.

Nicotinic acid is the most effective medicine for the increase of HDL-C (Table 23.2), but its utilization in DM is problematic due to the increase of insulin resistance that it causes and the consequent deterioration of metabolic control. In addition, more often than not, it is not well tolerated because of facial flushing. It should also be noted that nicotinic acid is the most effective medicine for the reduction of the atherogenic lipoprotein Lp(a).

Bile acid sequestrants (e.g., cholestyramine) are positively charged resins that are bound to biliary acids in the gastrointestinal tract, preventing their absorption. Since > 95 percent of the bile acids that enter the intestine with the bile are ultimately reabsorbed, this action of resins 'empties' the hepatic pool of bile acids and causes an increase of their synthesis in the liver. Simultaneously a reduction of cholesterol in the liver occurs, which leads to an up-regulation of hepatic LDL receptors and removal of LDL from the blood. Because of the multiple gastrointestinal side effects (bloating, abdominal aches) and the difficulty of patients' compliance with the treatment, the utilization of these resins has been very limited in clinical practice.

A new category of medicines – the selective inhibitors of cholesterol absorption, the first representative being *ezetimibe* – offers a new pioneering approach in the treatment of hypercholesterolaemia. This medicine (at a dose of 10 mg daily) selectively inhibits the absorption of cholesterol at the brush border of the small intestine, without impairing the absorption of triglycerides, fat-soluble vitamins, fatty acids or bile acids. Ezetimibe can decrease serum LDL-C by roughly up to 18 percent and when combined with statins, the reduction of LDL-C is definitely longer. Furthermore, this allows the avoidance of possible side effects from the increase of the dose of statins. At the present, there are no large studies in DM or investigating the action of this medicine with regards to cardiovascular events.

Phytosterols (plant sterols) are steroid substances found in large concentrations in plant oils, seeds and walnuts. They differ from the cholesterol molecule by having an additional methyl or ethyl group in a side chain. They appear to decrease the solubility of cholesterol in the oily and micyleal phase and thus they displace cholesterol from the micylia of bile salts, preventing its absorption. Phytosterols can be considered as complementary factors in the reduction of cholesterol achieved with the proper diet. At present there are no good studies in diabetic patients.

Finally, treatment with oestrogen replacement therapy in postmenopausal women is no longer recommended for the reduction of lipids and cardiovascular risk, because of the revelation that the cardiovascular risk actually increases initially, together with the risk for breast cancer.

CASE STUDY 1

A 58 year old man with a history of Type 2 DM for the last four years presents to the Diabetes Clinic for a routine follow-up visit. His blood sugar is at a relatively good level (HbA_{1c}: 7.0 percent), with morning levels at home usually around 110 mg/dl (6.1 mmol/L) and evening levels around 160 mg/dl (8.9 mmol/L). The physical examination is unremarkable, with the exception of slight obesity (BMI: 30.5 kg/m²). Blood pressure is 128/78 mmHg, and the fundoscopy is without appreciable findings. Recent laboratory examinations show the following: urea 22 mg/dl (3.65 mmol/L); creatinine 0.9 mg/dl (79.6 μmol/L); total cholesterol (TC) 236 mg/dl (6.1 mmol/L); triglycerides (Trigl) 300 mg/dl (3.4 mmol/L); HDL-cholesterol (HDL-C) 34 mg/dl (0.9 mmol/L); and LDL-cholesterol (LDL-C) 142 mg/dl (3.7 mmol/L). The 24-hour urine albumin excretion is 14 mg. His pharmaceutical regimen includes a sulfonylurea and metformin. What you would advise the patient in this visit?

The main problems faced by this patient include slight obesity and dyslipidaemia, as well as blood sugar control. All of these together need to be managed in order to decrease substantially the cardiovascular and the microvascular risk. The patient should be given advice for a hypocaloric and hypolipidaemic diet, together with instructions to increase his physical activity. The blood lipid profile should be repeated in a week or two, in order to confirm the presence of dyslipidaemia (because of the relative variability presented by its measurement). The serum transaminases should also be measured so that a baseline value will be recorded (for likely future comparative use in a hypolipidaemic regimen). Since the blood sugar control is at a relatively good level (HbA_{1c}: 7.0 percent), the patient should be encouraged to make further changes in diet and physical activity and to continue blood sugar monitoring at home. Moreover, after it is ascertained that there are no contraindications, aspirin in small doses should be prescribed to prevent cardiovascular complications (although this treatment is not uniformly accepted).

Ten days later the patient returns with normal serum transaminases levels and unchanged blood lipids levels. What would you advise the patient now?

Since the presence of a typical dyslipidaemia in the frame of Type 2 DM was confirmed (increased triglycerides, low HDL-C levels and normal to slightly elevated levels of TC and LDL-C, but most probably with 'small and dense' molecules of low-density-lipoproteins), and since weight loss with diet and exercise usually improves the dyslipidaemia, but does not restore it to normal levels, as previously mentioned, there exists an indication to begin hypolipidaemic treatment. The current guidelines determine that the concentration of LDL-C should be taken into consideration first before beginning therapeutic treatment. A statin is considered to be the medicine of first choice (Table 23.3), initially at low doses with adjustment of the dose every 2–3 months, until the achievement of the target LDL-C < 100 mg/dl (2.59 mmol/L).

The patient was given advice on lifestyle changes concerning his diet and physical activity and an initial dose of a statin was prescribed (see Table 23.3). Two months later his lipid levels were as follows: TC 215 mg/dl (5.56 mmol/L); HDL-C 35 mg/dl (0.91 mmol/L); Trigl 250 mg/dl (2.82 mmol/L); LDL-C 130 mg/dl (3.36 mmol/L). The transaminases remained within normal limits. What you would suggest now?

Since none of the blood lipid targets has yet been achieved, the LDL-C level should continue to be our first priority. The statin dose should be increased (or be changed to a more effective statin – see Table 23.3). The periodic monitoring of transaminases should be continued and the possible symptoms of myositis-rhabdomyolysis should be explained to the patient (muscular pains, change in the colour of urine) if this has not already been done at the previous visit.

Two months later a repeat of blood lipid measurement showed: TC 182 mg/dl (4.71 mmol/L); HDL-C 36 mg/dl (0.93 mmol/L); Trigl 239 mg/dl (2.7 mmol/L); LDL-C 100 mg/dl (2.59 mmol/L). What you would recommend now?

The LDL-C target has been achieved, but since the triglycerides levels are still high and the HDL-C low, on condition that the glycaemic control is satisfactory, a fibrate could be added (gemfibrozil or fenofibrate) to the existing regimen with the statin. It should be emphasized here that the risk for rhabdomyolysis will be increased slightly with this combination. However, it has been shown that the fibrates increase the size of the LDL molecules and decrease the mortality of diabetic patients with normal LDL-C levels. Consequently, despite the small myositis risk, their use has important benefits. Fenofibrate seems to be superior to gemfibrozil when combined with a statin, because of a smaller probability of interaction and increase of the statin levels in the blood.

The patient received fenofibrate (micronized fenofibrate 200 mg daily) together with the statin, the aspirin and the antidiabetic pills that he was already receiving. Two months later examination of blood lipids showed the following: TC 176 mg/dl (4.55 mmol/L); HDL-C 40 mg/dl

(1.03 mmol/L);   Trigl   190 mg/dl   (2.15 mmol/L);   LDL-C   98 mg/dl (8.66 mmol/L). The cardiovascular risk of the patient has now been considerably decreased.

CASE STUDY 2

A 67 year old woman with a history of DM and hypertension for the last 15 years, obesity (BMI: 31 kg/m², presents at the Diabetes Clinic for a regular visit. She reports that she has smoked 10 cigarettes a day for 35 years. Recent laboratory examinations show total cholesterol 300 mg/dl (7.76 mmol/L), triglycerides 685 mg/dl (7.74 mmol/L), HDL-cholesterol 34 mg/dl (0.88 mmol/L) and LDL-cholesterol 129 mg/dl (3.34 mmol/L). Her renal and hepatic functions are normal and the blood sugar is at a relatively good level, with HbA$_{1c}$ 7.4 percent. The patient reports that her mother, who also suffered from DM, had died at the age of 72 years from a myocardial infarction and she expresses concerns for her own prospects. What you would advise this patient at this visit?

It should first be noticed that the level of LDL-C is not usually directly measured in daily practice, but is instead calculated, based on the Friedewald formula:

$$[LDL\text{-}C] = [TC] - [HDL\text{-}C] - [Trigl/5] \text{ (all values in mg/dl)}$$

This formula is only valid, however, for triglycerides levels < 400 mg/dl (4.52 mmol/L), and consequently the laboratory that measured the blood lipid levels in this patient should not have reported a level for the LDL-C, because based on these data it cannot be calculated. The direct measurement of LDL-C is possible but laborious and complex and is not part of a routine laboratory measurement. The treating clinician should contact the biochemical laboratory for clarification of the matter. The physician should also confirm with the patient that the measurement of blood lipids was performed after an overnight fast of 12–14 hours, in order to ensure that this high triglycerides level does in fact represent fasting hypertriglyceridaemia (an increase of VLDLs) and not post-prandial (increase of chylomicrons).

There is no proof at this point from well performed clinical studies that blood sugar control in diabetic patients decreases substantially the risk of cardiovascular complications in Type 2 DM. The treatment, however, of hypertension and dyslipidaemias, as well as the cessation of smoking, have been proven to decrease this risk. The first priority in the treatment of dyslipidaemia in a diabetic patient, as was mentioned before, is for the level of LDL-C to be < 100 mg/dl (2.59 mmol/L). Usually, however, Type 2 diabetic patients do not have high concentrations of total and LDL-C, but manifest high levels of triglycerides with low levels of HDL-C, precisely as with the patient in our case. The problem is also that these patients have 'small and dense' LDL molecules (type B dyslipidaemia), which renders them more atherogonic. In this particular case, the therapeutic management of such high levels of triglycerides and of low HDL-cholesterol has priority. It is obvious from the very high fasting triglycerides levels that the serum VLDL lipoproteins are significantly elevated, which will inevitably also cause an increase of cholesterol that is contained in this VLDL molecule. The reduction of triglycerides is very likely to have a beneficial effect on the cholesterol level as well. It should also be emphasized that the nutritional treatment of individuals with hypertriglyceridaemia aims at first to reduce the body weight – when this is obese – but also to reduce or prohibit the consumption of alcohol and simple sugars. It is also noticeable that the reduction of blood sugar often brings about a reduction in the elevated triglycerides levels. For this reason, before any hypolipidaemic medicines are administered, it is prudent first to try and achieve glycaemic control as far as possible. If, despite all these measures, the triglycerides levels remain high, it is recommended to start medication. The time of therapeutic lifestyle changes and the effort of blood sugar control is usually individualized, depending on the level of risk for the particular patient, but should not usually exceed 3–6 months. Medicines that mainly decrease the trigly-cerides are the fibrates (gemfibrozil, fenofibrate) and nicotinic acid (see Table 23.2).

The patient was given advice on a hypolipidaemic diet and exercise. Because she was not compliant with the advice, after six weeks she was prescribed gemfibrozil at a dose of 600 mg twice daily, with directions to repeat a fasting blood lipid profile in 6–8 weeks. She was also advised to interrupt the medicine and contact her physician immediately in the event of myalgias or dark urine appearance (for diagnosis of myositis/rhabdomyolysis). Cessation of smoking and monitoring of the arterial pressure and blood sugar at home were also recommended. Two months later the blood lipids levels were as follows: total cholesterol 255 mg/dl (6.59 mmol/L); triglycerides 340 mg/dl (3.84 mmol/L); HDL-C 41 mg/dl (1.06 mmol/L); and LDL-C 146 mg/dl (3.78 mmol/L). The serum transa-minases and creatinine levels were within normal limits.

Since the target for LDL-C (< 100 mg/dl) has not been achieved, and becames the triglycerides levels still continue to be quite elevated, a more powerful hypolipidaemic medicine should be prescribed for their reduction. The combination of a statin with a fibrate once again appears to be the proper combination, even if there are still no studies that confirm the beneficial effect of this combination in cardiovascular events. The replacement of gemfibrozil by fenofibrate should also be considered (for reduction of the risk for myositis). Fenofibrate is generally a very well tolerated medicine, with minimal side effects, which has also been shown to decrease the angiographic progression of coronary heart disease (DAIS study), contributing to the increase in size of LDL molecules. The target for HDL-C (> 50 mg/dl [1.29 mmol/L) in women) is also likely to be approached with this combination. The cessation of smoking and the control of hypertension also constitute equally important factors for this patient.

Further reading

American Diabetes Association. (2004) Dyslipidemia management in adults with diabetes. *Diabetes Care* **27**(Suppl 1): S68–S71.

Athyros, V.G., Papageorgiou, A.A., Athyrou, V.V., Demitriadis, D.S., Kontopoulos, A.G. (2002) Atorvastatin and micronized fenofibrate alone and in combination in Type 2 diabetes with combined hyperlipidemia. *Diabetes Care* **25**: 1198–202.

Colhoun, H.M., Betteridge, D.J., Durrington, P.N. *et al.* (2004) Primary prevention of cardiovascular disease with atorvastatin in Type 2 diabetes in the Collaborative Atorvastatin Diabetes Study (CARDS): Multicentre, randomized, placebo-controlled trial. *Lancet* **364**: 685–96.

Collins, R., Armitage, J., Parish, S., Sleigh, P., Peto, R. (2003) MRC/BHF Heart Protection Study of cholesterol lowering with simvastatin in 5963 people with diabetes: A randomized placebo controlled trial. *Lancet* **361**: 2005–16.

Effect of fenofibrate on progression of coronary-artery disease in Type 2 diabetes: (2001) the Diabetes Atherosclerosis Intervention Study, a randomised study. *Lancet,* **357**, 905–10.

Executive summary of the third report of the National Cholesterol Education Program (NCEP) Expert Panel on Detection, Evaluation and Treatment of High Blood Cholesterol in Adults (Adult Treatment Panel III). (2001) *JAMA* **285**: 2486–97.

Ginsberg, H.N. (2004) Diabetic dyslipidemia, in *Therapy for Diabetes Mellitus and Related Disorders*, 4th edn, American Diabetes Association, (ed. H.E. Lebovitz), pp. 293–309.

Katsilambros, N. (1995) Post-prandial triglyceridaemia (letter). *Diabet Med* **12**: 451.

Poirier, P., Despres, J.P. (2003) Lipid disorders in diabetes, in *Textbook of Diabetes*, 3rd edn, (eds J. Pickup and G. Williams), Blackwell Science Ltd, Oxford **54**: pp. 1–21.

Rubins, H.B., Robins, S.J., Collins, D., *et al.* (1999) Gemfibrozil for the secondary prevention of coronary heart disease in men with low levels of high-density lipoprotein cholesterol. Veterans Affairs High-Density Lipoprotein Cholesterol Intervention Trial Study Group (VA-HIT). *N Engl J Med* **341**: 410–8.

24

Diabetes and driving

Panagiotis Tsapogas

CASE STUDY 1

A 25 year old man, who has had driving licence for car and motorcycle for four years, presents typical symptoms of Type 1 DM and begins intensive insulin treatment. Who is responsible for advising him regarding driving and what advice should he be given?

The physician who makes the diagnosis and begins treatment is obliged to recommend to the newly diagnosed and insulin-treated patient with Type 1 DM that he temporarily interrupt both car and motorcycle driving, until both doctor and patient are as certain as possible that the risk of hypoglycaemias is minimal. Driving *per se* has effects that can cause a reduction of blood sugar levels. In a study, patients with Type 1 DM who were submitted to a driving-simulation test, needed more glucose infusion, presented more autonomic nervous system symptoms, had more tachycardia and more often needed to receive carbohydrates, than control subjects (also with Type 1 DM) who simply watched a driving videotape. Moreover, the perception of hypoglycaemias differs from person to person and so it is essential that the patient knows this complication of treatment with insulin. Hypoglycaemia inhibits the correct estimation of the risk from driving.

When DM is under control and the patient is familiarized with the effects and nature of hypoglycaemias, he can start driving again. Before he starts, he should measure his blood sugar level. His training should include detailed instructions on rapid action carbohydrates intake when hypoglycaemia is imminent. Similarly, alcoholic beverages should be avoided. The recordings of the patient's blood sugar levels should

---

Diabetes in Clinical Practice: Questions and Answers from Case Studies.   Nicholas Katsilambros *et al.*
© 2006 John Wiley & Sons, Ltd.

be regularly checked by the doctor. Furthermore, the patient should be warned that after physical activity or omission of a meal after an insulin injection, he could have a hypoglycaemic event.

CASE STUDY 2

A 25 year old woman with Type 1 DM from the age of 6 years, and who has had several episodes of hypoglycaemia that she always easily perceives, becomes pregnant. Should she be advised not to drive?

Despite the frequent episodes of hypoglycaemia, the patient can recognize and treat them. Pregnancy is not a reason to stop driving. In the case of a patient with gestational DM, who would be supposed to begin insulin treatment for the strict control of DM, the instructions could differ. It would, however, be wise for the patient not to drive until she is familiarized with the hypoglycaemias and with their prevention.

In a patient with insulin-treated DM who drives, it should be repeatedly stressed that before driving she should measure her blood sugar level and correct it with carbohydrate intake in the case of low values (below 70 mg/dl [3.89 mmol/L] according to some authors). Intermediary rests for blood sugar measurements are also obligatory every one or two hours, when the journey is long.

In any case, particular attention should be given to the complications involving the eyes of patients with long-standing DM. Visual disturbances can present in the early stages, when blood sugar fluctuations are large, as well as when diabetic retinopathy is present. It should also be emphasized that vision is not satisfactory for a few hours following the instillation of a mydriatic medicine. Cases of patients who caused car accidents when they drove from the hospital, after undergoing fundoscopy, have been reported.

CASE STUDY 3

A 55 year old man reports a recent car accident. While driving, he lost control of his car, ending up on the pavement, and was unable to explain what happened. He had not drunk any alcohol. The patient is being treated with an intensive insulin-therapy regimen and has satisfactory glycated haemoglobin (6.2 percent). He does not consider the hypoglycaemias to be a serious problem. Would you advise him to stop driving?

Yes. The loss of hypoglycaemia awareness that occurs in a diabetic individual, who is strictly controlled as in our example, is reason to stop driving until the condition is corrected. The frequent hypoglycaemias lead to unawareness of the precursors of hypoglycaemic symptoms, and this situation is often corrected with a change in blood sugar targets for DM control. Specifically, relatively higher blood sugar and glycated haemoglobin levels are acceptable.

The physician should insist on asking the patient for any possible change in the way in which he perceives the hypoglycaemias. Potentially, other members of the patient's family could be asked for their own observations. At the regular follow-up of the patient, the recording of the self-monitored blood glucose values should be checked.

CASE STUDY 4

A 50 year old man, working as the driver of a personnel-transport bus in a company, with typical symptoms of DM for the last year that is not sufficiently controlled with antidiabetic tablets (HbA$_{1c}$ 10.2 percent), refuses to begin treatment with insulin, because he is afraid that he will lose his job. Who is responsible for a possible car accident? Should the company that employs the patient be informed?

The physician should inform the patient and advise him, presenting the scientific medical opinion. The patient should be advised to stop driving until his DM is under control and he is familiar with the hypoglycaemias.

The European legislation reports, regarding driving and DM, that where a new driving licence or renewal of an existing one is requested by diabetic individuals, this should be issued after a medical examination by a specialist doctor, when no complications exist and when road safety is not endangered.

In 2003 the European committee convened a team of experts so that 'they could determine diseases that can influence the mental stability of driving licence holders, such as epilepsy, diabetes, cardiovascular disorders, etc.' Afterwards, it reports that existing studies have already shown that these diseases render a person incapable of riding a motor cycle or driving a mechanically-driven vehicle and awaits the publication of this study in order to adapt the corresponding guidelines.

In Great Britain (Table 24.1) the regulations are prohibitory for insulin-treated patients with regard to certain types of driving licences (C1: vehicles weighing 3.5–7.5 tons), and they impose that the patient can recognize the precursor symptoms of hypoglycaemia. An analytical presentation of the regulations was published recently. The organization

Table 24.1. The British regulations on the driving licences of individuals with DM from the Driver and Vehicle Licensing Authority (modified from DVLA)

	Group 1 (motorcycles and passenger cars)	Group 2 big trucks (category C) and buses (category D)
Insulin treatment A detailed letter is sent to drivers with DM with regards to their licence	The patient should be able to recognize the symptoms of hypoglycaemia and be competent with regard to vision. Licence issued for one, two or three years	Applications for the issuance of driving licences or renewal of authorization in patients who receive insulin are not given for driving certain types of vehicles from 1st April 1991. Drivers with licences prior to 1st April 1991 are dealt with on an individual basis and authorizations are given after a satisfactory exam. Changes that became effective in April 2001 allow exceptions for applications or renewal of applications for vehicles of type C1 (weight: 3.5–7.5 tons) after an annual medical examination. The authorization can be removed according to the law and the patient should make a new application if insulin is interrupted.

Temporary insulin treatment For example: gestational diabetes, after a myocardial infarction, participating in clinical studies with insulin	The patient can maintain the driving licence but he or she should stop driving if a hypoglycemia occurs that does not allow him or her to function. The DVLA should be informed if the treatment continues for more than three months	
Diet and tablets	The patient can maintain the licence up to the age of 70 years unless complications occur, e.g., diabetic damage to the eyes, influencing visual acuity or the optic fields, or if insulin is required for treatment	The drivers can receive a licence unless complications occur, e.g., diabetic damage to the eyes influencing visual acuity or the optic fields, in which case it will either be recommended that the licence issuspended, or a new application can be made, or they can receive a permit for a limited time. If they start insulin, rejection of the application will be recommended or a new application will be completed later
Diet only	The patients do not need to inform the DVLA unless they manifest complications, e.g., diabetic damage to the eyes influencing visual acuity	The patients do not need to inform the DVLA unless they manifest complications, e.g., diabetic damage to the eyes influencing visual acuity or the optic fields, or

(continued)

Table 24.1. (Continued)

	Group 1 (motorcycles and passenger cars)	Group 2 big trucks (category C) and buses (category D)
	or the optic fields, or if insulin is required for treatment	if insulin is required for treatment
Complications of diabetes		
Frequent hypoglycaemic episodes that are likely to influence driving in a negative way	Interruption of driving until satisfactory diabetic control is achieved, after a medical report	The same as insulin-treated persons. Rejection of the application or a new application is recommended
Hypoglycaemia unawareness	If this is confirmed, driving should stop. The patient can restart driving when a medical report assures that hypoglycaemia awareness has been restored	The same as insulin-treated persons. Rejection of the application or a new application is recommended
Complications from the eyes that influence visual acuity or the optic fields	Particular table for disturbances from the eyes is used by DVLC	The same as insulin-treated persons. Rejection of the application or a new application is recommended
Renal complications	Particular table for diseases of the kidneys is used	Particular table for diseases of the kidneys
Disturbances of the extremities e.g., peripheral neuropathy	Particular table is again used	Particular table

responsible for authorizing driving licences (DVLA, Driver and Vehicle Licensing Authority) has judged precisely that a patient with DM, who begins insulin for the first time, should interrupt driving until the diabetes is under control and he or she is familiarized with hypoglycaemia. This is in effect for both people manifesting Type 1 DM for the first time, as well as for people with known Type 2 DM who begin treatment with insulin after initially receiving tablets. The driving licence should be issued for one, two or three years and the patient is re-examined.

Final decisions by the Greek State and the European Union have not been taken, and the same situation exists in the USA. It is obvious that the dilemma for the legislators is large, as expressed in all publications concerning this subject.

Further reading

Arent, S. (2003) The role of health care professionals in diabetes discrimination issues at work and school. *Clinical Diabetes*, **21**, 163–7.

Clarke, W.L., Cox, D.J., Gonder-Frederick, L.A., Kovatchev, B.P. (1999) Hypoglycemia and the decision to drive a motor vehicle by persons with diabetes. *JAMA*, **282**, 750–4.

Cox, D.J., Gonder-Frederick, L.A., Kovatchev, B.P., Clarke, W.L. (2002) The metabolic demands of driving for drivers with Type 1 diabetes mellitus. *Diabetes Metab Res Rev*, **18**, 381–5.

Cox, D.J., Penberthy, J.K., Zrebiec, J., Weinger, K., Aikens, J.E., Frier, B., Steton, B., De Groot, M., Trief, P., Schaechinger, H., Hermanns, N., Gonder-Frederick, L., Clarke, W. (2003) Diabetes and driving mishaps: Frequency and correlations from a multinational survey. *Diabetes Care*, **26**, 2329–2334.

Flanagan, D.E.H., Watson, J., Everett, D., Cavan, D., Kerr, D. (2000) Driving and insulin-consensus, conflict or confusion? *Diabetic Med*, **17**, 316–20.

Gill, G., Durston, J., Johnston, R., MacLeod, K., Watkins, P. (2002) Insulin-treated diabetes and driving in the UK. *Diabetic Med*, **19**, 435–9.

Marrero, D., Edelman, S. (2000) Hypoglycemia and driving performance: A flashing yellow light? (Editorial) Diabetes Care, **23**, 146–7.

MacLeod, K.M. (1999) Diabetes and driving: Towards equitable, evidence-based decision making. *Diabet Med*, **16**, 316–20.

25

Diabetes and travelling

Stavros Liatis

Why do diabetic individuals have to take special precautions when they are going to travel?

Diabetes mellitus should not be considered as an obstacle to travel. However, particular attention is required, because often during a journey situations arise that may lead to possible decompensation of the blood glucose control. Of course, during short, local travels, the problems are usually minimal. However, every long journey should be planned carefully. For very distant travels, the patient should discuss with the doctor, probably in a visit that is exclusively dedicated to this subject, the particular measures and precautions that should be taken. During this visit, the general blood glucose control of the patient is considered and the usual problems that can result during a journey are discussed as well as how these problems should be managed. Things to consider are the type of DM, the therapy being followed, the duration of the journey, the possible time difference, the means of transportation and the place of destination (climate conditions, endemic diseases, level of medical services).

What should the diabetic individual carry on a journey?

- Diabetic identity. It is recommended that this should be clearly visible when worn and that it should report that the individual suffers from DM. This is particularly important for individuals who use insulin. Unfortunately, in our experience (in Greece), very few individuals with DM agree to wear one.

Diabetes in Clinical Practice: Questions and Answers from Case Studies.   Nicholas Katsilambros *et al.*
© 2006 John Wiley & Sons, Ltd.

- Medicines (pills/insulin, syringes, pen(s), backup pen, glucagon kit). The patient should carry at least double the quantity of medicines that is usually required for the time interval of the travel, since significant delays may sometimes occur (extended stays in harbours, airports etc.). It is prudent that the proper quantity of insulin for the whole duration of the stay abroad is carried, since in some countries, problems with the supply of certain insulins may exist. Moreover, care should be taken that direct access to the medicines is available (placement in carrying bags that are not stowed away), both in case of delays, as well as for (the non-infrequent) case of loss, transfer to the wrong destination or theft of the baggages. Individuals who use insulin pumps should pay attention to consumable materials. Also, these individuals should carry with them pen(s) or syringes with the appropriate kind of insulin, in the event of pump dysfunction.
- A doctor's prescription and description of the therapeutic regimen used. During travels abroad, these elements should be written in English and, if possible, in the local language of the country of destination.
- Glucose meter, glucose measurement strips, lancets and acetone strips, in adequate quantities and probably for the entire time period of absence, since consumable materials may not be available abroad.
- Simple carbohydrates for the management of hypoglycaemias should be (glucose candies are recommended) easily to hand and taken in adequate quantities to allow for the possibility of delays.
- Plans that cover the possibility for a modification of the therapeutic regimen during the travel (mainly applies to long air journeys).

How should the insulin be transported?

The vials that contain insulin should be carefully stored, so that the possibility of breakage is minimized. There is no need for ice or special equipment for the transport of insulin, because it can be maintained for a long period at room temperature. However, its exposure to extreme temperatures should be avoided. Thus, during air travels, insulin should not be placed in the baggage storage area of the plane, since very low temperatures prevail that can cause crystallization and a decrease in its activity. Also, long exposure of insulin to solar radiation should be avoided, for example during a summer day at the beach.

What common situations during a journey can cause problems in the control of DM?

Dietary habits should be maintained, as much as possible, during a journey. The food offered in the plane is sometimes inappropriate for diabetics, either because it is very low or very rich in carbohydrates. When travelling abroad, there is often no familiarization with the various local foods (content in carbohydrates) so a problem with glycaemic control can occur. Thus, in the beginning at least, it is wise to stick to international cuisine, if available, and to try unfamiliar foods in small quantities.

Traveller's diarrhoea constitutes a frequent and significant problem for diabetics. Instructions for preventing this should be given (use of bottled water only, avoidance of raw vegetables, fresh juices, and less well-cooked meat, etc.).

Particular attention should be exercised when the destination is a country with hot climate. In such climates, it is possible that a reduction in the dose of insulin is needed. The attention of the diabetic should be drawn to the problems of increased perspiration, the balance of fluids and the protection of the skin from the sun.

More often than not, during a vacation journey, situations of increased physical activity occur. Often, as pont of tourist tours, much more walking than usual is required. Proper directions should be given for adequate hydration and adaptation of the antidiabetic regimen especially to individuals not used to such situations. The physically unfit diabetic should avoid intense physical exercise (e.g., mountaineering, rowing, long swimming) because serious complications can result.

It is particularly important for the diabetic to check the feet daily, since problems due to wounds caused by shoes are more frequent when travelling. It is recommended not to wear new shoes on a journey, because as a rule more walking than usual in involved.

What particular precautions should be taken during long air journeys, when a time difference exists?

The problem with time difference concerns primarily individuals who use insulin treatment and is connected mainly with the injections of long acting insulin. In these travels, when the plane flies from east to west, the

24-hour day 'is elongated'. Thus, the first long-acting insulin injection in the destination, if based on the local time, will be later after the previous one (that was injected in the place of departure) than usual. If the difference of time is small (< 4 hours), no significant problem usually occurs. If, however, the time difference is larger, a modification in the therapeutic regimen is needed. The modification depends on the type of treatment. Usually, the dose of insulin is given on time (based on the new time) and if a significant time gap exists, it is covered with rapid-acting insulin, depending on the blood sugar levels. The same policy is also usually followed when only one dose of long-acting insulin per day is administered (e.g., insulin Glargine). In any case, during long air-travels, frequent measurements of the blood sugar level (every 2–3 hours) are recommended. In insulin-treated Type 2 diabetics there is usually no need for intermediary administration of rapid-acting insulin, even if the dose is delayed for several hours. Instead, it is recommended that these individuals reduce the intake of carbohydrates at the hours of 'insulin gap'.

When the direction of the air travel is from the west to the east, the 24-hour day is 'shortened'. Thus, the first long-acting insulin injection in the destination will be sooner after the previous one (that was administered in the place of departure) than usual. In these cases, a reduction of the last long-acting insulin dose (before departure) is programmed beforehand (usually by 25–50 percent) and administration of the next injection is given regularly, based on the new time at the destination.

In any case, during such a long journey, a less strict glucose control is preferred: the main objective is to avoid hypoglycaemias, which under these conditions can cause more serious problems.

CASE STUDY 1

A Type 1 diabetic patient is going to travel from Athens, Greece, to Los Angeles, USA. There is a 9-hour time difference and the direction of travel is to the west. The patient is treated with an intensified insulin regimen, with insulin Glargine, 24 units, before bedtime and a very-rapid-acting insulin analogue before each meal. The programme of travel is as follows (Greek time): 08.00: departure from Athens; 17.00 arrival in New York; 18.45: departure from New York; 23.30: arrival in Los Angeles. The local time at arrival is 14.30. What instructions should be given to this patient regarding the administration of insulin?

First of all, the administration of the very-rapid-acting insulin analogue is to be continued as before (i.e., before each meal, depending on the blood glucose levels and the carbohydrates content of the meal). As regards insulin Glargine, two alternative solutions were proposed to the patient:

- *Option 1.* Administer Glargine regularly (before bedtime and always based on the local time). In this way, there is an insulin gap without coverage with basic insulin of roughly nine hours duration, from the time of arrival in Los Angeles (14.30 local time/23.30 time in Greece – when the patient was supposed to inject his Glargine insulin dose normally, had he not travelled) until the evening of the same day (when the injection will finally be performed). This gap will be covered using very-rapid-acting insulin analogue every three hours, depending on the blood sugar level (Figure 25.1a).
- *Option 2.* The evening before the departure, split the insulin Glargine dose, aiming at covering the next 33 hours (24 hours of the usual cover + 9 hours of the time difference). Administer half the dose (12 units) at the programmed time (i.e., around 22.00–23.00 hours) and the remainder dose 12 hours later (i.e., 2–3 hours after the departure for New York). The total dose of Glargine can be increased by 25–30 percent because the time period to be covered is increased. Administer the next dose normally, before bedtime, at the day of arrival in the place of destination, based on the local time (Figure 25.1b). In any case, frequently measure blood sugar levels and, if required, correct possible hyperglycaemia with a few units of very-rapid-acting insulin.

CASE STUDY 2

A 61 year old woman with Type 2 DM is treated with a mixture of rapid/medium action insulin at a proportion of 30/70, with a dose of 38 units in the morning and 18 units in the evening, before breakfast and dinner, respectively. Her glucose control is satisfactory (HbA$_{1c}$: 7.2 percent). She is to travel from Greece to Thailand. The schedule of her travel is as follows: 06.00: departure from Athens; 15.30: arrival in Ban-gong (local time: 21.30). Before she travels she asked for instructions from her treating physician with regard to the insulin regimen and its adaptation to the time difference.

The time difference causes the following problem: if the second dose of insulin on the day of travel is done at the local time of the country of arrival (i.e., Thailand's time), the injection will be actually performed six hours earlier (due to the time difference between Greece and Thailand). In order to avoid the accumulation of insulin, it was proposed that the

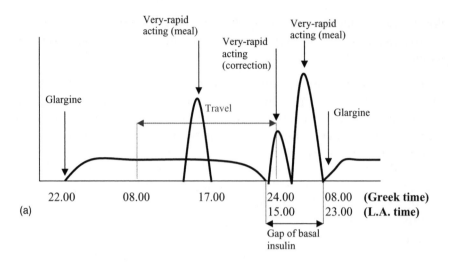

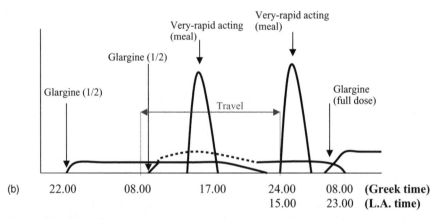

Figure 25.1. Adaptation of insulin regimen in a patient with Type 1 DM who travels to the west by plane: a) Option 1; b) Option 2 (See text).

patient reduce the morning dose by 25 percent (i.e., administration of 28 units instead of 38) and administer the second dose regularly, at Thailand local time. A small reduction of the consumed calories (corresponding to the reduction of insulin) was also proposed to her during the journey, so that the blood glucose does not get out of control, as well as intake of a regular dinner after arrival and the injection of the 'evening' insulin dose.

Further reading

Dewey, C.M. and Riley, W.J. (1999) Have diabetes, will travel. *Postgrad Med*, **105**, 111–3, 117–8, 124–6.

Frier, B.M. (2003) Diabetes mellitus and lifestyle: driving, employment, prison, insurance, smoking, alcohol and travel, in *Textbook of Diabetes*, 3rd edn (eds J. Pickup and G. Williams), Blackwell Science Ltd, Oxford, **68**, pp. 1–18.

Gill, G.V., Redmond, S. (1993) Insulin treatment, time zones and air travel: A survey of current advice from British diabetic clinics. *Diabet Med*, **10**, 764–7.

26

Nutrition and diabetes

Konstantinos Makrilakis and Ioannis Ioannidis

What are the general nutritional principles in DM?

The nutritional recommendations for diabetic patients have been the object of various studies, discussions and revisions over the last 80 years. Before the discovery of insulin in 1921, the nutritional recommendations concerned 'hunger-diets' and an almost complete deprivation of food. After the discovery of insulin, the fear that 'sugar is bad' in DM led to diets of low carbohydrate and high fat content, until it was realized that the high content of fat in the diet, and particularly saturated fat, was what really harmed diabetic patients and led to the complications of the disease, mainly from the cardiovascular system. Today the recommendations for DM have been re-evaluated and include a more liberal approach with regard to carbohydrates and mono-unsaturated fat (basically olive-oil), but more limited with regard to saturated (animal) fat. Also, the supply of plenty of dietary fibre in the diet is considered very important.

The intense research activity of the last decades has contributed considerably to the understanding of the relationship between diet and health, not only for diabetic individuals but for everyone. The positive effect on health of a traditional *Mediterranean diet* has led to it being acknowledged as the very model of a healthy diet. A Mediterranean diet features the following 10 characteristics:

- preferential consumption of olive-oil (in combination with other fats)
- small consumption of animal fats
- large consumption of vegetables

Diabetes in Clinical Practice: Questions and Answers from Case Studies. Nicholas Katsilambros *et al.*
© 2006 John Wiley & Sons, Ltd.

- large consumption of fruits
- large consumption of cereals (preferentially unrefined)
- large consumption of legumes
- moderate consumption of fish
- moderate consumption of dairy products, with emphasis on cheese and yoghurt
- small consumption of meat and meat products
- small to moderate consumption of wine, mainly at meals

A schematic depiction of the above items is presented in Figure 26.1.

It has become increasingly more widely accepted that several aspects of the Mediterranean diet, and more specifically the consumption of olive-oil in combination with vegetables and legumes, can offer, to a large extent, protection from a wide spectrum of chronic diseases (cardiovascular, cancer, etc.). Since olive-oil constitutes a central part of the Mediterranean diet, it is considered important that it be highlighted here. Olive-oil is the main source of mono-unsaturated fat, which is considered particularly beneficial for the body. Recently, emphasis has also recently been given to the micro-constituents of olive-oil, which amount to up to 3 percent of the raw product. Their importance for health seems to be large. At the moment, the antioxidant action of only some these micro-constituents of has been studied, but the research in this sector is intensive and extensive. Olive-oil has 200 micro-constituents, many of which have not been studied yet. Virgin olive-oil, which is extracted without the mediation of high temperatures, has the highest concentration of micro-constituents. In Greece, 85 percent of the produced olive-oil is pure virgin olive-oil. Olive-oil and the complex carbohydrates that are derived from legumes, whole-grain bread and cereals, which appear in abundance in the Mediterranean diet, contribute very little to post-prandial hyperglycaemia, which could prove to be important in the appearance and development of metabolic and other diseases, for example, diabetes mellitus.

There is no doubt that the Mediterranean diet constitutes the cornerstone of the therapeutic management of DM, both of Type 1 (characterized by dependence on insulin) and Type 2 (characterized by insulin resistance and usually accompanied by obesity).

The main objectives of the nutritional approach in DM are to:

- help in the maintenance of blood glucose levels as close to normal as possible;

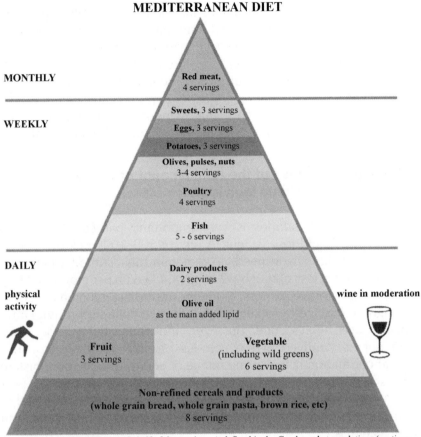

MEDITERRANEAN DIET

MONTHLY — Red meat, 4 servings

WEEKLY — Sweets, 3 servings; Eggs, 3 servings; Potatoes, 3 servings; Olives, pulses, nuts 3-4 servings; Poultry 4 servings; Fish 5 - 6 servings

DAILY — Dairy products 2 servings; Olive oil as the main added lipid; Fruit 3 servings; Vegetable (including wild greens) 6 servings; Non-refined cereals and products (whole grain bread, whole grain pasta, brown rice, etc) 8 servings

physical activity

wine in moderation

One serving equals approximately half of the portions as defined in the Greek market regulations (portions served in restaurants)

Also remember to:
 • drink plenty of water
 • avoid salt and replace it by herbs (e.g. oreganon, basil, thyme, etc)

Source: Supreme Scientific health Council, Hellenic Ministry of Health

Figure 26.1. Schematic depiction of the Mediterranean diet.

- minimize the risk of hypoglycaemias in those who use insulin or insulin secretagogues;
- produce desirable weight loss in the obese and maintenance of a good nutritional status in the young or the elderly;
- help in the control of blood lipids and the arterial blood pressure;
- decrease the future risk of long-lasting complications, like hypertension, dyslipidaemias, nephropathy and primarily the cardiovascular diseases.

It is essential that these objectives take into consideration particular conditions and preferences (cultural, national, individual) as well as the coexistent conditions or illnesses (pregnancy, acute or chronic illness, etc.) of every individual, in order to ensure a better long-lasting adaptation and compliance to the nutritional recommendations. Due to the complexity of the nutritional recommendations, it is considered prudent that a specialized dietitian participates in the therapeutic team that counsels the patient, together with the physician and nursing staff.

What is the importance of the total amount of calories in the diet of the diabetic individual?

The total intake of calories is very important, particularly in obese diabetics who should lose weight. A diet of 500–1000 calories per day less than what the person needs to maintain their current weight, will generally lead to a loss of roughly 2–4 kg (4.4–8.8 lb) per month, which is a healthy degree of weight loss and helps ensure the maintenance of the lost weight (the biggest problem in the management of obesity). During childhood and adolescence, however, individuals with Type 1 DM should not be deprived of the calories essential for their growth. A temporal correlation between the intake of energy and the administered insulin should exist. In general, diabetic individuals who make use of insulin need to synchronize their meals with the administration and the type of insulin, so that they avoid large fluctuations of blood sugar and hypoglycaemias.

What are the main sources of nutritional components of food and what is their caloric value?

The main sources of nutritional components of food are carbohydrates, proteins and fats. Carbohydrates are generally separated into simple (monosaccharides, disaccharides [simple sugars]) and complex ones (polysaccharides, e.g., starch), based on the number of monosaccharide units in their chemical composition. The structural component of proteins is amino-acids. Fats constitute a heterogeneous group of substances with the main characteristic that they are insoluble in water. They are separated into simple fats (cholesterol, fatty acids) and complex ones (triglycerides [glycerin with three molecules of fatty acids], cholesterol esters [cholesterol with fatty acids], phospholipids [glycerin with fatty acids and phosphorus] and sphingolipids [ceramides, sphingomyelins]). Depending on the number of double bonds in the molecules of fatty acids that they contain, fats are separated into saturated, mono-unsaturated and poly-unsaturated ones (with none, one or more than one double bonds, respectively).

The caloric value of the nutritional components is as follows: for carbohydrates, 4 calories (kcal) per gram; for proteins, also 4 kcal/g; and for the fats, 9 kcal/g. It should also be stressed that the thermogenetic action of these nutritional components differs. The thermogenetic action is the energy that is spent by the body for the digestion, absorption and metabolism of foods (it is produced in the form of heat). It is maximal for the proteins, intermediate for the carbohydrates and minimal for the fats. It is therefore evident that fat has a very large potential for energy storage, because of its large caloric value and because of the minimal energy cost of its metabolism and storage. It should also be mentioned that alcohol has a significant caloric value (7 kcal/g).

What is the recommended consumption of carbohydrates by diabetic individuals?

According to current, but also older perceptions, particular preference should be given to the complex carbohydrates (starches) that are rich in dietary fibre (for more on dietary fibre see below). More specifically, foods like whole-grain bread and cereals, fruits, vegetables, legumes, etc. are preferred. These should constitute 50–55 percent of the total energy intake. Alternatively, a lower carbohydrate intake is allowed (< 50 percent, potentially 40 percent) combined with increased intake of mono-unsaturated fatty acids (olive-oil). In any case, saturated (animal) fat intake should be relatively small. As regards the type of carbohydrates, the polysaccharides (complex carbohydrates, such as starch) are absorbed more slowly and do not cause large fluctuations in the blood glucose levels, whereas large quantities of simple carbohydrates (such as common sugar) should generally be avoided because of the fast absorption rate and the effect on glycaemia. Small quantities of simple carbohydrates, however, especially when taken in the context of mixed meals, do not unfavourably influence the glycaemic control and are not contraindicated.

What is the Glycaemic Index and what is its importance?

Food carbohydrates (CHOs) differ in their ability as regards digestion and absorption from the intestine. This depends on various factors, related to the carbohydrates themselves (nature of starch, etc.), the cooking method of the food, its fibre, fat and protein content, as well as other factors – intrinsic or extrinsic to the intestine – that influence the gastrointestinal motility and function. Therefore, consumption of equal quantities of CHOs that are contained in different foods will cause a different glycaemic response in the blood. The concept of the Glycaemic Index (GI) was developed to provide a numerical classification of the post-prandial increase of the blood glucose level after the intake of various CHO-containing foods. The GI denotes the mathematical expression of the increase in blood glucose that is achieved when the test food is compared (regarding glycaemia) with a reference food, when consumed in quantities that contain the same amount of CHO (initially the reference food was glucose, but this was later substituted by white bread).

As shown in the mathematical formula below, the GI is defined as the incremental area under the blood glucose curve (above baseline value) usually two hours after the consumption of 50 g CHO from a test food, divided by the area under the curve after eating a similar amount of CHO of a reference food (usually white bread, which is given a GI value of 100).

$$GI = \frac{\text{Area under blood glucose curve, above baseline value, of the CHO} - \text{containing testfood (2 hours)}}{\text{Area under blood glucose curve, above baseline value, of the reference food (whitebread, 50g)}} \times 100$$

The higher the GI of a food, the faster and higher the blood glucose would be expected to rise after ingestion of the food. The GI depends mainly on the rate of digestion and absorption of the carbohydrate of the food and varies widely among the various foods (Table 26.1).

Although, for the calculation of the GI of a food, a certain amount of CHO in that food (50 g) is always used, in practice it is known that the amount of CHO in the foods consumed daily, varies widely. Because the glycaemic and insulinaemic response depends both on the quality and the quantity of the CHO of the food, the concept of the Glycaemic Load

Table 26.1. Glycaemic Index (GI) and Glycaemic Load (GL) of various foods

Food	GI	Portion	Carbohydrates	GL
White rice	125	1 cup	53	67
Roasted potato	121	1	51	61
Breakfast corn	119	1 cup	24	29
French fries	107	113 g	35	37
Honey	104	1 teaspoon	17	18
Watermelon	102	1 piece	17	17
Carrots	101	½ cup	8	8
White bread	100	1 slice	12	12
Raisins	91	28 g	22	20
Ice-cream	87	½ cup	16	14
Orange juice	81	170 g	20	16
Brown rice	78	1 cup	45	35
Banana	75	1	27	20
Grapes	61	½ cup	14	9
Orange	61	1	16	10
Apple juice	58	170 g	22	13
Spaghetti	58	1 cup	40	23
Apple	51	1	21	11
Chick peas	47	1 cup	45	21
Lentils	40	1 cup	40	16
Whole milk	38	1 cup	12	5
Fructose	33	2 spoonfuls	31	10
Cherries	31	1 cup	24	7

1 cup = 225 ml

(GL) has been introduced, which determines the total glycaemic effect of the consumed food. The GL is defined as the product of the GI with the total dietary CHO composition (per portion) of the test food. Each unit of GL represents the equivalent glycaemic effect of 1 g CHO from white bread, which is used as the reference food. The concept of the GL probably has larger biologic significance than the isolated values of the GI of foods, because it takes into consideration both the quality and the quantity of the CHO of the foods. In this way, foods with small quantities of CHO per portion will cause a small rise of glucose in the blood, even if their GI is high, because their GL will be low. Carrots represent a typical example. Carrot has a relatively high GI (around 101), but the quantity of CHO in a portion of carrots (1/2 a cup) is small (8 g), which yields a small

GL (around 8). So the consumption of a portion of carrots will have a small effect on plasma glucose and insulin concentrations (see Table 26.1).

The GI has only been studied for research purposes so far, but many advocate its use in clinical practice as well. It should be emphasized that there is generally a relative lack of large randomized clinical studies and it is only during the last few years that large epidemiologic and clinical studies have emerged in the literature, examining the relation of the GI with various diseases. Several of these studies have shown the beneficial effects of diets with low-GI foods regarding the prevention or treatment of DM, obesity, cardiovascular diseases, some forms of cancer (especially of the large intestine) and general well-being.

Although it seems reasonable that low-GI foods should be unequivocally preferred as part of a healthy diet, especially by diabetic patients, it should be mentioned that some of the low-GI foods are quite dense in calories, mainly due to their high fat content. Furthermore, there are many factors, besides the food itself, that make its use in clinical practice difficult. For example, the method of preparation, the acidity, the other foods that are served together, the type and content of food in terms of dietary fibre, fat and proteins all influence the GI. Dietary fat can decrease post-prandial glucose levels by delaying gastric emptying. The physical form of the food also has significant effects on post-prandial hyperglycaemia and inulinaemia (generally, the rawer the food, the lower the glycaemic response). The variability of the GI can be very high even in carefully controlled studies the variability (measured as the coefficient of variation) can be as high as 30 percent, which complicates its generalized and uniform use.

At the present time, therefore, the GI has not enjoyed universal acceptance and is not widely used in clinical practice. Despite the up-to-date positive data from its use, it is certain that more long-term studies are needed, in order to reveal the likely beneficial contribution of the adoption of this index in the daily dietary practice of diabetic and non-diabetic individuals.

What are the quantity and type of recommended fat in the diet of diabetic individuals?

The total fat intake should not exceed 35 percent of total energy intake. For obese individuals, this quantity should not exceed 30 percent.

Especially for saturated fat, however, it should not exceed 10 percent of the daily calories (<8 percent if the LDL-cholesterol is increased). The poly-unsaturated fat should not exceed 10 percent of total calories. As was already mentioned, particular emphasis is placed today on the mono-unsaturated fats (main representative, olive-oil), which, together with carbohydrates, are recommended to constitute 60–70 percent of the total energy intake (mono-unsaturated fat may constitute 10 –20 percent of the total energy, on condition that the total fat intake does not exceed 35 percent). The dietary intake of cholesterol is also recommended to be decreased (no more than 300 mg daily – and no more than 200 mg/day for individuals with dyslipidaemia. The trans-fatty acids, which emanate from hydrogenated fats (fried oils, etc.), are very detrimental (equally as saturated fat) and should be avoided. The n-3 fatty acids, found mainly in fish or administered as dietary supplements, are beneficial as regards the reduction of triglycerides, which are often increased in diabetic individuals, but because of the increase in LDL-cholesterol that they cause, they should be used with caution. Two to three portions of fish per week contain an adequate quantity of n-3 poly-unsaturated fatty acids and are generally recommended in the diet of diabetic patients.

What are the guidelines regarding the intake of proteins?

Proteins are recommended to constitute 10–20 percent of total calories, as long as the renal function is normal. In the case of renal insufficiency, a reduction of protein intake to 0.8 g/kg/day is recommended, as well as reduction in the dietary intake of phosphorus and potassium. Moreover, the intake of high biological value protein, from fish, chicken, meat, eggs, etc., is preferred.

What are the recommendations concerning the intake of dietary fibre, vitamins, salt and alcohol?

The intake of an adequate amount of dietary fibre is considered very important. Soluble dietary fibre (pectins, comea, etc.) found in fruits and vegetables is more beneficial than insoluble fibre (cellulose, hemicelluloses) found in cereals, because it decreases the post-prandial glycaemia and acts favourably on blood lipids. It is recommended that the diet of a diabetic person contains at least 20–30 g of dietary fibre daily.

The essential vitamins and trace-elements are usually contained in a balanced diet and it is not necessary for extra quantities to be consumed, except for special situations like pregnancy, old age or coexistent illnesses, when the diabetic individual should consult a registered dietitian and the treating physician (e.g., for addition of folic acid, calcium, vitamins etc.).

The recommendation for salt restriction in the diet concerns all individuals today, since foods contain a much bigger quantity of sodium than humans need. For diabetics this recommendation is even more imperative, since as a whole they constitute a group of people generally considered to be 'salt sensitive', particularly if hypertension coexists (as it frequently does) or, even more crucially, nephropathy. It is recommended that salt intake does not exceed 6 g (i.e., one teaspoon) daily.

Alcohol in small quantities (up to two glasses of wine daily for men and one for women [or equivalent quantities of other alcoholic drinks]) is considered beneficial for the cardiovascular system of diabetic individuals. Larger quantities can be detrimental. The type of alcohol (red wine or other) does not appear to have particular importance.

CASE STUDY 1

A 52 year old woman suffers from Type 2 DM. The diagnosis was made recently (three months ago). Her weight is 83 kg (183 lb) and her height 1.65 m (5 ft, 5 in). Her family doctor recommended that she loses weight and she currently follows a special diet that would help in controlling the blood sugar. She contacted a special centre where she asked, among others questions, if she could (and if she should) consume 'special' foods for diabetic individuals or 'light' products. What are the current opinions regarding these questions?

A frequent question regarding the diet of diabetic individuals concerns the use of sweetening substances that can substitute for sugar. These sweetening substances are classified into two categories:

- sweeteners with calories (fructose, maltodextrin, polydextrose, sorbitol, xylitol, mannitol, isomaltose);
- sweeteners without calories (saccharin, aspartame, cyclamic acid, acetosulphame potassium, sucralose). Note: Aspartame loses its sweetening properties when heated, whereas the remaining substances in this category maintain their sweetening properties with heating.

Fructose is a caloric sweetener that should not be used as a substitute for sugar, since it is converted into glucose very quickly, particularly in uncontrolled diabetic individuals. The other sweeteners of this category (mainly sorbitol or xylitol) are used in chewing gums and sugarless candies. The administration of large quantities of these sweetening substances can cause osmotic diarrhoea and diabetic children can be particularly sensitive to this side effect. It is useful to point out that *a product without sugar does not necessarily mean a product without calories or a product without carbohydrates.*

The second category of sweeteners has no calories and can be used freely. The refreshments known as 'light' contain such sweetening substances and can be consumed relatively freely.

As regards the consumption of special foods for diabetics, their use is not necessary and should not be encouraged. This is especially valid nowadays, when the strict restriction of carbohydrates and the complete avoidance of sugar are no longer recommended. Usually, special diabetic foods contain either fructose or sorbitol, substances that do not present, as already mentioned, any particular advantages. Moreover, many of these products contain a lot of fat, in particular saturated fat. In fact, their use often leads to over-consumption of food, because of the misleading reassurance provided by the spurious label 'special food for diabetics'. For this reason, when such substances are used, they should be included in the daily dietary schedule.

Finally, as regards the 'light' products flooding the market, one should be careful. In order for a product to be characterized as 'light', it should contain at least 25 percent less calories, or other component (e.g., fat), in relation to the corresponding regular product. This means that we need to read carefully the ingredients of these products in order to potentially incorporate them into a diabetic diet. Thus, if a cheese has 20 percent fat content, in comparison to a cheese that contains 40 percent fat, it can be characterized as 'light', but surely cannot be consumed freely by diabetics (it contains calories and a lot of fat!).

CASE STUDY 2

A 62 year old obese man has suffered from Type 2 DM for the last five years. Despite the fact that he follows certain dietary recommendations, his weight has not changed. This surprises and annoys him, because as he characteristically says: 'I've not eaten sweets or sugar for a long time, and I seldom eat spaghetti and potatoes'. Are his comments justified?

Type 2 diabetic individuals are in their vast majority obese. Weight loss constitutes the first and most essential objective of the dietary intervention. This can be achieved only with a hypocaloric diet: *One should eat less calories than one consumes.* In formulating a dietary schedule, therefore, the calculation of the energy needs of the individual has a fundamental role. These depend on age, gender, height and physical activity. The correct calculation of the energy needs of diabetic individuals is of utmost importance. Consequently, the type of macro-nutrient components included in the dietary plan are not decisive in weight loss. The total reduction of calories leads to a reduction of body weight, which involves a very important improvement of the metabolic control. *The diabetic individuals select what they eat but the doctor selects how much they should eat!*

CASE STUDY 3

A 27 year old man suffers from Type 1 DM. He exercises frequently (almost daily) and seeks our advice about changes that he should make in his diet so that it covers his needs while avoiding blood sugar fluctuations (mainly hypoglycaemias).

Whenever a diabetic individual takes on non-programmed muscular work (for example, gardening, sports, etc.), it is essential that he or she receives extra carbohydrates at the beginning or in the middle of the muscular effort. The quantity varies depending on the amount of physical activity (usually 10 to 30 g carbohydrates, for example, a small fruit or up to two slices of bread).

Prolonged exercise may require additional administration of carbohydrates (proportional quantity every 30–45 minutes of moderate to intense physical exercise).

If the exercise is performed on a regular basis, a readjustment of the insulin dose will probably be needed as well as a readjustment of the diet: individuals with increased physical activity have increased caloric needs (that can reach up to 45 calories per kilogram of ideal body weight daily).

In cases of occasional increased physical activity, as for example in the work of farmers, needs can vary depending on the physical activity of a particular day. In these cases it is prudent to recommend two dietary plans with different calorie content (one plan for days of relative rest and one for days of intense work).

Further reading

American Diabetes Association (2004) Nutrition principles and recommendations in diabetes. *Diabetes Care*, **27**(Suppl 1), S36–S46.

Chalmers, K.H., Peterson and A.E. (1999) *Myths of a 'Diabetic Diet'*. ADA, Alexandria.

Dally, A. and Powers, M.A. (2004) Medical nutrition therapy, in *Therapy for Diabetes Mellitus and Related Disorders*, 4th edn, American Diabetes Association, (ed. H.E. Lebovitz), pp. 124–35.

DNSG (2000) Recommendations for the nutritional management of patients with diabetes mellitus. The Diabetes and Nutrition Study Group (DNSG) of the European Association for the Study of Diabetes (EASD), *Eur J Clinic Nutrition*, **54**, 353–55.

Ha, T. and Lean, M.E.J. (1997) Diet and lifestyle modification in the management of non insulin dependant diabetes mellitus, in *Textbook of Diabetes*, 2nd edn, (eds J. Pickup and G. Williams), Oxford, **37**, 1–18.

Katsilambros, N. (2001) Nutrition in diabetes mellitus. *Exp Clin Endocrinol Diabetes*, **109**(Suppl 2), S250–S258.

Mann, J.I., De Leeuw, I., Hermansen, K., Karamanos, B., Karlstrom, B., Katsilambros, N., Riccardi, G., Rivellese, A.A., Rizkalla, S., Slama, G., Toeller, M., Uusitupa, M., Vessby, B. (2004) (on behalf of the Diabetes and Nutrition Study Group (DNSG) of the European Association for the Study of Diabetes (EASD)), Evidence-based nutritional approaches to the treatment and prevention of diabetes mellitus. *Nutr Metab Cardiovasc Dis*, **14**, 373–94.

Trichopoulou, A., Costacou, T., Bamia, C., Trichopoulos, D. (2003) Adherence to a Mediterranean Diet and survival in a Greek population. *N Engl J Med*, **348**, 2599–2608.

27

Treatment of diabetes with pills

Panagiotis Tsapogas

What are the categories of antidiabetic pills?

There are five categories of antidiabetic pills:

- sulfonylureas
- meglitinides
- biguanides
- thiazolidinediones
- alpha-glucosidase inhibitors

The mode of action of these medicines, as well as their therapeutic utilization, is analysed in the following sections.

What is the most important study available as regards the prevention of complications of DM in Type 2 diabetics?

This is the United Kingdom Prospective Diabetes Study (UKPDS) from 1998. This study concerned the roughly decennial follow-up of individuals diagnosed with Type 2 DM. A comparison was performed between conventional (with diet only) and intensive treatment of DM with pills (glibenclamide (glyburide), chlorpropamide, glipizide, metformin and acarbose) and/or insulin, with regard to the prevention of chronic diabetic complications (HbA_{1c} lower by 0.9 percent in the intensive treatment group). Only information received by patients who were treated with glibenclamide, chlorpropamide and metformin were statistically significant enough to allow conclusions to be reached regarding blood sugar control.

Diabetes in Clinical Practice: Questions and Answers from Case Studies. Nicholas Katsilambros *et al.*
© 2006 John Wiley & Sons, Ltd.

This study showed that the intensive treatment of DM with glibencla-mide, chlorpropamide, metformin or insulin can considerably decrease the morbidity of the chronic complications of DM, compared to conventional treatment, without indicating any particular advantage of any of these antidiabetic substances.

SULFONYLUREA

What are sulfonylureas and which type of DM are they indicated for?

These are substances with a chemical structure similar to the sulfonamides that have a hypoglycaemic effect. Initially (1956) tolbutamide was discovered, and then chlorpropamide (1957), acetohexamide (1963) and tolazamide (1966). These were called first generation sulfonylureas. Today these substances are barely used, since the second generation sulfonylureas are now available (Table 27.1), that is, glibenclamide (1969), gliclazide (1972), glipizide (1973) and glimepiride (1994). This latter substance is characterized by some researchers as a third generation sulfonylurea. An important difference of the second generation sulfonylureas is that they are more potent than the first generation ones; also, their metabolites are generally inactive. Therefore, their hypoglycaemic action is more predictable. Their duration of action ranges from 12–24 hours, except for chlorpropamide which reaches 60 hours (its elimination half-life is 36 hours). The binding to plasma

Table 27.1. Second generation sulfonylureas that are on the market. Differences of action and dosage

Substance	Content of tablet	Dosage/day	Tablets/day	Excretion kidneys-faeces (%)
Glibenclamide (Glyburide)	5 mg	2.5–15 mg	1 × 1–3	50–50
Gliclazide	80 mg	40–320 mg	1–2 × 2	70–30
Gliclazide MR	30 mg	30–120	1–2 × 1	
Glipizide	5 mg	2.5–20 mg	1 × 2	80–20
Glimepiride	1, 2, 3, 4 mg	1–6 mg	1 × 1	60–40

albumin is non-ionic in second generation sulfonylureas, whereas it is either ionic or non-ionic in first generation ones. For this reason, the second generation sulfonylureas have a lower probability of interacting with other medicines that compete with them for the binding sites.

Their indications include Type 2 DM, provided that sufficient secretion of insulin by the patient's pancreas exists. They are not indicated for the treatment of Type 1 DM or of secondary diabetes due to pancreatectomy, haemochromatosis or chronic pancreatitis. They should not be administered in pregnancy.

How do sulfonylureas act?

Sulfonylureas are bound to a part of the β-cell cytoplasmic membrane potassium channel, called the sulfonylurea receptor (SUR, see Figure 27.1). This binding causes inhibition of the exit of potassium ions from the β-cell and a change of the cell's resting potential. This results in the opening of special calcium channels of the cytoplasmic

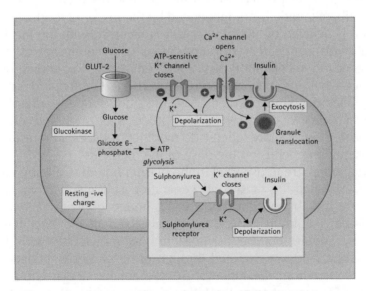

Figure 27.1. Mechanism with which glucose and sulfonylureas cause insulin secretion from the β-cell. (Reprinted from Textbook of Diabetes, 3rd edn., J. Pickup & G. Williams, Copyright 2003, with permission from Blackwell Science Ltd.)

membrane, the entry of calcium ions inside the cell and the stimulation of insulin secretion. This is the way in which the response of the β-cell to glucose and other insulin-secreting stimuli (amino-acids, etc.) is ultimately performed. It is obvious that sulfonylureas act only when the capacity of the β-cell to produce insulin is intact.

How is a sulfonylurea selected and how is it administered therapeutically?

The choice is based on the potency, the dosage (see Table 27.1), the method of metabolism and the probability of causing undesirable side effects. Benefits from their usage, apart from control of blood sugar, that differentiate the second generation sulfonylureas from each other, are discussed below.

Sulfonylureas should be administered 20 minutes before meals, since they achieve drastic levels in the blood circulation one hour after their absorption by the peptic system. In any case, during chronic use, this characteristic is weakened. According to some researchers, the absorption of glibenclamide is not influenced by the intake of food, and that of glipizide is delayed by 90 minutes if it is received with the meal. Their plasma levels are decreased in conditions of hyperglycaemia, perhaps because of the deceleration of stomach emptying. Depending on each substance's half-life, they are administered once (glimepiride) or twice daily (gliclazide, glibenclamide). A recent study supports administration of glibenclamide once a day. Newer products of modified release are administered once a day (gliclazide modified release). The result of the administration depends on the dose of the medicine.

Sulfonylureas are transported in the plasma bound to albumin at > 90 percent. The half-life of second generation sulfonylureas varies (glibenclamide 3–5 hours, gliclazide 8–12 hours, glipizide 2.5–5 hours, glimepiride 5–8 hours). They are metabolized in the liver (which is why they should not be administered to individuals with hepatic insufficiency) and are excreted through urine or stools (glibenclamide by 50 percent from the kidneys, 50 percent by stools, glipizide and gliclazide 70 percent from the kidneys and roughly 10 percent by the stools, glimepiride 58 percent and 35 percent, respectively).

Patients with impaired renal function or the elderly should avoid treatment with sulfonylureas of longer duration of action. Glibenclamide, the most frequently prescribed sulfonylurea, can have a total duration of hypoglycaemic action of 24 hours, since its metabolites maintain their potency at 25 percent that of the full compound and can cause prolonged hypoglycaemias. A similar duration of action has also been reported for gliclazide, the metabolites of which are, however, inactive (as are those of glipizide, which has a shorter duration of action). Glimepiride also has a long duration of action.

Despite its long duration of action, glimepiride does not manifest a significant difference in the pharmacokinetic behaviour between younger and older patients, and does not accumulate in patients with disturbed renal function.

What are the reasons why treatment with a sulfonylurea may fail?

Primary failure occurs when right from the beginning the β-cell is unable to secrete the proper quantity of insulin despite the effect of the medicine.

Secondary failure is manifested after a period of successful action of the medicines and is primarily due to an exhaustion of the β-cell capabilities, as DM progressively worsens.

Which medicines can worsen the control of DM treated with sulfonylureas?

The following medicines can exacerbate DM: medicines that accelerate the sulfonylurea metabolism, such as barbiturates or rifampin; medicines with hyperglycaemic action, such as thiazides and β-adrenergic blockers (they inhibit insulin secretion); and medicines that cause resistance to the action of insulin, like corticosteroids, catecholamines and growth hormones.

Apart from the potency, what other characteristics of insulin secretion differentiate the second generation sulfonylureas from each other?

The levels of insulin in individuals who use different sulfonylureas have been compared in many research studies, since hyperinsulinaemia has been incriminated for the appearance of events that can be related with insulin resistance (myocardial infarctions and strokes). The UKPDS study did not confirm the researchers' concern on this point and it is likely that hyperinsulinaemia constitutes only an indicator for the macrovascular complications and not the direct reason. The newer sulfonylureas glipizide, gliclazide and glimepiride bring about a smaller secretion of insulin than glibenclamide. The insulin secretion after ingestion of gliclazide and glimepiride varies during the day, following the post-prandial insulin requirements. Glibenclamide causes a slow, steadily increasing secretion of insulin from the isolated pancreas, and gliclazide causes a two-phase secretion of insulin and a more rapid return to baseline. In other studies, gliclazide inhibited the oxidation of LDL particles and caused an increase of the antioxidant properties of the plasma both in-vitro and in-vivo, in contrast to many other sulfonylureas.

Apart from their action on the pancreas, are there extrapancreatic actions of sulfonylureas?

Sulfonylureas directly or indirectly influence other metabolic indices as well. For example, glibenclamide was shown to improve post-prandial hypertriglyceridaemia, by decreasing chylomicron concentrations. It also restricts the post-prandial activation of coagulation, by decreasing fibrinogen, the thrombin-antithrombin complexes and the D-dimers. For gliclazide, a favourable action on the retina of diabetic patients has been reported.

Very interesting experimental data have also been reported with regard to the action of sulfonylureas on the heart. Glibenclamide for example does not allow, under experimental conditions, the so-called 'ischaemic preconditioning', a situation that protects, in varied degrees, against myocardial necrosis in the event of an infarction. More specifically, in myocardial ischaemia, when glibenclamide is administered the opening of the K_{ATP} channels does not take place, so that the necessary depolarization and opening up of the calcium channels, which protects the myocardial cell, does not happen. This phenomenon does not happen when glimepiride or gliclazide is administered. In this regard, these sulfonylureas are considered by many authors to be more advantageous compared to the other sulfonylureas. It should be noted, however, that in the UKPDS study, in which glibenclamide was compared with chlorpropamide and insulin, no differences were found with regard to the clinical importance of their use concerning the risk for cardiovascular events.

What are the undesirable effects of sulfonylureas?

The most important undesirable effect is hypoglycaemia, which is usually manifested after the omission of a meal or generally from the inability to eat food for various reasons. Old age and various coexisting diseases (like Addison's disease) are aggravating factors for the manifestation of hypoglycaemia and should be taken into account. Situations that prolong the excretion of the medicine's metabolites (renal or hepatic insufficiency) or other medicines that augment their actions can cause hypoglycaemia. However, studies regarding the safety of second generation sulfonylureas show, for this point, conflicting results. It should also be noticed that glimepiride causes noticeable fewer and milder episodes of hypoglycaemia compared to glibenclamide. This is due to the proportionally smaller insulin secretion that glimepiride causes.

The management of severe episodes of hypoglycaemia in patients treated with sulfonylureas is done in hospital and the patients should be monitored for 48–72 hours. Injections of repeated boluses of glucose solution 35 percent as well as iv infusions of 10 or 20 percent glucose solution are performed. The administration of glucocorticoids may also be required (see Chapter 5).

An increase of body weight, mainly because of blood sugar control and the restriction of glucosuria, is observed after the reception of most sulfonylureas, with differences that are likely due to the bigger or smaller insulin secretion. For this reason, glimepiride is considered preferable in overweight individuals compared to glibenclamide.

Other undesirable effects, however infrequent, are nausea, vomiting and non-specific gastrointestinal disturbances, as well as rashes. Very seldom, haemolytic anaemia, agranulocytosis (for first generation sulfonylureas), jaundice/cholestasis or granulomatous hepatitis and allergy have been reported. Most undesirable effects are expressed in the first 2–3 months of reception of the medicine.

Chlorpropamide has been reported as causing water retention and hyponatraemia (antidiuretic action), and also flushing after alcohol ingestion, a phenomenon that infrequently can also be caused by glibenclamide.

CASE STUDY 1

An 85 year old man, a nursing home resident, was transported to the emergency room because of communication disturbances and the inability to receive food and water. This had been observed for the previous 12 hours and had worsened gradually up to the point of coma. During the previous week, the patient had received bromazepam tablets (Lexotanil) because of insomnia. The patient suffered from Type 2 DM, treated for the last ten years with three doses of glibenclamide 5 mg daily. The last dose had been received in the morning of the same day, six hours before his presentation to the hospital, and the previous evening, together with glibenclamide, he had received two aspirin tablets because of lumbago. At the same time he was being treated with anticoagulants and allopurinol. Before the arrival of the ambulance, the nursing home personnel measured the blood glucose level which was found to be 'Low', (too low to measure). They tried to give him a solution of sugar by mouth, without success.

In the emergency room, the patient opened his eyes and reacted to pain but could not speak. His body weight was 60 kg (132.3 lb) and he was afebrile. The blood glucose meter showed a capillary blood glucose level of 55 mg/dl (3.05 mmol/L), and he was already receiving an infusion of glucose solution 10 percent. Five ampoules of 35 percent, 10 ml, glucose solution were injected intravenously. The serum creatinine was 3.2 mg/dl (282.9 μmol/L). Twenty minutes after the beginning of the infusion, the plasma glucose was 36 mg/dl (2.0 mmol/L). He was given 1 mg glucagon intravenously with a temporary response of his consciousness level and increase of the blood glucose to 90 mg/dl (5.0 mmol/L). During the next 24 hours, repeated blood glucose measurements showed levels between 60 mg/dl (3.3 mmol/L) and 90 mg/dl (5.0 mmol/L). The infusion of the 10 percent glucose solution was continued and at the end of the second day his blood sugar level ranged between 130 mg/dl (7.2 mmol/L) and 160 mg/dl (8.9 mmol/L). His consciousness was restored and he was given frequent carbohydrate-containing meals.

What risk factors for hypoglycaemia did this patient have?

The patient was elderly (> 65 years), potentially malnourished, had renal insufficiency (quite common in old age) and was receiving the most potent form of second generation sulfonylureas, with a prolonged duration of action. The tranquilizer may have meant that he was unable to receive food consequently his level of consciousness was affected. Moreover, he was receiving medicines that intensify the action of sulfonyluyreas.

How does the risk of hypoglycaemia increase in individuals receiving aspirin or other medicines?

Aspirin occupies the binding sites of sulfonylureas to the serum albumin. The problem usually concerns large doses of aspirin. With the same mechanism, fibrates and trimethoprim increase the action of sulfonylureas. Allopurinol and probenecid inhibit the excretion of sulfonylureas from the kidneys. Anticoagulants, alcohol and H_2-blockers prevent their metabolism in a competitive way, while the alcohol also exerts a distinct hypoglycaemic action. Beta-blockers inhibit the action of the counter-regulatory hormones for the hypoglycaemia.

MEGLITINIDES (MEGLITINIDE ANALOGUES)

What is the particular therapeutic characteristic of meglitinides?

Meglitinides have a rapid onset and rapid end to their hypoglycaemic action. This characteristic renders them useful for the control of post-prandial glucose levels and for the avoidance of hypoglycaemias several hours after a meal. Repaglinide and nateglinide tablets are recommended to be taken immediately before a meal. If a meal is skipped, the medicine should not be received. These characteristics are considered as advantages of meglitinides over sulfonylureas.

The main undesirable effect of meglitinides is hypoglycaemia, but this does occur less frequently than the hypoglycaemia caused by sulfonylureas. The increase in the body weight caused by meglitinides is also smaller than that of sulfonylureas.

What is the mechanism of action of meglitinides?

They are bound to the sulfonylurea receptor of the pancreatic β-cell membrane and cause secretion of insulin. The binding occurs at a different part of the receptor compared to sulfonylureas, but as with sulfonylureas, closing of the potassium channels follows, with a subsequent depolarization of the membrane, opening up of calcium channels and entry of calcium ions into the cell. The increased intracellular calcium ions concentration ultimately causes the mobilization of the secretory insulin granules towards the cell membrane and the exit of insulin. The effect of meglitinides restores to some degree the first phase of insulin secretion.

Their action depends on glucose levels. It is interrupted when these are low, and therefore the hypoglycaemias sometimes caused by the action of sulfonylureas, which is prolonged and independent from the glucose levels, are avoided. The action of meglitinides begins after 20–40 minutes and lasts roughly 3–4 hours (nateglinide has the quickest and shortest action of all insulin-secretagogues). There are no data concerning the effect of meglitinides on serum lipids.

In what dosage are meglitinides available?

Repaglinide is available in 0.5, 1 and 2 mg tablets. It is administered at a dose of 0.5–4 mg before each meal and has an elimination half-life of one hour. It is excreted in the stools. It can be used as monotherapy in individuals with Type 2 DM who cannot control their disease with diet alone, or it can be used in combination with metformin.

Nateglinide is available in 60, 120 and 180 mg tablets. It is usually administered at a dose of 60–120 mg before each meal and has an elimination half-life of 1.4 hours. 80 percent is excreted from the kidneys and 10 percent by the stools. It can be used in combination with metformin.

BIGUANIDES (METFORMIN)

CASE STUDY 2

A 40 year old man with a family history of DM comes to the Diabetes Clinic for the second time, three months after his first visit. At the first visit he had been diagnosed as having Type 2 DM, which had manifested after intense family problems, with typical symptoms (polyuria and polydipsia) and balanoposthitis. At that time the patient weighed 102 kg (224.9 lb) and had a body mass index of 33.6 kg/m^2. He had an office job, sitting for long hours, and smoked roughly 30 cigarettes a day. He drank 2–3 glasses of beer 2–3 times per week. His arterial blood pressure was 140/80 mmHg, his glycosylated haemoglobin (HbA$_{1c}$) 10 percent (normal values 4.8–6.2 percent) and his fasting blood glucose 200 mg/dl (11.1 mmol/L). The serum total cholesterol was 294 mg/dl (7.6 mmol/L) and the triglycerides 400 mg/dl (4.52 mmol/L). He had been recommended to follow a diet of 1,700 calories and to start exercising, as well as perform a cardiovascular system check up (exercise stress test, carotid ultrasound), 24-hour urine albumin excretion and serum TSH measurement. He was also prescribed a daily aspirin. The patient followed the diet, as well as a programme of relatively increased physical activity and lost 9 kg (19.8 lb), improving his blood examinations. During the last visit his arterial pressure was 130/80 mmHg, his fasting blood glucose 130–140 mg/dl (7.2–7.8 mmol/L), post-prandial glucose 190–210 mg/dl (10.6–11.7 mmol/L), HbA_{1c} 8.9 percent, serum total cholesterol 212 mg/dl (5.5 mmol/L) and triglycerides 201 mg/dl (2.3 mmol/L). The 24-hour urine albumin excretion and the serum TSH were within normal range, as was a complete chemistry profile. The symptoms had completely subsided. He did not give up smoking, but slightly limited it, and he stopped drinking beer.

After a review of his diet and his general health condition, metformin was recommended at a dose of 850 mg with lunch. Furthermore, a statin was prescribed. The importance of smoking cessation was pointed out to him.

Why was metformin recommended for this particular patient?

The patient did not manage to decrease his blood sugar to desirable levels with diet and exercise. This is the indication for metformin – the only biguanide available – as monotherapy. This particularly concerns obese individuals, since the administration of the medicine is not associated with weight gain (as happens with other medicines) and potentially causes a small weight loss. Metformin is also useful in patients that need to maintain the weight loss achieved with diet and exercise. It is an equally effective antidiabetic medicine in obese and lean individuals with DM.

Risk factors for atheromatosis (obesity, smoking, sedentary life-style, hyperlipidaemia) are also taken into consideration, without being specific indications. It appears that metformin acts beneficially on a lot of the metabolic syndrome parameters (insulin-resistance syndrome) apart from glycaemia. More specifically, it decreases fasting hyperinsulinaemia, moderately improves the lipid profile and has some antithrombotic action as well, decreasing the PAI-1, the fibrinogen and the platelet aggregation.

In the UKPDS study, metformin was administered as an initial antidiabetic monotherapy in overweight Type 2 diabetic patients. Its administration decreased the macrovascular complications and increased survival, compared to the sulfonylureas or insulin that had the same long-term hypoglycaemic effects (follow-up of 10 years).

The dosage of metformin is 850 mg with a meal, with gradual increase up to a maximum of 2,550 mg (usually one tablet before each main meal) per day.

What is expected by the administration of metformin in this particular patient? How does metformin act?

An improvement of blood glucose by 50–60 mg/dl (2.8–3.3 mmol/L) and of HbA_{1c} by 1.5–2 percent is expected. Various clinical studies have shown that the higher the initial levels of hyperglycemia, the bigger the decrease of blood glucose levels, with the use of metformin.

It appears that the effect of metformin is more intense on pre-prandial glycaemia, and smaller on post-prandial glycaemia, which potentially conflicts with older perceptions.

The action of metformin is only expressed in the presence of insulin, since this substance does not cause an excretion of insulin. Metformin decreases fasting hyperglycaemia via a reduction of hepatic gluconeogenesis, potentiating the action of insulin in the liver. It also increases the uptake of glucose from the muscles via a mobilization of the glucose transporters. The increased cellular uptake of glucose is combined with an increased activity of glycogen synthase and increased storage of glycogen.

Metformin also represses the lipid acid oxidation, a process that is dependent on insulin, and decreases hypertriglyceridaemia. In the intestine, metformin increases the metabolism of glucose, thus contributing to the stabilization of the body weight, in addition to its hypoglycaemic action.

The precise mechanism of action of metformin, however, is not completely clear. Perhaps this substance activates a protein kinase that is activated by the AMP.

With which antidiabetic medicines can metformin be combined?

Metformin can be combined with all the other antidiabetic medicines (insulin-secretagogues: sulfonylureas or meglitinides), a-glucosidase inhibitors (acarbose), thiazolidinediones (rosiglitazone or pioglitazone) and with insulin. The combination of metformin with sulfonylureas decreases the blood sugar more than each medicine separately.

In Greece, there is a fixed combination of metformin with glibenclamide (Normell) and with rosiglitazone (Avandamet), and in the USA, there are combinations of metformin with glyburide (glibenclamide), glipizide, pioglitazone and rosiglitazone.

The coadministration of metformin with other antidiabetic medicines can cause hypoglycaemia. If there is sufficient pancreatic β-cell function, the hypoglycaemic action of metformin further augments the corresponding action of the other antidiabetic substances, as well as that of insulin. The regular monitoring of blood sugar levels is more imperative in patients receiving a combination of metformin with other antidiabetic substances.

The intake of cimetidine (H-2 blocker) can increase the concentration of metformin in the blood, since cimetidine competitively inhibits the tubular excretion of metformin.

What are the contraindications for the administration of metformin?

Metformin is strongly contraindicated in situations that can constitute a background for the appearance of lactic acidosis (see below for more details). The medicine is also contraindicated in patients with impaired renal function (serum creatinine ≥ 1.5 mg/dl [132.6 µmol/L] in men or ≥ 1.4 mg/dl [123.8 µmol/L] in women). In elderly patients, the decision whether to administer metformin is based on the creatinine clearance (metformin should not be prescribed if this is < 60 ml/min/1.73 m^2). The renal function should be evaluated every year. In patients who need contrast media intravenously for radiologic examinations, metformin should be discontinued 1–2 days before and after the examination. Apart from these situations, the administration of metformin is also contraindicated in:

- acute or chronic cardiac insufficiency
- respiratory insufficiency
- septicaemia
- very old age (> 80 years)
- significant hepatic insufficiency

- alcohol abuse
- history of lactic acidosis
- pregnancy and lactation
- conditions of shock
- serious illness and surgical interventions (anaesthesia): temporary discontinuation

In the patient under discussion, the frequent consumption of beer concerns the treating physician.

After the gradual increase of the dose (two 850 mg tablets daily), the patient comes back complaining of epigastric pains, manifested around half-an-hour after the intake of the metformin tablet. **Are epigastric pains a side effect of metformin?**

The undesirable side effects of metformin emanate mainly from the peptic system. It can cause epigastric pains, nausea, anorexia, metallic taste in the mouth, flatulence and diarrhoea. Some patients complain of a feeling of easy fatiguability. The undesirable side effects are more frequent at the beginning of the treatment (some authors report rates of 30 percent) but they often subside after a few days or after a transient decrease of the dose. It is reported that 5–10 percent of the patients receiving metformin are forced to interrupt it because of its undesirable side effects (mainly due to diarrhoea).

The epigastric pain in this particular patient may also be due to the aspirin or statin that he receives. Also, smoking causes gastritis.

Another side effect of metformin also reported is a decrease of vitamin B12 levels in the blood of the patients, although this does not yet have a proven clinical significance.

The worst undesirable side effect of metformin – albeit rare – is *lactic acidosis* which is manifested in patients that receive metformin despite contraindications. The mechanism of lactic acidosis in those receiving the medicine is not absolutely elucidated. Biguanides are bound to the mitochondrial membranes and inhibit the aerobic metabolism. Secondarily, an increase of the anaerobic metabolism is caused, and consequently lactic acid production increases. Although the incidence of lactic acidosis with metformin is around 0.03 cases per 1000 patient-years of treatment, the mortality rate is high, roughly 50 percent. Lactic acidosis can also happen in diabetics who do not receive metformin, and also in patients who deliberately consume excessively big doses of the medicine without contraindications.

After two years of good control with metformin, the current patient had not managed to stop smoking and the lipid profile still remained abnormal. He visits the Diabetes Clinic looking obviously weak and reports recent hospitalization in a cardiologic unit because of an acute myocardial infarction. He now uses treatment with insulin. **Can the patient once again begin metformin?**

Metformin is contraindicated, as was mentioned before, in every situation of hypoxia, such as chronic congestive heart failure, which causes an increase in lactic acid production. The recent development of myocardial infarction, unless it is accompanied by cardiac insufficiency with haemodynamic instability, is no longer considered to be a contra-indication for the administration of metformin. Previous guidelines definitely excluded these patients for the six months following the infarction.

The patient wonders why his sister, who does not have DM, also receives metformin from her doctor. **What are the indications for metformin administration other than for Type 2 DM?**

Metformin is also prescribed for women for conditions often associated with polycystic ovary syndrome (which is frequently accompanied by insulin resistance). These include oligomenorrhoea, infertility because of anovulation, hirsutism, obesity and DM. There are small studies that refer to the prevention of gestational DM in women with polycystic ovary syndrome, but no double blind study.

The administration of metformin is contraindicated during pregnancy.

Metformin is allowed in adolescents and children with Type 2 DM.

THIAZOLIDINEDIONES

What are the thiazolidinediones and how do they act?

A new category of antidiabetic medicines consists of thiazolidine-diones (TZDs) or glitazones. the main action of which is the reduction of insulin resistance in the peripheral tissues (mainly the adipose tissue, but also the muscles and less so the liver). The first medicine of this category (troglitazone) came out in the USA in 1997, but was withdrawn in 2000 because of serious hepatotoxicity. Today two substances of this category are available, pioglitazone and rosiglitazone.

TZDs bind to special nuclear cell receptors, called PPAR-γ (Peroxisome Proliferator Activated Receptor-γ), which are found all over the body, but with higher concentration in the adipose tissue, the muscles and the liver. After binding to the receptor, the complex interacts with the Retinoid X Receptor (RXR) so that an activated heterodimer complex is produced, that then causes transcription of genes of various proteins. The manifestation of the action of TZDs is expressed via these proteins. The presence of insulin is essential for the hypoglycaemic action of TZDs, which actually potentiate its action. This fact renders these medicines useful in Type 2 DM, since it is characterized by insulin resistance.

Concisely, TZDs have the following effects:

- they cause an increase of glucose transporters GLUT1 (in the adipose tissue) and of GLUT4 (in muscles), resulting in an increase of the intracellular transport of glucose;
- they increase the phosphorylation of the insulin receptor after the binding of insulin, so that the message of binding is transmitted more rapidly into the cell;
- they decrease the hepatic gluconeogenesis;
- they inhibit lipolysis and thus decrease the free fatty acids, which are incriminated in the development of insulin resistance, and they potentiate the action of lipoprotein lipase, via which the chylomicrons and endogenous triglycerides are removed from the circulation;
- they cause redistribution of adipocytes, so that more small adipocytes – sensitive to insulin – are distributed in the periphery, and less intra-abdominal;
- they promote the expression of the adiponectin gene and inhibit the resistin gene, thus increasing the sensitivity of the adipose tissue to insulin.

However, several aspects of the mechanism of action of TZDs, both in muscles and in the adipose tissue, still remain elusive.

TZDs manifest other actions as well. These include an improvement in endothelial function, reduction of the carotid intima-media thickness and inhibition of the proliferation of smooth muscle cell fibres, as well as the decrease of fibrinogen, CRP (C-reactive protein), PAI-1 (plasminogen activator inhibitor-1), tumour necrosis factor-a (TNF-a) and small-dense atherogenic LDL. They also cause a reduction in the urine albumin excretion rate and the arterial pressure. These effects most likely exert an antiatheromatous effect and are the subject of continuing research. If these preliminary, very encouraging effects of TZDs on the atherosclerotic risk factors are to be translated to a reduction of cardiovascular events, this will become clear in the near future, from the results of ongoing large studies. The multiple effects of TZDs in the various tissues and multiple genes (> 100) that these influence, currently renders precise determination of their mechanism of action impossible with regard to their hypoglycaemic effect.

What are the indications for TZDs?

TZDs are indicated in diabetic individuals with insulin resistance, either as monotherapy or in combination with a sulfonylurea or with metformin. In the USA their combination with insulin has also been approved (in Europe, for the present moment at least, this has not received approval, because of fears of undesirable side effects in individuals with cardiac insufficiency). A particular indication for coadministration with metformin is the failure of diet and exercise while the maximal dose of metformin is already being received. An indication for coadministration with a sulfonylurea is the failure of diet and exercise while the maximal dose of sulfonylureas is being administered and there is a contraindication of prescribing metformin or an intolerance to metformin. If the combination of a sulfonylurea with metformin fails, then either the addition of a TZD or the replacement of one of the two medicines with a TZD is recommended. TZDs can be administered as monotherapy in individuals with Type 2 DM if diet and exercise fail to control the blood sugar. Modern studies propose the use of TZDs in combination with metformin or with a sulfonylurea early in the development of DM, or in combination with meglitinides, and also in triple combination with insulin-secretagogues and metformin.

TZDs have also been tried in women with polycystic ovary syndrome, with up to now beneficial results as regards ovulation, hirsutism, hyperandrogenaemia and insulin resistance. At present, however, TZDs have not been approved for this condition.

How much is the glycosylated haemoglobin expected to decrease when a TZD is administered?

With the administration of a TZD the glycosylated haemoglobin (HbA$_{1c}$) is expected to decrease by about 1.0–1.6 percent (especially if the initial level is over 8 percent), and the fasting blood glucose level is expected to decrease by 50–70 mg/dl (2.8–3.9 mmol/L). The maximal recommended dose of rosiglitazone is 4 mg twice a day and of piogli-tazone 45 mg once a day, independent from the intake of food. The usual initial dose is 2–4 mg daily for rosiglitazone and 15–30 mg daily for pioglitazone.

How fast do TZDs act and how soon do they exhibit secondary failure?

The onset of action of TZDs is delayed, not because of prolonged elimination half-life (3–7 hours for pioglitazone and 3–4 hours for rosiglitazone), but because of their mechanism of action that involves the activation of genes. Thus their metabolic effects are not expressed before 3–6 weeks of treatment, contrary to the other modern antidiabetic medicines. If they are administered alone, the peak action is expressed after three months, and if they are administered with a sulfonylurea or metformin, after roughly one month. In contrast with the other antidia-betic medicines that manifest secondary failure relatively quickly, several authors support the notion that the action of TZDs remains constant for at least two years.

When is the use of TZDs contraindicated?

TZDs are contraindicated when hepatic insufficiency exists or when the initial level of the serum transaminases is higher than 2.5 times the upper limit of normal. They one also contraindicated when there is cardiac insufficiency of any stage (although some authors recommend that they are not given only in stages III and IV of cardiac insufficiency). TZDs are not contraindicated when there is moderate renal insufficiency, but only when the creatinine clearance is < 10 ml/min. Because of the findings in experimental animals that speculate a neoplastic action of the TZDs, it has been proposed that they are avoided in individuals with a family history of adenomatous polypodiasis or other cancers. They are also contraindicated in pregnancy, because there is no experience of their use in humans, and studies in animals have shown a delay in foetal growth.

What are the main undesirable side effects of TZDs and with what mechanisms have they been explained?

Ankle oedema constitutes an undesirable side effect of TZDs manifesting at a rate of 4–5 percent of patients. Fluid retention, which is partly responsible for the increase of body weight that is observed in patients treated with TZDs, can decompensate preexisting cardiac insufficiency, or cause the development of cardiac insufficiency that was not previously diagnosed. In this case, diuretics do not help and discontinuation of the TZD is imperative. If insulin is coadministered, the oedema can be more intense and more frequent (roughly 15 percent). The patients should be informed about the possibility of the increase of body weight and be stricter with their diet. Various mechanisms for the appearance of oedema have been proposed: increase of plasma volume, increased renal sodium reabsorption, activation of the sympathetic reflex, disturbances of intestinal reabsorption of ions and increased production of vascular endothelial growth factor.

Apart from water retention, an increase of the total body fat can also contribute to the increase of body weight, as has been shown in many studies. The increase of body weight is around 2–4 kg (4.4–8.8 lb) in the first 6–12 months of treatment and concerns the increase of peripheral and not splanchnic fat. When combined with sulfonylureas the increase of weight is usually larger and is highest in combination with insulin (5–6 kg [11.0–13.2 lb]). There have been infrequent cases of weight gain up to 20 kg (44.1 lb) on treatment with TZDs, with no explanation why. When this increase is very large, several authors recommend interruption of TZDs.

Fluid retention can also cause anaemia because of haemodilution. The haematocrit can be decreased by 1–2 percent and the haemoglobin by around 1 g/dl. This reduction presents in the first 12 weeks of treatment and appears to reflect an increase in the volume of blood, since the red blood cells mass remains stable. Some authors report a small reduction of white blood cells and platelets.

Hepatic damage can occasionally present as a side effect of TZDs. In reality, because of the reduction of insulin resistance, these medicines are expected to decrease the intrahepatic fat concentration and the fat infiltration that is observed in obesity and DM. As a matter of fact, recent studies have shown an improvement of clinical and pathologic characteristics of patients with non-alcoholic steatohepatitis after treatment with TZDs, without increase of the transaminase levels. The transaminases should in any case be regularly monitored (before therapy and every two months in the first year, and less frequently thereafter). Troglitazone, the first TZD that was used for treatment, was withdrawn because of significant hepatic complications. The latest experience with the available TZDs is reassuring as regards the probability of hepatocellular damage.

Most writers also stress the increased cost of TZDs compared to other antidiabetic pills.

What is the effect of TZDs on serum lipids?

Most studies agree that TZDs increase HDL-cholesterol by 10–14 percent, decrease free fatty acids and contribute to the increase in size of small-dense LDL molecules, which has a beneficial effect on the risk for atherosclerosis. Moreover, they do exert a mild hypotriglyceridaemic effect when the triglycerides are > 200 mg/dl (2.3 mmol/L). It should also be mentioned that modern pharmaceutical research is directed towards the development of products that are simultaneously PPAR-γ and-α agonists, affecting both the metabolism of glucose and lipids.

CASE STUDY 3

A 48 year old woman with a 10 year history of Type 2 DM that has been treated for six years with metformin (at an escalating dose reaching 850 mg three times per day during the last year), presents to the Diabetes Clinic for a regular visit. She feels well and denies any dyspnoea, orthopnoea or ankle oedema, or any undesirable effect of metformin. Her weight is stable, as is her diet (roughly 1,400 kcal/day). Because of her work she does not exercise regularly, except for walking 300 metres every day. Her dietary habits and her activities have not altered during the last 7–8 years, and she does not predict that she will be able to exercise more in the future, because of family and professional responsibilities. She does not smoke. On physical examination there are no murmurs in her heart, no jugular distention, or lower extremity oedema. Her liver edge is palpable and soft. She has a body mass index of 30 kg/m^2 and slight hypertension (recent measurement 146/88 mmHg), for which she receives an angiotensin converting enzyme inhibitor. Her renal and liver function tests are normal. She has been treated with a statin for two years and the recent levels of total cholesterol are 213 mg/dl (5.51 mmol/L), of HDL-cholesterol 42 mg/dl (1.09 mmol/L), LDL-cholesterol 131 mg/dl (3.39 mmol/L) and triglycerides 199 mg/dl (2.25 mmol/L). Usual morning fasting blood glucose levels are 140–160 mg/dl (7.8–8.9 mmol/L) and post-prandial 200–230 mg/dl (11.1–12.8 mmol/L). Her glycosylated haemoglobin level is 8.4 percent, increased by 1.2 percent from the previous measurement five months ago. Her urine albumin excretion rate is at the upper limits of normal (27 mg/24 h). An abdominal ultrasound showed fatty infiltration of the liver, but the remainder of the abdominal organs are without abnormalities. The patient was advised to have a stricter diet and more exercise and was prescribed a small dose of a thiazide diuretic as well as rosiglitazone at a dose of 4 mg per day.

Why was a thiazolidinedione (TZD) added to the regimen of this particular patient?

The metformin that this patient has continuously been receiving for the past few years cannot sufficiently control her blood sugar any langer, as proven by the latest progressively increasing glycosylated haemoglobin levels. This particular patient manifests insulin resistance, as is evident from the obesity, and the presence of diabetes, hypertension and dyslipidaemia. With this in mind, a substance was selected that manages insulin resistance as a whole and not an insulin secretagogue medicine.

After three months the patient comes back for her regular examination. The blood sugar levels are slightly improved (fasting usually 115–140 mg/dl [6.4–7.8 mmol/L], post-prandial 145–180 mg/dl [8.1–10.0 mmol/L]). Her physical examination is unchanged, without oedema. Her body weight has increased by 2 kg (4.4 lb), and her blood lipid levels are as follows: total cholesterol 235 mg/dl (6.08 mmol/L), HDL-cholesterol 46 mg/dl (1.19 mmol/L), LDL-cholesterol 146 mg/dl (3.78 mmol/L) and triglycerides 197 mg/dl (2.23 mmol/L). The glycosylated haemoglobin is 7.9 percent. The arterial pressure is 130/80 mmHg. The liver function tests remain within normal levels, albeit increased compared to the previous ones. The dose of the statin and rosiglitazone is doubled (rosiglitazone to 8 mg/day).

Since there was an improvement of the metabolic control with the addition of the TZD but not yet complete achievement of the targets, and since the medicine was well tolerated, it was decided to give the patient more time to allow the full effect of the medicine. It is reminded that sometimes many months are needed (up to 8–9) for the full manifestation of the metabolic effects of TZDs.

After another three months, the glycosylated haemoglobin level subsided to a level of 7.0 percent, but the patient now complains of ankle oedema. A further increase of her body weight by 2 kg (4.4 lb) was observed, and the blood lipid levels definitely improved, reaching near normal levels. The liver function tests were unchanged. The TSH level is normal. The urine albumin excretion rate is 18 mg/24 h. An echocardiogram is normal.

The achievement of good glycaemic control (HbA$_{1c}$ 7 percent) with the administration of the maximal TZD and metformin doses proves that the patient did have insulin resistance. The small increase of body weight can be managed with a better attention to the diet and potentially with anti-obesity medicines.

ALPHA-GLUCOSIDASE INHIBITORS

Which alpha-glucosidase inhibitors are available on the market?

There are three alpha-glucosidase inhibitors: acarbose, miglitol and voglibose. Of these, acarbose has been studied most extensively.

Why were these medicines created?

During the process of digestion, monosaccharides pass from the mucosal to the serosal surfaces of the small intestine and enter the mesentery venous and the portal system. Monosaccharides are the form with which the food carbohydrates can be absorbed. The absorption occurs mainly in the upper half of the small intestine. Monosaccharides result from the hydrolysis of the complex carbohydrates, which are mainly α-glucose-bound residues, and form di-, oligo- and poly-saccharides, like sucrose, dextrins and starch. The split occurs in the brush border of the intestinal lumen, in the presence of special enzymes, the glucosidases (maltase, isomaltase, glucoamylase, dextrinase, saccharase).

In individuals with DM, the regulatory mechanism of a sufficient and timely insulin secretion from the β-cell that controls the rapid postprandial rise of blood glucose is impaired. Also, as is known, the severity of hyperglycaemia can, in some degree, be controlled with the restriction of dietary carbohydrates.

For this reason substances that decrease the rate of monosaccharide absorption from the small intestine were created. They achieve this by impeding the split of di-, oligo- and poly-saccharides to easily digestible monosaccharides. The decrease in the percentage of carbohydrates of food involves an increase in the percentage of fat, which is contrary to the guidelines of diabetic scientific organizations, which resulted from observations with regard to a healthy diet.

What is acarbose chemically and how does it act?

Acarbose is a pseudo-tetrasaccharide, a biotechnology product. It contains acarbiosine, which resembles a disaccharide, connected with a maltose residue via an α-glucosidic bond. Acarbiosine is recognized and gets bound to the glucosidases of the intestinal brush border. This results in the inhibition of carbohydrate hydrolysis and the delay of their digestion in the duodenum and jejunum during the first two hours after the meal. This effect is dose-dependent. Acarbose is excreted unaltered by the kidneys, and less than 2 percent is absorbed by the intestine.

What is the fate of undigested carbohydrates and what undesirable effects can be produced by their presence in the lower gastrointestinal tract?

Undigested carbohydrates are removed with the stool. However, in the large intestine, the normal intestinal flora causes fermentation of the redundant carbohydrates and local excessive production of the products of this fermentation (lactic acid, hydrogen, carbon dioxide, etc.). As a consequence, those substances that are not absorbed cause flatulence, abdominal aches, diarrhoea or excessive production of gases. To some degree these complaints can be avoided with progressive increase of the dose and they generally subside completely after the first weeks or months. However, if a large quantity of sugar is consumed and the recommended diet it is not followed, the diarrhoea can be intense.

What are the indications and contraindications for acarbose?

Acarbose is indicated first of all in the prevention of post-prandial hyperglycaemia in individuals with Type 2 DM. Its effectiveness is limited to a decrease of glycosylated haemoglobin by 0.5–1.0 percent when used as monotherapy. It can be combined with a sulfonylurea, metformin, insulin and with the combination of two or even three substances (see the first footnote in Figure 27.1). In all cases, however, its effectiveness is most apparent when the severity of the disease is relatively small. Its indications also include its administration in insulin-dependent individuals (Type 1 DM) in combination with insulin.

Acarbose is contraindicated in pregnant and nursing women and when there are chronic intestinal diseases with definite disturbance in digestion and absorption. Great caution should be exercised when the patient has large hernias as well as ulcers or stenoses of the intestine. Individuals with constipation due to DM should better avoid the intake of acarbose, because the neuropathy of the autonomous nervous system that causes constipation can intensify flatulence and abdominal aches.

Can acarbose cause hypoglycaemia? Are there other undesirable side effects?

Acarbose, when administered as monotherapy, does not cause insulin secretion and consequently does not cause hypoglycaemia. When it is administered together with a sulfonylurea or insulin, the hypoglycaemia that can be caused by these substances is probably more severe and cannot be corrected with administration of sugar (sucrose), because, as a disaccharide, this cannot be absorbed in the presence of acarbose. Hypoglycaemia in individuals who use acarbose is managed by administering glucose and not sugar (which is a mixture of glucose and fructose).

The possibility of asymptomatic increase of the transaminases has also been reported, but this subsides with the discontinuation of acarbose. Individual incidents of severe pharmaceutical hepatitis have also been reported.

Are there other beneficial effects of acarbose apart from the decrease of post-prandial hyperglycaemia?

A meta-analysis of seven long-term studies showed that acarbose can protect, to a significant degree, from the development of myocardial infarction. A positive effect of acarbose (albeit not statistically significant) was found for the prevention of angina, cardiac insufficiency, the process of revascularization after an infarction, peripheral vascular disease and stroke. This result is probably due to the decrease in the post-prandial glucose levels, since no other mechanism has so far been found. However, a newer meta-analysis of 41 studies with α-glucosidase inhibitors (30 with acarbose) did not show any beneficial effect of these medicines on morbidity and mortality, although there was a decrease in the glycosylated haemoglobin, the fasting and post-prandial plasma glucose as well as the level of post-prandial insulin. Generally, the question of protection (with regard to mortality) of these medicines in DM is not completely clear and the results of many ongoing studies with newer medicines (e.g., glitazones) are expected with interest.

COMBINATIONS OF ANTIDIABETIC MEDICINES

Is the treatment with combinations of antidiabetic medicines prudent?

Such combinations are a prudent treatment, since each different type of antidiabetic medicine aims at a different mechanism of the pathophysiology of DM.

The combination of a sulfonylurea with metformin in various doses is considered classic. Nateglinide and repaglinide can be combined with metformin. An initial indication for glitazones was the coadministration with metformin and then with sulfonylureas, and later they were approved as monotherapy. Recently the triple combination of glitazones (rosiglitazone) with metformin and a sulfonylurea was allowed. Acarbose can be combined with a sulfonylurea or metformin.

How much do the antidiabetic medicines decrease glycosylated haemoglobin?

The degree of glycosylated haemoglobin reduction is, apart from any other factor, also dependent on the correct indication for the administration of each medicine separately. As was mentioned before,

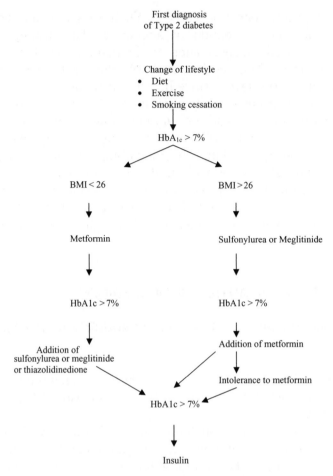

First diagnosis
of Type 2 diabetes

Change of lifestyle
- Diet
- Exercise
- Smoking cessation

HbA$_{1c}$ > 7%

BMI < 26   BMI > 26

Metformin   Sulfonylurea or Meglitinide

HbA1c > 7%   HbA1c > 7%

Addition of
sulfonylurea or meglitinide
or thiazolidinedione   Addition of metformin

Intolerance to metformin

HbA1c > 7%

Insulin

- Long acting insulin at bedtime combined with pills (except TZDs)

- Mixture of insulin (rapid acting with slow-acting) twice a day. Discontinuation of pills or continuation of metformin

- Multiple injections regimen if flexibility is required

At any site of the algorithm, acarbose can be added in a progressively higher dose. The same medicine can be administered initially as monotherapy, especially when postprandial hyperglycaemia is more evident.

Note: In cases of obesity, anti-obesity medicines can potentially be prescribed

Figure 27.2. Algorithm of therapeutic approach of a patient with Type 2 DM (Modified from Wallace T.M. and Mastthews D.R.,)

sulfonylureas and metformin decrease the glycosylated haemoglobin by 1.5–2 percent, acarbose by 0.5–1 percent, meglitinides by 0.7–2 percent and glitazones by 1–1.5 percent. The results are dose-dependent and the decrease is usually bigger (> 2 percent) when the initial value of glycosylated haemoglobin is higher.

There are differences when the patient receives antidiabetic treatment for the first time or changes treatment due to failure of a previous treatment (smaller decrease in the latter situation). In the second case, the combination of a sulfonylurea with metformin has been calculated to decrease glycosylated haemoglobin by 1.7 percent, the combination of sulfonylurea with acarbose to decrease by 0.9 percent, of meglitinide with metformin by 1.4 percent, of glitazone with metformin by 0.5–1.5 percent and of glitazone with sulfonylureas by 0.5–1.5 percent.

The combination of a sulfonylurea with rapid-acting insulin decreases the glycosylated haemoglobin by 0.5–1.8 percent, of metformin with rapid-acting insulin by 1.7–2.5 percent, of acarbose with medium-duration insulin by 0.4–0.5 percent, of meglitinides with insulin by 0.7 percent, and of glitazones with insulin (a combination that still has not received approval in Europe) by 0.8–1.4 percent.

It should be noted, however, that these percentages can be used only as general statistical conclusions and not as the necessarily expected response of particular individuals who receive some antidiabetic treatment. This is because the regulation of blood sugar is also the result of proper nutrition and physical activity in addition to pharmaceutical treatment, which should therefore be individualized.

An algorithm for the therapeutic management of DM is shown in Figure 27.2

Further reading

Bailey, C.J., Metformin (2004) in *Therapy for diabetes mellitus and related disorders*, 4th edn, American Diabetes Association, (ed. H.E. Lebovitz), pp. 196–191.

Benbow, A., Stewart, M., Yeoman, G. (2001) Thiazolidinediones for Type 2 diabetes. All glitazones may exacerbate heart failure. *BMJ*, **322**, 236.

Buse, J.B., Tan, M.H., Prince, M.J., Erickson, P.P. (2004) The effects of oral anti-hyperglycaemic medications on serum lipid profiles in patients with Type 2 diabetes. *Diabetes Obes Metab*, **6**, 133–56.

Chiasson, J.-L., Josse, R.G., Gomis, R., Hanefeld, M., Karasik, A., Laakso, M. (2003) Acarbose treatment and the risk of cardiovascular disease and hypertension in patients with impaired glucose tolerance. The STOP-NIDDM Trial. *JAMA*, **290**, 486–94.

Dimitriadis, G., Boutati, E., Lambadiari, V., Mitrou, P., Maratou, E., Brunel, P., Raptis, S.A. (2004) Restoration of early insulin secretion after a meal in Type 2 diabetes: effects on lipid and glucose metabolism. *Eur J Clin Invest.*, **34**, 490–7.

Fuhlendorff, J., Rorsman, P., Kofod, H., Brand, C., Rolin, B., MacKay, P., Symko, R., Carr, R. (1998) Stimulation of insulin release by repaglinide and glibenclamide involves both common and distinct processes. *Diabetes*, **47**, 345–51.

Gribble, F.M., Reimann, F. (2003) Sulphonylurea action revisited: the postcloning era. *Diabetologia*, **46**, 875–891.

Hanefeld, M., Cagatay, M., Petrowitsch, T., Neuser, D., Petzinna, D., Rupp, M. (2004) Acarbose reduces the risk for myocardial infarction in Type 2 diabetic patients: Meta-analysis of seven long-term studies. *European Heart Journal*, **25**, 10–16.

Ioannidis, I., Tsoukala, C., Panayotopoulou, C., Skrapari, I., Maglara, E., Anastasopoulou, Y., Mandalaki, T., Katsilambros, N. (1999) Effects of glibenclamide on post-prandial coagulation activation. *Nutr Metab Cardiovasc Dis*, **9**, 204–7.

Lebovitz, H. (2004) Insulin secretagogues: Sulfonylureas, Repaglinide, and Nateglinide, in *ADA's Therapy for Diabetes Mellitus and Related Disorders*, pp. 164–75.

Nesto, R.W., Bell, D., Bonow, R.O., Fonseca, V., Grundy, S.M., Horton, E.S., Le Winter, M., Porte, D., Semenkovich, C.F., Smith, S., Young, L.H., Kahn, R. (2004) Thiazolidinedione use, fluid retention, and congestive heart failure: a consensus statement from the American Heart Association and American Diabetes Association. *Diabetes Care*, **27**, 256–63.

Ovalle, F. and Bell, D.S. (2002) Lipoprotein effects of different thiazolidinediones in clinical practice. *Endocr Pract*, **8**, 406–10.

Raptis, S.A. and Dimitriadis, G.D. (2001) Oral hypoglycemic agents: insulin secretagogues, alpha-glucosidase inhibitors and insulin sensitizers. *Exp Clin Endocrinol Diabetes*, **109**(Suppl 2), S265–S287

Raptis, S.A., Hatziagelaki, E., Dimitriadis, G., Draeger, K.E., Pfeiffer, C., Raptis, A.E. (1999) Comparative effects of glimepiride and glibenclamide on blood glucose, C-peptide and insulin concentrations in the fasting and post-prandial state in normal man. *Exp Clin Endocrinol Diabetes*, **107**, 350–5.

Skrapari, I., Perrea, D., Ioannidis, I., Karabina, S.A., Elisaf, M., Tselepis, A.D., Karagiannacos, P., Katsilambros, N. (2001) Glibenclamide improves postprandial hypertriglyceridaemia in Type 2 diabetic patients by reducing chylomicrons but not the very low-density lipoprotein subfraction levels. *Diabet Med*, **18**, 781–5.

Santiago, J.V. (1996) Glucose control in diabetes mellitus: role of acarbose in reducing post-prandial hyperglycemia. *Drug Benefit Trends*, (supp 8E), 27–35.

Tentolouris, N., Kolia, M., Tselepis, A.D., Perea, D., Kitsou, E., Kyriaki, D., Tambaki, A.P., Karabina, S.P., Sala, C., Fragoulopoulos, E., Katsilambros, N. (2003) Lack of effect of acute repaglinide administration on post-prandial lipaemia in patients with Type 2 diabetes mellitus. *Exp Clin Endocrinol Diabetes*, **111**, 370–3.

UKPDS Study Group (1998). Intensive blood glucose control with sulfonylurea or insulin compared with conventional treatment and risk of complications in patients with Type 2 diabetes (UKPDS 33), *Lancet*, **352**, 837–53.

van de Laar, F.A., Lucassen, P.L., Akkermans, R.P., van de Lisdonk, E.H., Rutten, G.E., van Weel, C. (2005) α-glucosidase inhibitors for patients with Type 2 diabetes. Results from a Cochrane systematic review and meta-analysis. *Diabetes Care*, **28**, 154–63.

Wallace, T.M. and Matthews, D.R. (2003) The drug treatment of Type 2 diabetes, in *Textbook of Diabetes*, 3rd edn, (eds J.C. Pickup and G. Williams), Blackwell Science Ltd, Oxford, pp. 45.1–45.18.

Yki-Järvinen, H. (2004) Thiazolidinediones. *NEJM*, **351**, 1106–18.

28

Treatment of diabetes with insulin

Stavros Liatis

How is insulin that is used therapeutically produced?

Human insulin is produced in the β-cells of the pancreatic islets. The two peptide chains of insulin are initially produced as a high molecular weight precursor molecule, pre-proinsulin. Then the pre-peptide (signal peptide) is cleaved away from the primary peptide chain, while this is still in the rough endoplasmic reticulum, and pro-insulin is formed. Pro-insulin is cleaved by proteases into insulin and C-peptide inside the secretory granules of the β-cell. Finally, when needed by the body, insulin and C-peptide are released into the circulation.

The insulin products available today contain human insulin, which is produced with the technology of recombinant DNA. With this technique, a gene that produces human pro-insulin is inserted into a bacterium (or fungus). Insulin is afterwards isolated with enzymatic cleavage of the C-peptide. The companies that produce insulin use different individual techniques.

How do commercially available insulin preparations differ from each other?

Commercially available insulin preparations are separated into five main categories (Table 28.1) depending on time of onset and duration of their action:

1. Insulins of very rapid onset and very brief duration of action, which include only insulin analogues (insulin Lispro, insulin Aspart and insulin Glulisine).

Diabetes in Clinical Practice: Questions and Answers from Case Studies.   Nicholas Katsilambros *et al.*
© 2006 John Wiley & Sons, Ltd.

Table 28.1. Characteristics of insulin preparations

Insulin preparations	Onset of action	Peak of action	Duration of action
Very-rapid-acting insulin analogues			
Insulin Lispro	5–15 min	30–90 min	3–5 hours
Insulin Aspart	5–15 min	30–90 min	3–5 hours
Insulin Glulisine	5–15 min	30–90 min	3–5 hours
Rapid-acting insulin			
Soluble (regular) insulin	30–60 min	2–3 hours	5–8 hours
Insulins of intermediate action			
Isophane insulin (NPH)	2–4 hours	4–10 hours	10–16 hours
Zinc insulin (Lente)	3–4 hours	4–12 hours	12–18 hours
Insulins of delayed action			
Insulin Glargine	2–4 hours	It does not exist	20–24 hours
Insulin Detemir	2–4 hours	6–14 hours *	16–20 hours
Zinc insulin of extended action (Ultralente)	6–10 hours	10–16 hours	18–24 hours
Mixtures of insulin			
90/10 (90% intermediate, 10% rapid)	30–60 min	Two-phase	10–16 hours
80/20 (80% intermediate, 20% rapid)	30–60 min	Two-phase	10–16 hours
75/25 (75% protamine lispro, 25% Lispro)	5–15 min	Two-phase	10–16 hours
70/30 (70% intermediate, 30% rapid)	30–60 min	Two-phase	10–16 hour
70/30 (70% protamine Aspart, 30% Aspart)	5–15 min	Two-phase	10–16 hours
60/40 (60% intermediate, 40% rapid)	30–60 min	Two-phase	10–16 hours
50/50 (50% intermediate, 50% rapid)	30–60 min	Two-phase	10–16 hours

*The peak of action of this insulin is mild

2. Insulins of rapid onset and short duration of action, including soluble insulin, which is often reported in the international literature as insulin 'Regular'.
3. Insulins of medium (or intermediary) action, which include the isophane insulin or insulin NPH (Neutral Protamine Hagedorn) and the zinc-containing insulin (Lente).

4. Insulins of slow onset and prolonged duration of action, which include newer insulin analogues (Glargine, Detemir) as well as the (older) zinc-containing insulin of prolonged action (Ultralente).
5. Mixtures of insulins that contain two types of insulin, one with very rapid or rapid action and the other of intermediary action, in different proportions.

What are insulin analogues?

These are peptides that result from the transformation of the insulin molecule through the addition or exchange of certain amino-acids. These transformations give the insulin molecule certain desirable characteristics concerning the speed and stability of its absorption. The need for production of insulin analogues resulted from the fact that the pharmacokinetics of the available insulins did not sufficiently match the physiologic secretion of insulin, both during fasting as well as postprandially.

The currently existing insulin analogues are separated into those that have a very rapid onset and short duration of action, and those that have long and steady action (Table 28.2).

Why are there so many different insulin preparations?

Every insulin product from those reported in Table 28.1 has particular characteristics that provide particular pharmacokinetic attributes. The

Table 28.2. Insulin analogues

Insulin analogues	Modifications in the molecule of insulin
Very rapid onset – short duration of action	
Lispro	Switch of proline-lysine at positions B28–B29
Aspart	Replacement of proline by aspartate at position B28
Glulisine*	Replacement of proline by glutamate at position B29
	Replacement of asparagine by lysine at position B3
Slow onset – long duration of action	
Glargine	Replacement of asparagine by glycine at position A21
	Addition of 2 arginine molecules at position B30
Detemir*	Addition of a fatty acid chain (myristic acid) at position B29

*Insulin Detemir was approved by the FDA in June 2005 and insulin Glulisine in April 2004.

insulin molecule is basically the same in each product. Even in the insulin analogues that, as mentioned before, have in their molecule certain transformations in the sequence of their amino-acids, the region of the molecule that is bound to the insulin receptor remains unchanged and identical with the molecule of human insulin. The reason for the existence of so many commercial products lies in their various pharma-cokinetic attributes, mainly in the different speed of absorption from the site of subcutaneous injection.

The choice of insulin compound depends on the therapeutic regimen in which it is included. The therapeutic regimen is individualized and is planned taking into consideration a series of factors, such as the type and the duration of DM, the age, the wishes and the compliance of the patient, as well as any possible coexisting diseases, financial factors, etc. (see below).

What does the speed of insulin absorption after a subcutaneous injection depend on?

After the injection, a reservoir of insulin is created at the point of infusion, which is then progressively absorbed from the capillaries of the region and enters the circulation. The speed of absorption of the subcutaneous reservoir depends on a number of factors:

- *The insulin compound.* Every type of insulin has a different profile of absorption. The rapid acting soluble insulin (reguar insulin) is injected subcutaneously in the form of insulin hexamers. These are diffused in the subcutaneous tissue and are split progressively into smaller complexes (trimers → dimers → monomers) which are more easily absorbed by the capillaries. Isophane insulin (NPH) contains protamine in stoicheiometric proportion with insulin (i.e., it contains the same amount of protamine as insulin), which renders the formed hexamers more stable in the subcutaneous tissue, so that their absorption is delayed. The insulins that contain zinc are absorbed more slowly, because of higher stability of the hexamers, caused by the presence of zinc. In very rapid acting insulin analogues, the change that has occurred in the insulin molecule renders the hexamers unstable, resulting in an accelerated absorp-tion of insulin. In the slow acting Glargine analogue, however, the change of the molecule, and also the addition of zinc, renders the hexamers more stable in the subcutaneous tissue, with as a consequence its slower and constant absorption. The slow action of the insulin analogue Detemir is achieved partly via binding of its molecule with albumin, from which it is progressively released, achieving the characteristic action profile of this particular insulin.

- *Concentration and dose of insulin.* The concentration of insulin is identical in all the available products: 100 units (IU)/ml. The insulin dose definitely influences the speed of absorption with higher doses leading to its extension.
- *Site of injection.* The density of the capillary network is higher in the abdominal wall in comparison to the arm or the thigh. Consequently, the speed of absorption is, for the vast majority of insulin products, higher in the abdomen than other sites.
- *Local blood flow.* The factors that influence blood flow in the region of injection also influence the speed of insulin absorption. Thus, heat (sunbathing, a hot bath), muscular exercise and massage increase the speed of absorption whereas the cold decreases it.
- *Technique of injection.* The speed of insulin absorption is markedly influenced if, by mistake, the injection is performed intramuscularly or intradermally. The speed of absorption after an intramuscular injection is considerably accelerated. The possibility of error is more likely in lean individuals, especially if longer needles ($> 10\,mm$) are used, or if an erroneous technique is performed (no folding of skin).

Certain insulins (those found in a suspension form that are 'turbid', for example, isophane insulin and the mixtures that containing it) should be shaked before the injection. If shaking is omitted or if it is performed wrongly, the concentration of insulin in the subcutaneous tissue can be very different from what is desirable.

What does insulin bioavailability depend on?

This depends, on the one hand, on its speed of entry into the circulation (see previous question) and, on the other hand, on the hepatic and renal function. Also, but seldomly, it depends on the existence of anti-insulin antibodies in very high concentrations.

Is the injection of insulin with a pen preferable?

Insulin pens, as a means of subcutaneous insulin injection, are an important breakthrough in insulin therapy. They constitute a more practical and easier way of insulin transport and administration compared to the conventional syringes, and they achieve more precision in the administered dose. Moreover, they can function with very thin needles (usually 31G). Their use is relatively simple, especially those that are only used once (prefilled pens-syringes). One relative disadvantage, compared to the classic insulin syringes, is that they do not allow the mixture of insulins (usually rapid- and slow-acting) in varying proportions, based on the changing needs of the particularly unstable individuals with Type 1 DM. The pens should not be given to patients without sufficient training, and it should be ascertained that their operation has been completely understood.

What are the side effects of insulin treatment?

The main undesirable side effect of insulin therapy is hypoglycaemia. The probability of its appearance is increased with a more intensified form of treatment (see Chapter 5).

Individuals who receive insulin usually gain weight. This can be due to better glycaemic control (and the consequent reduction of glucosuria), and to the appearance of hypoglycaemias (even light ones) that lead to an increase of caloric intake. In the DCCT study (Diabetes Control and Complications Trial), individuals with Type 1 DM who received intensified insulin therapy increased their weight by 4.5 kg (9.9 lb) more than those who received conventional treatment, during the 9.5 years of follow-up. In the UKPDS study (United Kingdom Prospective Diabetes Study), individuals with Type 2 DM who received intensified insulin therapy increased their weight by 1.4–2.3 kg (3.1–5.1 lb) more than those who were treated with a sulfonylurea or metformin, respectively.

Allergic reactions following the administration of human type insulin are infrequent. They are separated into local (more frequent) and systematic (more infrequent) reactions.

Treatment with human insulin can cause the creation of small concentrations of antibodies against insulin. These create problems in the activity of the hormone only when they circulate in high concentrations in the blood, which is exceptionally infrequently.

The phenomenon of lipodystrophy used to constitute a non-infrequent problem in the past. Today, however, this is practically non-existent because of cleanliness and the type of insulin (human).

How many types of insulin therapy exist and what are they?

The answer to this question is very difficult because treatment with insulin is individualized. We could, however, first separate the treatment of insulin replacement into two main categories:

- Intensified regimens that imitate the physiologic insulin secretion from the pancreas, which are used mainly in Type 1 DM.
- Simpler regimens of insulin replacement that are administered either in cases where residual endogenous insulin secretion exists (as in Type 2 DM or during the honeymoon phase of Type 1 DM), or when the intensified regimens cannot be applied (as in cases when patients will not collaborate or cannot comprehend the treatment, or when they refuse multiple injections, self-monitoring, etc.).

How are the types of insulin therapy that imitate the physiologic secretion of insulin planned?

The physiologic secretion of insulin consists of two independent components. The first concerns the basic secretion of insulin, which occurs continually all day and is almost constant, with the exception of two peaks, one a little before waking in the morning and the second in the afternoon hours. The second component concerns the insulin that is secreted every time that the individual receives food (Figure 28.1). The

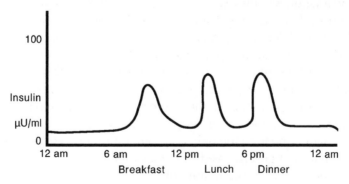

Figure 28.1. Secretion of insulin in a normal subject during a 24-hour period

quantity of 'prandial' insulin that is secreted depends mainly on the carbohydrate content of the meal.

In order for the treatment to imitate the physiologic secretion of insulin, it is clear that both of the above components should be taken into consideration. Therefore, two types of insulin are required; one type that imitates the basal insulin secretion and a second type, with every meal, that imitates the 'prandial' insulin. Thus, the so-called intensified basal-prandial insulin therapy regimens were created (basal-bolus regimens).

Reviewing what was previously mentioned regarding the types of insulin products, we can conclude that for the imitation of basal insulin secretion, intermediate and slow-acting insulins are to be used (in one or two injections daily), whereas before meals the rapid- and very rapid-acting insulins are to be used (an injection before each meal). Thus, various combinations result, each one of which constitutes a therapeutic regimen.

What are the advantages and disadvantages of an intensified insulin regimen?

The main advantage is better glucose control which leads to a reduction of diabetic complications. The largest prospective study ever conducted in individuals with Type 1 DM was the DCCT study, which showed that the appearance of microvascular complications is decreased dramatically when good glycaemic control is achieved. In the same study it was shown that intensive insulin therapy with the administration of basal-bolus insulin leads to better glycaemic control.

Apart from better control, the intensive basal-bolus insulin regimens give diabetics more comfort of movement, since they acquire more freedom as regards the schedule and content of their meals. Diabetics can have a meal whenever they want and in any quantity they want, on condition of course that they inject some insulin before the meal. The dose of insulin is adapted depending on the content of the meal in carbohydrates. These regimens are mainly applied to Type 1 DM, and as individuals with this type of DM are in the majority young and active, this freedom is an important motivation for selecting these types of therapeutic regimens.

The basic disadvantage is the increase of hypoglycaemias. In the DCCT study, the frequency of serious hypoglycaemias (that is, ones in which the patient needed the help of another individual to recover) in the intensive treatment group was three times higher compared to the group who received conventional treatment.

Other disadvantages are relative complexity, bigger weight gain, more frequent incidence of hypoglycaemia unawareness and higher financial cost.

Are there conditions for the application of basal-bolus insulin regimens?

Provided there is an indication for their administration, the basic condition is the acceptance of the regimen by the patient, after of course his or her thorough and objective briefing with regard to the necessity, functionality and precise way of application. The details of the treatment should be analysed and it should be emphasized that, together with the multiple injections, it is absolutely essential that the patient regularly monitors (at least four times a day) the glucose levels in the capillary blood. Acceptance by the patient assumes that a powerful incentive exists to achieve the best blood sugar control. This motivation is based on correct briefing and on factors such as age, maturity, educational level and psychological situation of the individual. Often, more than one meeting with the doctor is required before the individual with Type 1 DM is convinced that the intensive regimen constitutes the best choice for managing the disease.

How is the substitution of basal insulin secretion done?

The substitution of basal insulin secretion is achieved by administering one or two insulin injections of intermediate or slow duration of action daily. More precisely:

- *Isophane insulin (NPH).* An injection before bedtime is first administered. The reason for this particular time lies in the avoidance of nighttime hypoglycaemia (if the injection is given earlier, the peak of action will coincide with the first morning hours of high insulin sensitivity, when the risk of hypoglycaemia is increased). The pre-bedtime injection aims at placing the peak of action near the waking time, when higher needs of insulin usually exist (a period of low insulin sensitivity because of counter-regulatory hormones secretion). If only one injection of isophane insulin is administered, there is often a lack of basal insulin after the noon of the following day (because of its relatively short duration of action, see Table 28.1). The problem can be managed

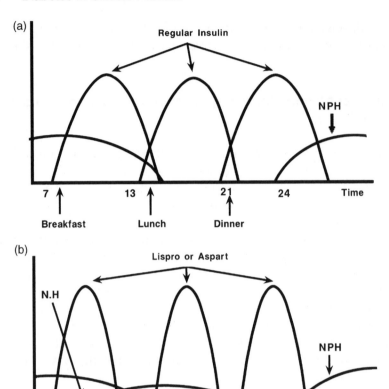

Figure 28.2. Schematic representation: a) Therapeutic scheme with one injection of isophane insulin (NPH) before bedtime and regular insulin 30 minutes before each meal. Large part the lack of basal insulin for a interval of the day is covered by the relatively prolonged action of the repeatedly injected regular insulin. b) Therapeutic scheme with two injections of isophane insulin (before breakfast and at bedtime) and one injection of very rapid-acting insulin analogue before each meal. Notice the frequent overlaps among the insulins.

either using only rapid-acting insulin as 'prandial' insulin (and not very rapid-acting analogues), whereby the relatively extended action of this kind of insulin is used to some degree as basal insulin, or by adding a second NPH injection (in smaller dose) in the morning (Figure 28.2). In this case it is preferable to use a very rapid-acting insulin analogue (Lispro or Aspart) as 'prandial' insulin, so that the overlap between the insulins is decreased. Moreover, the peak of the morning NPH dose should probably be taken into consideration and the dose of the noon 'prandial' insulin be decreased.

- *Zinc insulin (Lente).* Generally the same procedures mentioned above for isophane insulin are in effect. Zinc insulin has a slightly more extended action than isophane. These kinds of insulin are no longer used much in clinical practice.
- *Zinc insulin of extended action (Ultralente).* This insulin has a wide peak (12–16 hours after the injection) and increased variability (in the same patient as well as among different patients) in its action profile. Theoretically, it was constructed to cover the basal secretion administered once a day. However, the increased variability in its absorption often leads to unanticipated hyper- and hypoglycaemias.
- *Insulin analogues.* Glargine is the first insulin analogue of slow action to be used in clinical practice. It differs at the molecular level compared to human insulin both in chain A as well as in chain B (Table 28.2). Glargine is soluble in the slightly acidic environment of the solution in which it is supplied. After its injection in the subcutaneous tissue it is absorbed at a slow and constant rate. Its duration of action after subcutaneous injection is almost 24 hours (22 ± 4 hours) and, in contrast to the other slow-acting insulins, it does not have a peak. Moreover, it was found that its serum levels present smaller variability in the same and/or in different patients compared to isophane insulin. These characteristics allow the substitution of the basal secretion of insulin in the forms of basal-bolus treatment to be achieved. Thanks to its long action, the insulin Glargine can be administered only once a day, either after rising in the morning or before bedtime (Figure 28.3). Mixing with other insulins is not, for the time being at least, recommended.

Insulin Detemir is a slowly-acting analogue, the extended action of which is achieved mainly via connection of the molecule with plasma albumin. This analogue is derived after acylation of human insulin at position B29 (see Table 28.2). Detemir presents a slower onset and smaller peak of action compared to the isophane insulin. Its duration of action reaches up to 20 hours. This often renders essential its administration twice a day in intensified types of insulin therapy (morning and

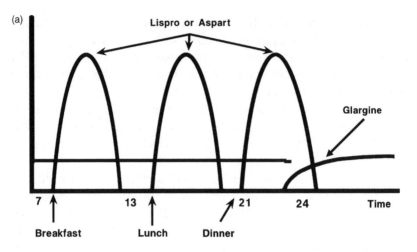

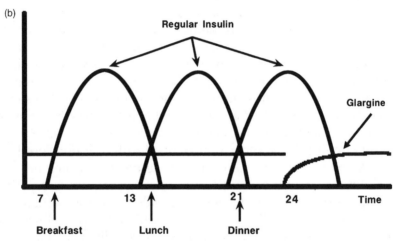

Figure 28.3. Schematic representation of a therapeutic scheme with administration of the insulin Glargine before bedtime and a) very rapid-acting-insulin analogue or b) regular insulin before each meal. Notice the flat action profile of Glargine and the absence of overlap among the insulins (particularly in scheme a) contrast to Figure 28.2.

before bedtime). An advantage of Detemir is the considerably smaller variability and higher reproducibility of its plasma levels compared to other insulins, after subcutaneous injection, both in the same individual and among different patients.

Which is the most preferable basal insulin?

Clinical studies, in which isophane insulin (NPH) is compared with zinc insulins (of simple or extended action) in Type 1 diabetics, are relatively few. In the studies that have been done, no essential differences between these insulins were found, both as regards glycaemic control and for the number and severity of hypoglycaemias.

In the past few years, a significant number of clinical studies have been performed comparing isophane insulin (NPH) (in one or two injections daily) with Glargine (in one injection daily) in individuals with Type 1 DM, who receive intensive insulin treatment. Most of these studies showed a reduction in the episodes of hypoglycaemia (especially during the night) with Glargine. Most studies did not show any difference in HbA_{1c} levels between the two types of insulin therapy, although in some studies the insulin Glargine achieved better fasting glucose levels than isophane insulin. The comparison of Glargine with zinc insulin of extended action (Ultralente), in combination with a very rapid-acting insulin analogue (as 'prandial' insulin), showed a larger reduction of HbA_{1c} and less hypoglycaemias in the insulin Glargine group.

Isophane insulin and the insulin Detemir have been compared less often, since Detemir is a newer analogue than Glargine. In one study, in patients with Type 1 DM, it appeared that Detemir, administered twice a day (either before breakfast and before bedtime, or simply every 12 hours), caused less night-time hypoglycaemias compared to isophane insulin, while at the same time it led to lower levels of premeal glucose. The total variability of glucose levels was smaller in the group of patients who received Detemir.

Studies are in progress comparing Glargine to Detemir and the results are eagerly awaited.

From the above data, we can conclude that the flat level and extended profile of action of Glargine simulates more with the physiologic basal secretion of insulin, compared to the older insulins. The advantages of Glargine are mainly less hypoglycaemias (especially at night), lower fasting glucose levels and the sufficiency (usually) of a once a day dose. Insulin Detemir, is administered twice a day and presents a profile of action with smaller a peak than the older insulins but definitely also, as was already mentioned, smaller variability of plasma levels after a subcutaneous injection.

How is the substitution of 'prandial' insulin done?

The 'prandial' insulin is substituted by administering an injection of rapid- or very-rapid acting insulin before the meal. If rapid-acting insulin is administered (i.e., soluble insulin), the injection should be given 30–45 minutes before the meal. If the administration of a very-rapid acting insulin analogue is preferred, the injection should be given immediately before the meal.

What is the most preferable 'prandial' insulin?

The choice is between rapid-acting insulin (regular insulin) and very rapid-acting insulin analogues (Lispro, Aspart or Glulisine). Examining the pharmacokinetic properties of these insulins, it is obvious that very rapid-acting insulin analogues imitate the physiological prandial secretion of insulin more efficiently, since they have a more rapid onset of action, more acute peak and shorter duration of action compared to regular insulin. Another advantage of insulin analogues is their immediate pre-prandial administration, since the necessary time interval between the injection of regular insulin and the meal is very often not observed by the patients, resulting in poor post-prandial glucose control. Clinical studies have shown that the administration of analogues is accompanied by fewer hypoglycaemias (both post-prandial as well as night-time) compared to the usual, rapid-acting regular insulin. The administration of insulin analogues in the meals presupposes complete coverage with basal insulin, because their duration of action is short. Thus, their administration is not recommended when only one injection of isophane insulin is used as basal insulin before bedtime (Figure 28.2a) The usage of analogues in combination with Glargine or Detemir is continuously gaining ground and tends to constitute the regimen of choice for Type 1 DM.

When is basal insulin administered and how is its dose determined?

When the substitution of basal secretion is done with one injection daily, it is administration before bedtime is usually preferred, because it has been proven that in this way the night-time hypoglycaemias are decreased. Insulin Glargine has also been given in the morning, after rising, with good results. When two injections of basal insulin are used (as with isophane insulin, insulin Lente and insulin Detemir), one of the two injections is usually given before bedtime and the second in the morning, after rising.

Most people with Type 1 DM, with body weight that does not deviate more than 20 percent from their ideal weight, need in total 0.5–1 unit of insulin per kg of body weight daily. This dose is usually smaller during the honeymoon period (i.e., usually for a few months after the diagnosis of DM), whereas it is bigger in periods of acute illness or intense psychological stress. Out of this total dose, roughly 50 percent is given as basal insulin. This percentage is valid when the insulin used as basal exclusively has this role, as is the case with insulins Glargine and Detemir. However, if the basal secretion is replaced by two injections of isophane insulin (or zinc-containing – Lente), their peaks often also substitute part of the meal insulins, with the result that their percentage of the total of administered units is higher than 50 percent (60–70 percent).

The precise percentage that the basal insulin occupies has to be calculated (on an) basis individual. The dose is mainly regulated based on the morning fasting glucose, depending on the targets, which are also individualized.

How are doses of 'prandial' insulin determined?

One of the main advantages of the basal-prandial insulin regimens is, as already mentioned, the liberation of the schedule and the content of the diabetic's meals. The first objective is achieved thanks to the action profile of the newer insulin analogues. The liberation of the content of the meal is achieved thanks to the calculation of a suitable dose of 'prandial' insulin, depending on the carbohydrate content of the meal. A prerequisite for the application of a system of carbohydrate measurement is the right training of the diabetic in the basic principles of the diet, so he or she learns to calculate the number of 'equivalent' carbohydrates of each meal. Each 'equivalent' constitutes roughly 10–15 grams of carbohydrates. As an example, a slice of bread (30 g) contains one equivalent. In the beginning, the patient is helped by special charts. The next step is the determination of the units of insulin that are required in order to absorb each equivalent, without disturbing the glucose homeostasis.

The number of units that are required per carbohydrate equivalent is individualized and often varies in the same individual depending on time of day, psychological condition, possible preceding or following physical exercise, and type of carbohydrates consumed. In any case, the usual dose is 1–2 units of insulin per carbohydrate equivalent. At the same time, a blood glucose measurement before the injection of prandial insulin and 'correction' of the dose depending on the result is always recommended (Table 28.3). The evaluation of the dose of 'prandial' insulin is based on the post-prandial blood glucose values (usually 2 hours after the meal), which should consequently be determined at regular time intervals.

Ultimately, every patient explores his or her blood sugar 'behaviour' in various situations, having as a basis the measurement of food carbohydrates and blood glucose, which he or she performs both pre- as well as post-prandially. The evaluation of these measurements, in collaboration with the treating physician, leads to improvements and transformations of the doses, which aim at the best possible glucose control.

Table 28.3. How is the dose of 'prandial' insulin determined?

Calculate 1–2 units per carbohydrate equivalent and measure capillary blood glucose. If the result is:

70–120 mg/dl (3.9–6.7 mmol/L) → no change in the dose
120–160 mg/dl (6.7–8.9 mmol/L) → administer 1 more unit
160–200 mg/dl (8.9–11.1 mmol/L) → administer 2 more units
(For every increase of blood glucose by 40 mg/dl (2.2 mmol/L)[*], administer 1 more unit of insulin)

> 300 mg/dl (16.7 mmol/L) → apart from the increase of the dose, delay the beginning of the food by 15–20 min and check the urine ketones. If they are positive, increase the intake of fluids and increase (by 1–2 units) the insulin dose. Recheck the blood glucose and urine ketones in two hours.

50–70 mg/dl (2.8–3.9 mmol/L) → decrease the dose by 1–2 units. Give the injection after the beginning of eating.

< 50 mg/dl (2.8 mmol/L) → decrease the dose by 2–3 units. Give the injection after eating. Include at least 10 g rapidly absorbable carbohydrates in the meal.

[*]This value is placed in the table somehow arbitrarily. In reality, it is individualized and determined by collaboration between the doctor and patient, depending on the course of DM control.

What are the indications for insulin administration in Type 2 DM?

Patients with Type 2 DM manifest a disturbance both in the action of insulin (insulin resistance) and in its secretion, which is decreased. During the natural course of the disease, the disturbance of insulin secretion progressively worsens. Ultimately, most Type 2 diabetics will need exogenous insulin administration. In the UKPDS study, 80 percent of the patients who were initially treated with a sulfonylurea, needed insulin after nine years.

The main indication for insulin administration in Type 2 DM is the secondary failure of treatment with oral antidiabetic medicines: that is, when a patient is receiving the optimal treatment with tablets and the HbA_{1c} is at levels approaching 8 percent, the administration of insulin is rendered necessary. Several experts recommend beginning insulin therapy even earlier (when HbA_{1c} steadily exceeds 7 percent). Other indications for insulin administration in individuals with Type 2 DM are reported in Table 28.4.

What insulin therapy regimens are used in Type 2 DM?

Type 2 DM is characterized, as mentioned, by variable residual functioning of the β-cell, which usually regulates good glycaemic control by substituting only the basal secretion of insulin. We can separate the forms of insulin treatment in Type 2 DM into three main categories:

- Substitution of only the basal insulin secretion, usually with simultaneous administration of antidiabetic pills. This scheme is preferred during the switch of treatment from pills to insulin, when there is evidence that the residual endogenous insulin secretion is relatively satisfactory. Such evidence exists when fasting plasma glucose is < 200 mg/dl (11.1 mmol/L), the HbA_{1c} is < 9 percent and the patient does not lose weight because of uncontrolled DM.

Table 28.4. Indications for treatment of Type 2 DM with insulin

Failure of the treatment with antidiabetic pills
Periods of stress (surgery, wound, infection, acute myocardial infarction)
Pregnancy
Serious hepatic or renal damage
In selected cases at diagnosis

- In more severe cases, when there is significant impairment of insulin secretion, the substitution alone of basal insulin no longer suffices and substitution of the 'prandial' insulin is also required. In these cases, schemes that also contain, apart from insulin of intermediate/slow action, rapid (or very-rapid) acting insulin, are usually administered, often in the form of ready-made mixtures. These mixtures are administered, for the most part, in the morning and in the evening preprandially. Sometimes a third injection is also added (usually rapid or very-rapid acting insulin) before lunch. At the same time, metformin can be prescribed in order to also decrease insulin resistance and limit the increase of body weight.
- In certain cases, the administration of a scheme of basal-bolus insulin can be required, as in Type 1 DM.

Apart from these three main categories, various other schemes are also used, since individualization is a basic rule in insulin therapy. Thus, in certain cases (as for example in steroid-induced DM) a long-acting sulfonylurea for substitution of the basal insulin secretion is administered along with regular insulin (or very-rapid acting insulin analogue) preprandially. Moreover, particularly in very obese patients with high insulin needs, schemes with three injections of insulin mixtures (usually 30/70 or 40/60) have also been tried before each meal.

In each one of the above cases, a corner-stone of treatment in Type 2 DM remains lifestyle modification, including the right diet, aimed at the intake of only the necessary calories from the most advisable foods (see Chapter 26) and the increase of physical activity.

What is the regimen of choice for the initiation of insulin therapy in individuals with Type 2 DM?

As already mentioned, the initial regimen of insulin therapy in these individuals is determined after many factors have been appreciated, the most important of which are the age and intellectual situation of the individual (ability to respond to the requirements of complicated schemes), possible coexisting diseases and preceding glucose control. A general rule is that the bigger the disturbance of insulin secretory ability, the more complicated are the schemes required to achieve the objectives.

Several writers, and also clinical doctors, recommend schemes of a basal insulin injection (usually before bedtime) in combination with tablets as the first choice in transition of patients with Type 2 DM to insulin therapy. A lot of studies have shown that these schemes are superior compared to insulin therapy alone, both for the achieved HbA_{1c}, as well as for the appearance of hypoglycaemias, the increase of weight and also – particularly important – the acceptance of the treatment by the patients. A very recent study showed that the initiation of insulin therapy with two injections of insulin mixtures of very-rapid/ intermediate acting insulin 30/70 (in combination with metformin) led to better control compared to an injection of insulin at bedtime (again in combination with metformin). In this study however, in individuals with $HbA_{1c} < 8.5$ percent, the two regimens led to similar control.

Ultimately, the most important thing is glycaemic control and achievement of the targets set by the doctor and the patient; the question of which means (which particular scheme) is selected to achieve this, is of course less important.

What constitutes the schemes of basal insulin-pills?

Any one of the intermediate- or slow-acting insulins can be administered, in one dose, before bedtime. Studies conducted in the past few years showed that the insulin Glargine causes fewer night-time hypoglycaemias, improves fasting plasma glucose and causes a slightly smaller weight gain compared to isophane insulin. However, there was no difference in the levels of HbA_{1c}. Moreover, Glargine can be administered in the morning, after rising, with the same results.

The coadministration of metformin limits the weight gain. If the desirable metabolic control with the combination of an evening insulin injection and metformin is not achieved, a sulfonylurea can be added. Some authors recommend maintenance with the sulfonylurea (together with metformin) from the beginning, when evening insulin is added. The combination of insulin with a sulfonylurea decreases the insulin needs and limits (to a smaller degree than metformin) the increase of body weight. The combination of insulin with meglitinides has not been tried in clinical studies. The coadministration of insulin with glitazones is expected to be approved soon in the European Union.

The dose of insulin is individualized. A generally acceptable rule is the administration of 10 units (or 0.1 U/kg of body weight) of slow-acting insulin before bedtime and the progressive titration of the dose until the

Table 28.5. Adjustment of the insulin dose injected at bedtime, in patients with Type 2 DM and fasting morning blood glucose target (FBG) 80–120 mg/dl (4.4–6.7 mmol/L)

Initial dose: 10 units
Adjustment of the dose each week
Mean value of FBG measurements of 4 last days:
> 180 mg/dl (10.0 mmol/L) → increase by 6 units
140–180 mg/dl (7.8–10.0 mmol/L) → increase by 4 units
120–140 mg/dl (6.7–7.8 mmol/L) → increase by 2 units
80–120 mg/dl (4.4–6.7 mmol/L) → no change in the dose
< 80 mg/dl (4.4 mmol/L) → return to the previous dose
Episode of hypoglycaemia → reduction by 2–4 units

desirable fasting morning glucose is achieved. The initial dose can be bigger (0.2–0.3 U/kg of body weight) when the individual is obese and/or the DM is out of control ($HbA_{1c} > 9$ percent). The titration of the dose depends on the morning fasting glucose levels. A simple titration algorithm is shown in Table 28.5

How do the schemes with premixed insulin preparations work?

In these schemes, individualization again constitutes the golden rule. The choice of the most suitable mixture, but also the dosage of insulin, depends on many factors, including the age of the patient, his or her nutritional programme, his or her physical activity, renal and hepatic function, etc. The most 'popular' mixtures are those that contain 30 percent rapid or very rapid-acting insulin and 70 percent intermediate-acting insulin (Figure 28.4). Usually, 2/3 of the total dose are given in the morning and 1/3 in the evening, pre-prandially (30–45 minutes before the meal) if the mixture contains regular insulin or immediately before the meal if it contains a very rapid-acting insulin analogue. However, the proportion of morning/evening dose varies considerably among patients. In certain cases the administration of a different mixture in the morning and in the evening may be required.

Most patients with Type 2 DM need 0.5–2 units of insulin per kilogram of body weight daily. When there is high insulin resistance, the dose can be much bigger. The onset of the treatment is done with the lowest dose in order to achieve metabolic control progressively and to avoid possible

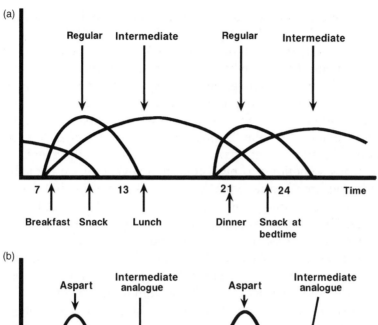

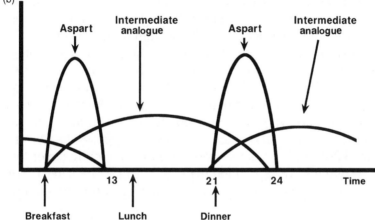

Figure 28.4. Schematic representation of a therapeutic scheme with administration of a) mixture of insulin (30% regular insulin, 70% intermediate acting insulin) in the morning and evening pre-prandially and b) mixture insulin of (30% very-rapid-acting insulin analogue, 70% intermediate acting insulin analogue) in the morning and evening pre-prandially. Notice the smaller overlaps among the insulins in scheme b) where there is usually no need for intake of additional snacks in between.

hypoglycaemias in patients with higher insulin sensitivity. The coadministration of metformin decreases the insulin needs.

The schemes with two injections of premixed insulin compounds are widely used because they are relatively simple and practical. However, in order for the blood sugar to get under control, the daily programme of the patients should be relatively stable, with only small divergences from day to day as regards the timing and content of meals and the level of physical activity. Patients who receive an insulin mixture that contains regular insulin in the morning, should usually eat a snack 2–3 hours after the injection to avoid hypoglycaemias (see Figure 28.4a). At the same time, lunch should be temporally placed when the peak of the morning intermediate-acting insulin begins (i.e., 5–6 hours after the morning injection). The administration of an insulin mixture in the evening before dinner, leads sometimes to night-time hypoglycaemia, especially if the dinner is consumed early, whereby the peak of the intermediate-acting insulin coincides with the early morning hours (1–3 a.m.) of high insulin sensitivity. This is avoided either by instructing the patients to receive a small quantity of carbohydrates (for example, a glass of milk with a rusk) before bedtime (if at that time the blood glucose level is < 140 mg/dl [7.8 mmol/L]), or by administering the regular insulin (pre-prandially) separate from the intermediate-acting insulin (before bedtime).

The mixtures containing very rapid-acting insulin analogues (see Figure 28.4b) have an advantage because they decrease the probability of hypoglycemia in the early afternoon hours and at night. This is due to the shorter duration of action of the analogue which leads to only a small degree of overlap with the intermediate-acting insulin. On the other hand, the administration of these mixtures presupposes the reception of a large breakfast, and sometimes they do not sufficiently cover the lunch needs, resulting in post-prandial hyperglycaemia. The latter is corrected by administering one dose of very rapid-acting insulin pre-prandially.

Are intensified regimens of basal-bolus insulin administered in Type 2 DM?

There are many factors that render such a solution difficult to apply. The majority of patients with Type 2 DM are elderly and it would be exceptionally difficult for them to adapt themselves to the requirements of such a scheme. Even if some of them could ultimately familiarize themselves, very few would accept injecting insulin 4–5 times daily. Furthermore, the cost of supplying an intensified insulin scheme would be overwhelming, just when there exist no explicit data supporting the supremacy of such schemes in Type 2 DM. However, in certain selected patients (including in the failure of other types of therapy, in young and active patients with significant impairment of the insulin secretory capacity, in renal or hepatic insufficiency, and in pregnancy), basal-bolus insulin schemes are administered for Type 2 DM, on condition of course that explicit motivation and the ability to respond to the requirements of this type of treatment are clearly present in the patient.

CASE STUDY 1

A 19 year old man was admitted to the hospital a week ago because of diabetic ketoacidosis; he was discharged three days ago. The regimen he received on discharge consisted of an insulin mixture, regular/NPH insulin 30/70 percent, 15 units in the morning and 10 units in the evening. He has now come to the Diabetes Clinic to receive advice from specialists in the care of diabetes. The patient had had the typical symptoms of hyperglycaemia for roughly 3–4 months before the diagnosis. He reports a weight loss of about 8–10 kg (17.6–22.1 lb). He had no significant past medical history. The physical examination was unremarkable except for a weight of 62 kg (136.7 lb), height of 1.83 m (6 ft) (BMI: 18.5 kg/m^2), capillary blood sugar level of 429 mg/dl (23.8 mmol/L) and HbA$_{1c}$ of 13.1 percent.

The patient and his family were informed about DM and the therapeutic possibilities. The concept of an intensive insulin regimen of basal-bolus insulin was explicitly explained to them. They had extensive discussions with a dietitian so that the elements of a right diet could be analyzed but also so patient could be informed about the carbohydrate equivalents. The need of self-monitoring of blood glucose at home with a portable glucose meter was stressed to the patient and the technique of measurement was explained to him.

It is explicit that in the first visit it is impossible for the patient to consolidate all this overwhelming new information, especially since he is under intense psychological stress because of the recent diagnosis of his disease. If feasible, discussion with a psychologist specialized in the subject is often very beneficial.

As already mentioned, from the very first visit the patient was informed about the advantages, but also the requirements, of an intensified insulin regimen. However, in order to give him time to consolidate and rehearse all the elements that compose the correct application of such a regimen, the scheme of the insulin mixture regular/NPH 30/70 was initially maintained, increasing the dose to 20 units in the morning and 14 units in the evening. Moreover, a very-rapid-acting insulin analogue was prescribed, with instructions to inject a few units (2–5, depending on the blood sugar levels) before lunch. The fact that significant insulin resistance coexisted (because of the recent ketoacidosis) as well as glucotoxicity (because of the prolonged and intense hyperglycaemia that preceded the diagnosis) was taken into consideration. A follow-up appointment was arranged for a week later.

At the follow-up, the patient brought the blood sugar measurements shown in the following table (the last four days are shown [in mg/dl (mmol/L)]):

	Breakfast		Lunch			Dinner	
Date	Pre	2 hrs	Pre	2 hrs	Pre	2 hrs	Bedtime
24/1	278	314	294	221	298	301	265
	(15.4)	(17.4)	(16.3)	(12.3)	(16.5)	(16.7)	(14.7)
25/1	264		194	205	355	298	
	(14.7)		(10.8)	(11.4)	(19.7)	(16.5)	
26/1	246	198	186		311	318	265
	(13.7)	(11.0)	(10.3)		(17.3)	(17.7)	(14.7)
27/1	199		254	186	299	256	
	(11.0)		(14.1)	(10.3)	(16.6)	(14.2)	

The blood sugar remains poorly controlled but fluctuates at lower levels than before (80 percent of the measurements are <300 mg/dl [16.7 mmol/L]), and the fluctuations are relatively small. As the patient moves away from the episode of ketoacidosis and the glucotoxicity is removed, he will very probably enter the honeymoon period, during which insulin needs decrease significantly.

At the second visit, new extensive discussion took place, focused on the resolution of various queries of the patient. He expressed the wish to start an intensified regimen of basal-bolus insulin. It was decided to start him on Glargine (basal insulin) before bedtime and a very-rapid acting insulin analogue (Lispro or Aspart) before each main meal. The dose of Glargine was calculated by dividing the total number of insulin units administered up to now by two:

$$20 \text{ (in the morning)} + 14 \text{ (in the evening)}$$
$$+ 4 \text{ (on average midday)} = 38/2 = 19 \text{ units.}$$

Another method of calculation is to subtract from the total intermediate/ slowly acting dose of insulin what the patient was receiving (in this case):

$$34 \times 70\% = 23.8 \text{ units} - 20\% \text{ (that is : } 23.8 - 4.76 = 19 \text{ units)}.$$

The patient's diet usually included 4–5 carbohydrate equivalents (bread) in the morning, 6–8 at lunch and 4–6 in the evening. He also receives a snack between breakfast and lunch time, which contains three carbohydrate equivalents. Consequently, the total number of carbohydrate equivalents is 18–21 daily. Thus, the remainding 17 units of insulin (that are intended for the 18–21 carbohydrate equivalents) were distributed first as one unit per equivalent. Moreover, the patient was given Table 28.3 so that he could correct his blood sugar pre-prandially. A new appointment was arranged for a week's time.

At this new visit, the patient brought the following measurements (the last four days are shown [in mg/dl (mmol/L)]):

	Breakfast		Lunch		Dinner		
Date	Pre	2 hrs	Pre	2 hrs	Pre	2 hrs	Bedtime
30/1	183	216	208	142	188	231	
	(10.2)	(12.0)	(11.5)	(7.9)	(10.4)	(12.8)	
	[3–5]*		[7–10]*		[5–7]*		
31/1	208	158	269	137	192		166
	(11.5)	(8.8)	(14.9)	(7.6)	(10.7)		(9.2)
	[3–6]*		[6–11]*		[4–6]*		
01/2	190		154	129	169	223	231
	(10.6)		(8.6)	(7.2)	(9.4)	(12.4)	(12.8)
	[3–6]*		[8–9]*		[6–7]*		
02/2	199	89	334	164	148	179	192
	(11.0)	(4.9)	(18.5)	(9.1)	(8.2)	(9.9)	(10.7)
	[4–7]*		[4–10]*		[7–8]*		

*The numbers inside the brackets (after each measurement) correspond, the first one to the number of carbohydrate equivalents, and the second one to the units of insulin that were administered.

There is definite improvement shown compared to the previous measurements. The morning fasting glucose level is quite stable and ranges between 180–200 mg/dl (10.0–11.1 mmol/L). Based on these levels it was recommended that the patient increase the basal insulin (Glargine) by 6 units. The post-prandial levels are, in the majority, within target in the morning and midday, but not in the evening. This is probably due to decreased evening levels of Glargine, since at that time 22–24 hours of administration are completed. An increase of the evening very-rapid-acting insulin analogue by 0.5 units per carbohydrate equivalent was recommended.

A few days later, the majority of the measurements were within target levels. Progressively, over the next three months, the doses of both the basal and 'prandial' insulin were decreased. The HbA$_{1c}$ was 5.9 percent, the patient was receiving 7 units of Glargine before bedtime and ½ unit of very-rapid-acting insulin analogue per carbohydrate equivalent. It is known that in Type 1 DM, the timely administration of insulin and good diabetic control extend the period of residual endogenous insulin secretion (honeymoon period, recession of DM) at which time insulin needs are small (sometimes minimal) and blood sugar control is of course easier. The administration of insulin should be continued so that the extension of the honeymoon period is achieved. During this period it is possible to maintain very good control even without an intensive insulin regimen [for example, with two injections of insulin (in small doses) of intermediate action or a mixture of insulins, in the morning and evening]. The patient under discussion opted to continue the intensified regimen. When his meal had a very small carbohydrate content he could omit the administration of 'prandial' insulin without a significant rise of his blood sugar. The honeymoon period in Type 1 DM usually lasts from several days to months, and more occasionally for more than a year.

CASE STUDY 2

A 28 year old man with Type 1 DM for four years receives intensive insulin therapy with isophane insulin (NPH) at bedtime (24 units) and regular insulin before each main meal. The latter dose is calculated depending on the content of the meal in carbohydrates. Usually, he receives two units per carbohydrate equivalent. At the same time, before the meal he measures the blood sugar and when the level exceeds 100 mg/dl (5.6 mmol/L) he adds one unit of insulin per 40 mg (2.2 mmol) glucose (for example, 140 mg/dl (7.8 mmol/L) → +1 unit, 180 mg/dl (10.0 mmol/L) → +2 units, and so forth). He is particularly regular in the taking of his meals and his DM control was up to recently excellent (HbA$_{1c}$ = 6.3 percent). During the last month, however, he experienced frequent hypoglycaemias that roused him in the early morning hours (3–4 a.m.). His DM control has been disturbed. This self-monitoring diary has the following measurements for the previous week (in mg/dl [mmol/L]):

Date	Pre-break-fast	Post-break-fast	Pre-lunch	Post-lunch	Pre-dinner	Bed-time	Notes
24/1 (Friday)	72 (4.0) [6]*		129 (7.2) [10]*		223 (12.4) [13]*		3.30 a.m.: 52 (2.9)
25/1 (Saturday)	321 (17.8) [12]*	199 (11.0) [3]*	55 (3.1) [6])	155 (8.6)	145 (8.1) [8]*	99 (5.5)	1 glass of milk + 1 rusk before bedtime
26/1 (Sunday)	124 (6.9) [8]*		88 (4.9) [10]*			135 (7.5)	½ glass of milk +1 rusk at bedtime
27/1 (Monday)	99 (5.5) [6]*		[10]*		194 (10.8) [12]*	214 (11.9)	4 a.m.: 48 (2.7)
28/1 (Tuesday)	298 (16.5) [11]*	176 (9.8)	204 (11.3) [13]*		276 (15.3) [14]*	223 (12.4)	4.10 a.m.: 67 (3.7)
29/1 (Wednes-day)	198 (11.0) [8]*		186 (10.3) [12]*		254 (14.1) [13]*	321 (17.8) [5]*	4.45 am.: 30 (1.7)
30/1 (Thursday)	355 (19.7) [13]*						

*In brackets are shown the numbers of the units of regular insulin administered. Every evening, at bedtime, the patient receives 24 units of isophane insulin.

The blood glucose control is not good. Episodes of hypoglycaemia at night-time are observed, which occur after the weekday days. The patient is aware of the hypoglycaemias and gets roused from his sleep, usually with intense perspiration and tachycardia, and on one occasion (early morning of the 30th January) he experienced orientation disturbances and required the help of his spouse. The patient, frightened from these symptoms, 'over-corrects' the hypoglycaemia, with the result that he has quite high blood glucose levels the next morning (25th January to 28th–30th January). It is also likely that the hyperglycaemia that follows the night-time hypoglycaemias is due to the described Somogyi phenomenon (counteractive hyperglycaemia, see Chapter 5). Afterwards, by increasing the morning dose of regular insulin, the blood sugar level is improved up to the lunch hours. Actually, on one occasion, hypoglycaemia occurred (25th January), obviously because of the accumulation of insulin (12 units before breakfast and three units more, without any food, two hours after breakfast). Before dinner, hyperglycaemia is observed (once again during the weekday days), which is followed by night-time hypo-glycaemia. On the 29th January, because of intense hyperglycaemia at bedtime, five more units of regular insulin were administered, resulting in the episode of severe hypoglycaemia. It is stressed that every day, 24 units of isophane insulin at bedtime were received.

The patient reported that during the last month he had undertaken afternoon work, and had transferred his evening dinner from 8 p.m. to between 10.30 p.m. and 11 p.m. Because of lack of time, he was injecting the evening regular insulin immediately before dinner and, roughly an hour later, he would sleep, after, as mentioned before, also injecting the 24 units of isophane insulin. Based on the above informa-tion we can notice the following points:

1. The high glucose levels before dinner during the weekdays are due to the large interval between lunch (around 1 p.m.) and dinner (10 p.m.). With his new programme, the patient remains without insulin from around 8 p.m. (when the action of the lunch-time regular insulin gets exhausted) until around 11 p.m. (when the action of the evening regular insulin begins). This happens because he only uses one injection of isophane insulin as basal insulin before sleep, the action of which is exhausted around 5–6 p.m. the next day.

2. n order to correct the hyperglycaemia before dinner-time, the patient injects a quite large dose of regular insulin, however, with erroneous timing (immediately before the meal), with the result, an hour later, that the hyperglycaemia remain or even intensify (29th January). This peak of action of insulin (around the early night hours, 1–2 a.m.) afterwards leads to a fall in the glucose levels, while at the same time there is overlap with the action of isophane insulin that continues for 2–3 more hours, resulting in the appearance of hypoglycaemia around 4 a.m.

3. On 29th January, at bedtime, because of the intense hyperglycaemia, the patient received five more units of regular insulin. This led to the appearance of even more severe hypoglycaemia.

4. It should be noticed that on Saturdays and Sundays, when the patient followed his old schedule, the injection of the evening 'prandial' insulin was done earlier and with correct timing as regards

the meal, so that no post-prandial hyperglycaemia is observed. On the contrary, at bedtime, the blood glucose levels were relatively low and the patient drank some milk with a rusk, according to the instructions previously given to him. No hypoglycaemia occurred on those nights.

The night-time hypoglycaemias and the hyperglycaemias before dinner constitute known 'weaknesses' of the above therapeutic regimen. The proposed solutions are:

1. Addition of a second injection of isophane insulin in the morning, before breakfast, at a smaller dose than the evening insulin, with simultaneous reduction in the dose of the latter injection. At the same time, replacement of the regular insulin with a very rapid-acting insulin analogue in order to decrease the overlap between the insulins (Figure 28.5).
2. Replacement of the evening isophane insulin with the long-acting insulin analogue Glargine. At the same time, the administration of a very-rapid-acting insulin analogue as 'prandial' insulin would be preferable, so as to achieve a correct timing with the meal (it is reminded that our patient is unable to wait for 30–45 minutes between the evening 'prandial' insulin and the dinner) and so that the action of

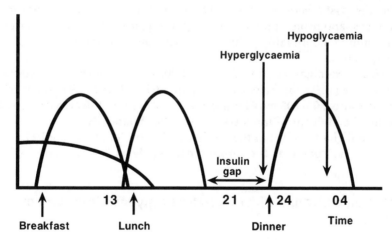

Figure 28.5. Graphic representation of a scheme of insulin therapy, which in combination with the dietary and lifestyle programme of the patient, caused the decompensation of blood sugar.

the evening 'prandial' insulin does not coincide with the night-time hours of high insulin sensitivity.
3. AS Solution 2, but with administration of two injections of the insulin Detemir instead of Glargine.

CASE STUDY 3

A 65 year old woman with Type 2 DM for the last 15 years presents for examination because of very high blood glucose levels. She is not regularly followed by a doctor and does not have a blood glucose meter at home. During the last months she has manifested polyuria, polydipsia and xerostomia. She has been receiving glibenclamide tablets for 10 years, the dose of which she increased progressively on her own, now receiving 15 mg daily (one tablet morning, midday, evening). She reports that in general she is careful with her diet and her weight is stable although during the previous months perhaps it has decreased by 2–3 kg (4.4–6.6 lb). She took the initiative to have some biochemical tests performed around 10 days ago, when the fasting plasma glucose level was 316 mg/dl (17.5 mmol/L). Alarmed by the result she had the measurement repeated two days later, when the result was 298 mg/dl (16.5 mmol/L).

The patient has had hypertension for 20 years treated with amlodipine, 10 mg daily. Otherwise she has no significant past medical history. She has not been evaluated for diabetic retinopathy for the last five years (she reports that in the past 'there was no problem') and does not know what micro-albuminuria and proteinuria are. She reports typical symptoms of peripheral sensory-motor neuropathy. She does not know what the glycosylated haemoglobin is.

Physical examination reveals the following: moderately overweight (weight 68 kg [149.9 lb]; height 1.59 m [5 ft 2.6 in]; BMI 26.89 kg/m^2); arterial blood pressure 165/105 mmHg; pulse rate 82 min; and decreased sensation (superficial and deep) of the lower extremities bilaterally.

The blood glucose level at the clinic was 278 mg/dl (15.4 mmol/L) and the HbA$_{1c}$ was 10.5 percent. The serum creatinine level was normal.

What should be done with regard to the glycaemic control of this patient?

The patient obviously manifests secondary failure of the oral antidiabetic drug treatment. The diagnosis of DM was done 15 years before, she receives almost the maximal dose of glibenclamide and her body weight is only slightly increased. The above data suggest a serious disturbance of insulin secretion. The addition of a second medicine (for example, metformin) is not expected to decrease HbA_{1c} more than 1.5 percent. The beginning of insulin treatment was recommended to the patient, but she explicitly refused. After instructions were once again given regarding proper diet and mild increase in physical activity, metformin was added to the treatment at an initial dose of 850 mg daily and later 1700 mg daily (one pill morning and evening, after the meal).

The patient returned after eight months. Her symptoms had not receded and her HbA_{1c} was 9.8 percent. She now accepted the treatment with insulin.

Due to the high level of HbA_{1c} and since it was considered that a significant degree of insulin secretory impairment from the pancreas exists, it was preferred to administer both basal and 'prandial' insulin right from the beginning, in the form of a fixed mixture, morning and evening. The choice of the mixture depends on the age of the patient, his or her compliance, the dietary schedule and the glucose levels as shown from the self-monitoring measurements. In this particular case a mixture of 30 percent regular insulin and 70 percent intermediate-action (NPH) insulin was initially preferred.

Calculation of the dose was as follows. 0.5 units insulin per kilogram of body weight were calculated to be necessary, that is 34 units of insulin (0.5×68), daily. Because it was decided to continue the metformin (at a dose of 850 mg daily), 15 percent of the insulin units were removed, that is five units, and finally 29 units of insulin were administered. Because the patient reports that her dinner is not particularly rich, the units were initially distributed as two thirds (19 units) in the morning, before breakfast, with the remainder (10 units) before dinner. It was stressed to the patient that the administration of insulin renders the self-monitoring of blood glucose with a meter essential (see Chapter 4). Proper advice on the suitable content and timing of the meals was given (Figure 28.4a). After discussion with the patient, the targets for the glycaemic control were set: for fasting glucose, <120 mg/dl (6.7 mmol/L); for post-prandial glucose, < 180 mg/dl (10.0 mmol/L); and for bedtime glucose, < 140 mg/dl 7.8 mmol/L), as well as HbA_{1c} < 7.0 percent.

The next meeting was arranged for one week, when the patient brought the following measurements (the values of the last three days are shown [in mg/dl (mmol/L)].

Date	Breakfast		Lunch		Dinner		
	Pre	**2 hrs after**	**Pre**	**2 hrs after**	**Pre**	**2 hrs after**	**Bedtime**
16/6	256 (14.2)	199 (11.0)	203 (11.3)	229 (12.7)	226 (12.5)		216 (12.0)
17/6	224 (12.4)		178 (9.9)		219 (12.2)		
18/6	230 (12.8)			218 (12.1)	198 (11.0)		207 (11.5)

Based on the above measurements, the dose of the morning insulin was increased by six units, so that the blood glucose levels two hours after the breakfast are improved (increase of the regular insulin by 1.8 units) as well as those after lunch (increase of intermediate-acting insulin by 4.2 units). The dose of the evening insulin was also increased by two units.

Twenty days later, the patient's measurements were as follows (the values of the last three days are shown [in mg/dl (mmol/L]):

Date	Breakfast		Lunch		Dinner		
	Pre	**2 hrs after**	**Pre**	**2 hrs after**	**Pre**	**2 hrs after**	**Bedtime**
7/7	145 (8.1)		148 (8.2)		177 (9.8)		165 (9.2)
8/7	148 (8.2)		132 (7.3)			156 (8.7)	
9/7	133 (7.4)			182 (10.1)			141 (7.8)

Most measurements now approach the set targets. Insulin was increased by two units in the morning and evening. A follow-up appointment was arranged for one month, when the measurements (of the three last days) were as follows (in mg/dl [mmol/L]):

Date	Breakfast		Lunch		Dinner		
	Pre	**2 hrs after**	**Pre**	**2 hrs after**	**Pre**	**2 hrs after**	**Bedtime**
29/7	**117** **(6.5)**		**99** **(5.5)**		224 (12.4)		**132** **(7.3)**

30/7	**99**	**178**	144
	(5.5)	**(9.9)**	(8.0)
31/7	**114**	**111**	200
	(6.3)	**(6.2)**	(11.1)

The vast majority of the measurements are now within therapeutic targets (bold letters). The patient notes that the high values are due to aberrations in diet. Three months after the beginning of insulin, the HbA$_{1c}$ was measured at 6.7 percent. The continuation of the same treatment and follow-up were recommended.

CASE STUDY 4

A 72 year old man with Type 2 DM for 12 years, who is obese (weight: 90 kg [198.4 lb], height: 1.70 m [5 ft 7 in], BMI: 31.2 kg/m^2), receives treatment with oral antidiabetic medicines: glimepiride 4 mg daily (in the morning) and metformin 2,550 mg daily (850 mg tablets morning, midday, evening). He regularly checks his blood sugar levels with a portable glucose meter. His DM control over the past few years has always been satisfactory (HbA$_{1c}$: 6.5–7.3 percent). However, over the last eight months he has observed a progressive increase in the blood glucose levels, and the last two HbA$_{1c}$ measurements, three months apart, were 7.8 percent and 8.3 percent (the most recent). His diet frequently deviates from the frame of instructions he has been given, because 'he likes good food'. He also has hypertension (under pharmaceutical treatment, with good control) and hyperlipidaemia (under treatment with a statin). His self-monitoring diary shows the following measurements for the last three days (in mg/dl [mmol/L]):

	Breakfast		Lunch		Dinner		
Date	Pre	2 hrs after	Pre	2 hrs after	Pre	2 hrs after	Bedtime
5/11	187		200			194	
	(10.4)		(11.1)			(10.8)	
6/11	223		188		227		
	(12.4)		(10.4)		(12.6)		
7/11	209		179		210		
	(11.6)		(9.9)		(11.7)		

The patient is receiving the maximal metformin dose together with a big dose of sulfonylurea and yet is not well controlled. Over the last six months he tried to decrease his weight by reducing the in- take of calories and by slightly increasing his walking time, but he failed.

This patient has an indication for insulin treatment. He has had known DM for 12 years, receives a combination of a sulfonylurea with metformin in large doses and his control is inadequate (HbA$_{1c}$ >8 percent). He has repeatedly received lifestyle intervention instructions, without any success. It was decided to stop glimepiride, to retain metformin and to add insulin of intermediate or slow action before bedtime. The evening insulin injection substitutes the basal secretion of insulin and usually suffices for the correction of hyperglycaemia when residual secretion from the β-cell exists, as often happens during the switch of treatment from antidiabetic tablets to insulin, especially in patients with HbA$_{1c}$ <9 percent and fasting plasma glucose not exceeding by far the 200 mg/dl (11.1 mmol/L) level. Moreover, the administration of only one insulin injection at bedtime is generally more easily accepted by patients, which is particularly important due to the frequent refusal of patients to accept the receipt of insulin.

Ten units of the insulin Glargine were prescribed at bedtime. It was explained to the patient that the adjustment of the dose would be performed based on the morning fasting glucose levels. The need for body weight loss with the correct diet was once again emphasized. One week later, the measurements of the three last days (in mg/dl [mmol/L]) were as follows:

| | Breakfast | | Lunch | | Dinner | | |
Date	Pre	2 hrs after	Pre	2 hrs after	Pre	2 hrs after	Bedtime
20/11	205 (11.4)			244 (13.5)		235 (13.0)	
21/11	239 (13.3)		255 (14.2)				
22/11	218 (12.1)				236 (13.1)		

It is obvious that the insulin dose is insufficient. The mean value of fasting plasma glucose is 220 mg/dl (12.2 mmol/L). The increase in the dose was determined to be six units (see Table 28.5). The following week, the mean value of fasting blood glucose was 192 mg/dl (10.7 mmol/L) and another increase of the dose by six units was recommended. The adjustment was continued (see Table 28.5) and one month later the dose of insulin was stabilized at 28 units. The majority of the measurements, both pre-prandial and post-prandial, were within targets. Three months after the beginning of insulin treatment, the HbA$_{1c}$ was 6.6 percent. The patient's weight remained stable. The same treatment was continued.

CASE STUDY 5

A 63 year old-man has suffered from Type 2 DM for 20 years. He has received isophane insulin (NPH) for three years, 26 units in the morning and 16 units in the evening. His control is moderate (the HbA$_{1c}$ level during the previous year ranged from 7.5 percent to 8.1 percent). One month ago he underwent a coronary artery bypass operation, after a myocardial infarction that he had suffered three months before. After the operation, he continued the same DM treatment. His body weight is normal (weight: 74 kg [163.2 lb], height: 1.72 m [5 ft 7.7 in], BMI: 25 kg/m^2). Recent laboratory evaluation showed a slightly increased creatinine level (1.5 mg/dl [132.6 μmol/L]). There exists background diabetic retinopathy and diabetic neuropathy. He reports that after the surgery his blood sugar control is worse than ever and he often manifests hyperglycaemic symptoms, despite the fact that he is particularly diligent with his diet. The latest HbA$_{1c}$ is 8.8 percent. He brings a diary with blood sugar measurements for the last three days indicatively shown below (in mg/dl [mmol/L]):

	Breakfast		Lunch		Dinner		
Date	Pre	2 hrs after	Pre	2 hrs after	Pre	2 hrs after	Bedtime
12/3	255 (14.2)				284 (15.8)		
13/3	231 (12.8)				299 (16.6)		
14/3	268 (14.9)				331 (18.4)		

Strict glycaemic control targets need to be set for this particular patient, since he already manifests both micro- as well as macro-vascular complications while he is still at a relatively young age. The fasting blood glucose level should be < 120 mg/dl (6.7 mmol/L), the post-prandial level < 150–160 mg/dl (8.3–8.9 mmol/L) and the HbA$_{1c}$ < 7 percent. At the same time, because of the recent heart surgery, there is significant, although transient, insulin resistance that is probably responsible for the further decompensation of his blood sugar. Post-prandial measurements are absent from his self-monitoring diary.

In this first approach with the patient, the dose of insulin was increased by four units in the morning and evening and a dietary program was recommended. The importance of the correct self-monitoring schedule, which includes both pre- as well as post-prandial measurements, was explained to him. A follow-up appointment was arranged for 10 days, when the following measurements were supplied (indicatively the last three days are shown [in mg/dl (mmol/L)]:

	Breakfast		Lunch		Dinner		
Date	Pre	2 hrs after	Pre	2 hrs after	Pre	2 hrs after	Bedtime
24/3	194 (10.8)	324 (18.0)					
25/3	200 (11.1)		279 (15.5)		249 (13.8)		
26/3	187 (10.4)			315 (17.5)		299 (16.6)	

The blood sugar control remains poor with only a small improvement in the morning fasting glucose levels. It was decided to administer a form of insulin therapy that included a fixed mixture of 30 percent very-rapid-acting-insulin analogue (Aspart) and 70 percent of intermediate-acting insulin analogue with protamine (Novomix), in the morning and in the evening, immediately before the meals. The dose of the evening insulin remained the same (20 units) and the morning insulin was decreased by six units (24 units), which were added at midday, immediately before lunch, in the form of very-rapid-acting insulin analogue. The therapeutic regimen was therefore as follows:

- morning: 26 units of a fixed insulin mixture 30/70 (very-rapid-acting analogue/intermediate-acting analogue);
- midday: 6 units of very-rapid-acting insulin analogue;
- evening: 20 units of fixed insulin mixture 30/70 (very-rapid-acting analogue/intermediate-acting analogue).

A new dietary programme with emphasis on the intake of a sufficient amount of breakfast was recommended. The administration of very-rapid-acting insulin analogue before lunch was considered necessary from the beginning, because the dose of the morning mixture could not be increased any further, since this would lead to hypoglycaemia 2–3 hours after breakfast (due to the simultaneous increase of the very-rapid-acting insulin analogue). It was emphasized to the patient that with this more intensified programme he should measure his blood sugar at least three times daily. A follow-up appointment was arranged for 15 days, when the following measurements were supplied (indicatively the last three days are shown [in mg/dl (mmol/L)]:

Date	Breakfast		Lunch		Dinner		Bedtime
	Pre	2 hrs after	Pre	2 hrs after	Pre	2 hrs after	
10/4	153	100		144		178	
	(8.5)	(5.6)		(8.0)		(9.9)	
11/4	140		99		126		151
	(7.8)		(5.5)		(7.0)		(8.4)
12/4	163			138		201	
	(9.1)			(7.7)		(11.2)	

The improvement is impressive. However, the morning values as well as those two hours after dinner remain above target. An increase of the evening insulin by four units was introduced, with the result that, at the following visit, the vast majority of the measurements were within therapeutic targets. Three months later, the HbA_{1c} was 6.6 percent. The same regimen was continued.

In relatively young patients with Type 2 DM, and with the presence of complications, more intensified forms of insulin therapy are required when there exists a serious disturbance in the secretion of insulin. Such a regimen was administered to this patient. Sometimes the administration of intensified regimens of basal-bolus insulin can be required, as in Type 1 DM, but usually this is avoided, because patients with Type 2 DM are usually less motivated and have a limited ability of corresponding to the requirements of these regimens.

Further reading

Barnett, A.H. (2003) A review of basal insulins. *Diabet Med* **20**: 873–85.
Bolli, G.B. (1997) Insulin treatment and its complications, in *Textbook of Diabetes* 2nd edn, (eds J. Pickup and G. Williams), *Oxford*, **43**: pp. 1–38.

Chan, J.L., Abrahamson, M.J. (2003) Pharmacological management of Type 2 diabetes mellitus: Rationale for rational use of insulin. *Mayo Clin Proc* **78**: 459–67.

Davidson, M.B. (2005) Starting insulin therapy in Type 2 diabetic patients: Does it really matter how? *Diabetes Care* **28**: 494–5.

De Witt, D.E., Hirsch, I.B. (2003) Outpatient insulin therapy in Type 1 and Type 2 diabetes mellitus. Scientific review. *JAMA* **289**: 2254–64.

De Witt, D.E., Dugdale, D.C. (2003) Using new insulin strategies in the outpatient treatment of diabetes. Clinical applications. *JAMA* **289**: 2265–69.

Diabetes Control and Complications Trial Research Group (DCCT) (1993) The effect of intensive treatment of diabetes on the development and progression of long-term complications in insulin-dependent diabetes mellitus. *N Engl J Med.*, **329**: 977–86.

Gerich, J.E. (2002) Novel insulins: expanding options in diabetes management. *Am J Med* **113**: 308–16.

Heinemann, L. (1997) Insulin pharmacology, in *Textbook of Diabetes* 2nd edn, (eds J. Pickup and G. Williams), *Oxford*, **42**:pp. 1-15.

Home, P., Bartley, P., Russell-Jones, D., Hanaire-Broutin, H., Heeg, J.E., Abrams, P., Landin-Olsson, M., Hylleberg, B., Lang, H., Draeger, E. (2004) Insulin Detemir offers improved glycemic control compared with NPH insulin in patients with Type 1 diabetes. *Diabetes Care* **27**: 1081–87.

Janka, H.U., Riddle, M.C., Kliebe-Frisch, C., Schweitzer, M.A., Yki-Järvinen. (2005) Comparison of basal insulin added to oral agents versus twice-daily premixed insulin as initial insulin therapy for Type 2 diabetes. *Diabetes Care* **28**: 254–9.

Raskin, P., Allen, E., Hollander, P., Lewin, A., Gabbay, R.A., Hu, P., Bode, B., Garber, A. (2005) (for the INITIATE Study Group) Initiating Insulin Therapy in Type 2 Diabetes: A comparison of biphasic and basal insulin analogs. *Diabetes Care* **28**: 260–5.

Ratner, R.E., Hirsch, I.B., Neifing, J.L., Garg, S.K., Mecca, T.E., Wilson, C.A. (2000) Less hypoglycemia with insulin Glargine in intensive insulin therapy for Type 1 diabetes. *Diabetes Care* **23**: 639–43.

Skyler, J.S. (2004) Insulin treatment, in *Therapy for Diabetes Mellitus and Related Disorders*, 4th edn. American Diabetes Association, (ed. H.E. Lebovitz) pp. 207–23.

UKPDS Study Group (1998). Intensive blood glucose control with sulfonylurea or insulin compared with conventional treatment and risk of complications in patients with Type 2 diabetes (UKPDS 33). *Lancet*, **352**, 837–53..

Yki-Järvinen, H., Ryysy, L., Nikkilä, K., Tulokas, T., Vanamo, R., Heikkilä, M. (1999) Comparison of bedtime insulin regimens in patients with Type 2 diabetes mellitus. A randomized, controlled trial. *Ann Intern Med* **130**: 389–96.

Yki-Järvinen, H. (2001) Combination therapies with insulin in Type 2 diabetes. *Diabetes Care* **24**: 758–67.

29

New therapies in diabetes

Panagiotis Tsapogas

INSULIN PUMPS

What is the continuous subcutaneous insulin infusion pump?

This is an appliance that continuously administers insulin subcutaneously. It is considered the best way of approaching the physiologic delivery of insulin in persons with Type 1 DM. The treatment with an insulin pump was initially introduced in the 1970s and the initial studies showed many advantages compared with the other methods of subcutaneous insulin administration. In the DCCT study, 42 percent of the participants with Type 1 DM received intensive treatment with insulin through a pump. Today, even more individuals with DM use an insulin pump, become more modern, easier to use appliances are available, with more capabilities. It is believed that the correct application of the pump contributes to better DM control, and to an improvement in the quality of life. More specifically, treatment with an insulin pump helps achieve the specific and individualized objectives as regards the desirable levels of blood glucose.

What kinds of insulin pumps are available?

Two kinds of pumps are available external pumps of continuous subcutaneous insulin infusion and internally placed ones. The former are widely used by people with Type 1 DM since they are significantly cheaper, and their effectiveness has been proven in large clinical studies. Internal pumps are expensive and need a small surgical operation. They have not been approved for wide-spread usage.

Insulin pumps do not measure the blood glucose level and do not have the capability of administering insulin without a given command from their user. For this reason, those who use pumps are obliged to measure their blood glucose at least before their meals and to know how much insulin they need for the correction of hyperglycaemia. A new pump that was recently approved (in April 2006) – the Minimed Paradigm Real Time insulin pump and continuous glucose monitoring system from the Medtronics Company. This pump has the capability of combining a glucose sensor in it, for continuous measurement of the interstitial space glucose level in real time (with five minutes lag time actually), which facilitates the monitoring of the blood glucose level continuously through the pump. Results of this approach concerning the long-term effects on DM control and diabetic complications are not yet available.

Insulin pumps from three different companies are available: the American Medtronics (Minimed), the Swiss Roche (former Disetronic) and the American Smiths (Deltec-Cozmo). These pumps differ from each other, in addition to their appearance, in the minimal quantities of insulin infusion, in the time of bolus infusion and in the software used. The candidate users should be informed by their doctors about the character-istics of each pump, as well as about their technological upgrades, so that they can select the pump that better facilitates their daily blood glucose regulation. It is emphasized, however, that for the best possible control, the most significant role is played not so much by the kind of the pump but by the elaborate (many times a day) measurement of blood glucose levels and the right application of instructions concerning self-monitoring and control.

How does the insulin pump function?

The pumps in common use are appliances that contain a quantity of rapid-acting insulin (usually a very-rapid-acting insulin analogue, Lispro or Aspart), which is administered in the diabetic individual via a thin catheter subcutaneously, usually in the abdominal wall. Rapid-acting regular insulin can also be used (Velosulin) since this type of insulin does not form crystal aggregates in the thin infusion catheter of the pump. The pump has the capability of administering: i) very small doses of insulin continuously (basal rate), that usually range between one tenth of an insulin unit (0.1 units) up to two units per hour; and ii) bigger doses of insulin at an interval of a few minutes (bolus). The decision to administer these doses rests on the user of the pump (see below). The small quantities of insulin that are administered subcutaneously as the basal rate every hour (tenths of an insulin unit up to two units per hour) are considered very advantageous (compared with the basal long-acting insulins given with a syringe or pen), because absorption from the subcutaneous tissue is smoother and more predictable.

The pumps are composed of an outer shell that usually has four keys and a screen for reading the doses or the basal rate. They contain a special syringe usually with 300 units of insulin, which is propelled by a piston. The movement of the piston is controlled by an electronic mechanism of high precision that takes energy from a battery. This mechanism is capable of propelling tenths of a unit of insulin to the catheter that is connected at one end with the syringe, while the other end is inserted (as mentioned before) by the pump user in the subcutaneous fat of the abdominal wall. The catheter should be changed every 3–4 days. All pumps have alarm mechanisms to show when the stored insulin or the battery is running low, or when no manipulations have occurred by the user for some time, etc. Moreover, each pump has certain particular technical characteristics.

How is the basal rate determined?

The basal rate is determined by the treating physician and is usually 50 percent of the total insulin needs of the pump user. The precise infusion is set depending on the needs of the individuals in a fasting state. The needs differ from person to person and from time to time (larger needs in the first morning hours due to the dawn phenomenon). There are different ways for the initial determination of the hourly basal rate. Some doctors divide the quantity they will administer as basal rate in 24 equal doses, while others use ready-made administration nomograms. In the following days, adaptation of the basal rate is done, depending on the results of the blood glucose measurements.

In extraordinary cases the user can alter the basal rate depending on the situation (decrease when there is increased physical activity, increase in situations of acute illness, etc.), returning at the usual basal rate when the extraordinary situation ends. Some patients use different basal rates on Sundays or on days when they have different physical activities.

How are the boluses determined?

The boluses (once only administration) of insulin that are administered before the meals (meal bolus) are often set as insulin needs per unit of carbohydrates. They are determined so that two hours after their administration and the meal, the insulin user has blood glucose values that are within targets. Special easy mathematical calculations are taught to the users to help individualize these needs. Usually 12–15 g of carbohydrates require one unit of insulin, but there are differences from person to person as well as in the morning or in the afternoon. Pump users should be educated at great length about their needs for insulin depending on the amount of carbohydrates of the meal, and they should be able to predict this amount with adequate precision.

Individuals that manifest delayed stomach emptying because of diabetic gastroparesis have the capability to receive an extended bolus with the pump or a percentage of this in the first minute and the rest slowly, for a time determined by their needs or the type of their food. Each company's pump offers different possibilities of administering a meal bolus.

Corrective boluses are set according to the experience of the user. For example, they may need one unit of insulin to decrease the blood glucose level by 30–50 mg/dl (1.7–2.8 mmol/L).

What are the indications for the use of an insulin pump?

According to the American Diabetes Association (ADA), the indications are as follows:

1. insufficient glycaemic control, that is $HbA_{1c} > 7$ percent, and/or dawn phenomenon, with fasting blood glucose $> 140–160$ mg/dl (7.8–8.9 mmol/L) in the morning, and/or significant fluctuations during the day;
2. hypoglycaemia unawareness or severe hypoglycaemic episodes;
3. requirements for a flexible life-style.

A pump is also indicated in pregnant woman with DM since it helps to achieve the strict targets set for the duration of the pregnancy.

The following indications for application of a continuous insulin infusion pump have been established:

1. Type 1 diabetics, in whom every effort to achieve satisfactory diabetic control with an intensified insulin therapy regimen fails (unsatisfactory HbA_{1c} level, intense fluctuations of blood glucose levels during a 24-hour period, intense 'dawn phenomenon').
2. Type 1 diabetics who manifest frequent and/or severe hypoglycaemias, especially in the night.
3. Type 1 diabetics who have developed decreased perception of hypoglycaemia (hypoglycaemia unawareness).
4. Type 1 diabetics who manifest high sensitivity to insulin and need a small total daily dose of insulin.
5. Type 1 diabetics who lead an erratic way of life, who have a circular work schedule, who are submitted to intense physical or mental lassitude at work, who for professional or personal reasons are not in a position to receive their main and intermediary meals at fixed hours, or who wish to omit a meal (particularly in the morning). In the same category, belong diabetics who wish to exercise more often for personal or professional reasons.
6. Type 1 diabetics who have developed complications, like generalized macrovascular disease (stroke or myocardial infarction) or nephropathy and proliferate (or even pre-proliferative) retinopathy. In these patients the 'as best as possible absolute control' of DM is sought. Special indications constitute the diabetic gastroparesis and the development and insistence of painful sensory neuropathy.
7. Diabetics with severe peripheral angiopathy – gangrene.
8. Patients who develop DM after pancreatectomy or after pancreatic transplantation.
9. Diabetics who are pregnant. Moreover, application of a pump is also advisable for the best possible control of DM in certain cases so that conception is achieved.
10. Other special situations, which also require, however, documented reasons for application of a pump.

Essential conditions for the application of pumps are that the users are able to handle the system of commands of the pump effectively, and that they have the mental motivation and intention to dedicate labour and time to their diabetic control. They should be determined to measure their blood sugar at least four times a day. Moreover, systematic teaching of the use of the pump is essential, while at the same time the responsible physician should have proven experience with the use of pumps. Consequently, it is obvious that it is not feasible, as well as not advisable, for all Type 1 diabetics to use pumps. Specialist doctors need to make strict choices based on the above criteria.

The use of pumps in diabetic children – or even infants – is continuously increasing, since the results of their use are encouraging.

Certain individual studies encourage the use of pumps in people with Type 2 DM; however, definitive data for this application are not yet available.

Why does hypoglycaemia unawareness constitute an indication for treatment with an insulin pump?

Insulin-treated persons, who manifest hypoglycaemia unawareness due to multiple hypoglycaemic episodes in the frame of very strict diabetic control, can correct this complication by setting slightly higher blood sugar targets. Treatment with an insulin pump helps the controlled achievement of these individualized targets.

What other requirements are therefor the use of an insulin pump?

The pump users should maintain basic conditions of hygiene where the catheter end connects to their skin. They should also know about the use of intensified treatment with insulin injections (in case this is needed), and have batteries and materials for the change of the catheter.

A 24-hour telephone service should be available that offers advice or solutions when problems with the use of the pump occur. All the companies that market the pumps have such services.

What undesirable effects can occur when using an insulin pump?

Local microbial infections at the point of catheter entry, hypoglycaemic or hyperglycaemic episodes and episodes of ketosis can occur if the pump is not used properly or if – and this is infrequent with the newer pumps – technical problems arise. These problems are usually prevented with the right education, the continuous psychological support of the users and regular visits to their physicians. With improvement in pump technology and the provision of more needs of the users in the software, undesirable effects are minimized. Moreover, the increasing international experience and rich literature gathered by the use of pumps, contribute to the reduction of undesirable effects.

Can insulin pump users remove the pump when they want?

They can disconnect the pump for a short period of time of 1–2 hours usually without consequences (for example, when they want to have a bath, etc.). If, however, they want to remove it for more time, they should receive extra insulin in order to cover the basal rate. If they do not want to use it for a day or more, they should apply an intensified regimen with subcutaneous insulin injections on these days.

How is the follow-up done of individuals with DM who carry an insulin pump?

These individuals should communicate with their doctor on an almost daily basis during the first weeks, until the blood sugar levels are controlled and there is certainty that the use of the pump and the measurement of the food carbohydrates are being performed correctly. Afterwards, these patients are followed in the same way as the other people with Type 1 DM, measuring their blood sugar levels at least four times daily and keeping records of the results and the units of insulin they receive.

If control is good, the insulin users should repeat their education on the measurement of the food carbohydrates after about one year.

Many patients who use an insulin pump feel that after a few months they can control their blood sugar levels without the help of their doctors and so they can omit visits. It should be stressed that this is wrong, because the follow-up of individuals with DM is not only limited to the regulation of the blood glucose levels, but also concerns the chronic diabetic complications that may potentially present.

What are the results of studies that compared treatment with a continuous subcutaneous insulin infusion pump to intensive treatment with multiple insulin injections?

As regards glycaemic control, the results are controversial. Some studies support the idea that treatment with pumps has an advantage and other studies show that the two treatments are equivalent. There is, however, a general consensus that the blood glucose fluctuations are smaller with the use of a pump, and the hypoglycaemic episodes are fewer. Moreover, a claimed increase in the percentage of ketoacidotic episodes with pump users, compared to those treated with multiple insulin injections, has not been proven. A lot of small studies agree that quality of life is better when a pump is used, and that microvascular complications occur less often. There is also evidence that diabetic neuropathy is improved with the use of an insulin pump.

There is no significant evidence that the incidence of macroangiopathy is reduced with the use of a pump compared with multiple insulin injections. Furthermore, the insulin needs are generally less (roughly by 15 percent) when a pump is used compared to multiple injections and some consider this element as a potential advantage for the prevention of atherosclerosis.

If the use of a continuous subcutaneous insulin infusion pump is considered as advantageous compared to the intensive regimen of multiple insulin injections, why isn't it imposed as a treatment for individuals with Type 1 DM?

Apart from the above mentioned conditions, the cost of the pump plays a significant role. In some countries, an unwillingness is observed concerning the use of pumps that stems from the conviction that their widespread application will adversely effect the insurance system. Studies in certain countries, however, have shown that treatment with insulin pumps is financially more beneficial, provided it is performed correctly, when the long-term economic benefits of the prevention of late diabetic complications are taken into account.

It should also be noted that psychological reasons deter some individuals with Type 1 DM from carrying the pump continuously. Provided that these individuals are sufficiently controlled with an intensive regimen of multiple insulin injections (which is not rare), and are satisfied with this treatment, obviously there is no reason to recommend treatment with an insulin pump.

INHALED INSULIN

What characteristics render the lungs an easy point of entry of insulin in the blood circulation?

- The lungs employ an extensive absorbent surface. Their extent in humans is 50–140 m^2, and they contain around 500 million alveoli. The alveolar-capillary barrier is thin.
- This surface is well perfused. The perfusion flow is about 5 litres per minute, and the pulmonary capillary blood volume is around 0.25 litres.
- Many peptidases are absent, and are infact encountered in the gastro-intestinal tract.
- The administered insulin does not immediately pass through the liver, unlike insulin physiologically secreted by the pancreas, which is channelled via the portal vein to the liver.

What are the pharmacotechnical forms of inhaled insulin?

Insulin can be inhaled in different forms, depending on how it has been prepared by various companies.

- *Dry powder*. This is inhaled with the Exubera system of inhalations, from Pfizer Inc. and Aventis Pharma, in collaboration with Nektar Therapeutics. This system is already evolving technologically and was very recently been approved (in January 2006) by the FDA for clinical use. It is soon expected to be available in Europe.
- *Aerosol (nebulized)* via the AERx inhalation system (produced by Aradigm) (in phase III studies).
- *'Artificial insulin spheres'* (Technospheres^{TM}/Insulin from MannKind), with their main characteristic being their precise resemblance to each other. The method is in phase II clinical studies.
- *Insulin connected to big porous particles*, stable in room temperature, which are inhaled with special appliances, from Alkermes and Eli Lilly.

These particles have a small density ($< 0.1\,g/cm^2$) and large 'geometrical' diameter (10–$20\,\mu m$) but their aerodynamic diameter is small (1–$3\,\mu m$). Also in phase II studies.

- *Crystalline insulin* from the KOS Company. It is administered via a simple metered dose inhalations appliance that functions mechanically (in Phase II).
- *Crystalline insulin* (Humulin R$^{®}$) in the preparation U500 from the Eli Lilly Company, with an inhalation appliance from Aerogen (in Phase I).

There is no consensus on whether dry powder or the solution is absorbed better, or is more effective, since there are no comparative studies.

What is the fate of insulin after its entry into the respiratory system?

1. Particles of $> 10\,\mu m$ in size remain in the mucosa of the mouth, the pharynx, the larynx and the bronchial tree. These particles contain a large quantity of insulin.
2. Particles of $< 1\,\mu m$ in size are exhaled.
3. Only particles of intermediate diameter (2 to $5\,\mu m$) enter the blood circulation.
4. Macrophages and peptidases degrade the insulin particles that remain in the alveoli.

How does the action of inhaled insulin differ from the action of the subcutaneously administered insulin?

The onset of action of the inhaled insulin is more rapid than that of subcutaneously administered rapid-acting regular insulin (but not than the onset of action of the very-rapidly acting insulin analogues). Its action has an intermediate duration between that of the very-rapid acting analogues and the rapid-acting regular insulin. Hence, this can be used before the meals, instead of the rapid-acting insulin.

What is the main benefit of the use of inhaled insulin?

Obviously, the main benefit is the avoidance of injections for the administration of rapid-acting insulin. From clinical studies up to now (which are small and of short duration so far), satisfaction from its use is definitely higher for patients, compared to the use of subcutaneous insulin. It can be expected that in particular patients with Type 2 DM who refuse treatment with subcutaneous insulin after secondary failure of oral antidiabetic medicines will be controlled better if they are persuaded to start inhaled insulin (compared to no insulin).

What problems exist with regard to the use of inhaled insulin?

- The existing inhalation appliances do not allow for an easy change of the dose of insulin.
- Only a small percentage (roughly 10 percent of the administered dose) is absorbed, since a quantity of insulin remains in the appliance (in the walls and the chamber), and, as mentioned before, particles smaller than 1 μm and larger than 10 μm are not absorbed.

  This characteristic renders the treatment with inhaled insulin *ten times more expensive* than treatment with subcutaneous insulin. The improvement, however, of glycaemic control in patients who refuse to start subcutaneous insulin, may possibly have more economic benefit as a whole, due to the expected reduction of chronic diabetic complications.
- Anti-insulin antibodies develop with the inhalation of insulin in larger proportions compared with the use of subcutaneous insulin, an element without clinical importance (so far).
- The respiratory function deteriorated in some individuals with Type 2 DM who inhaled insulin in a 6-month study with a specific appliance. The deterioration concerned the decrease of the diffusion capacity of CO (DLCO in ml/min/mmHg) and receded after the interruption of the inhalations. A similar deterioration was not observed in other studies, with different appliances.

How is the action of inhaled insulin influenced by smoking?

Chronic smoking accelerates the onset of action of inhaled insulin and causes a higher insulin concentration in smokers' blood compared to non-smokers. This is due to the increased permeability of the alveolar-capillary barrier of smokers.

The absorption of insulin from smokers' lungs is influenced by the time between the last smoke and the inhalation of insulin (also by the transdermal use of nicotine), rendering the action of inhaled insulin unpredictable to a large extent. For this reason the use of inhaled insulin should not be recommended in smokers with   DM.

Moreover, certain writers express scepticism because the action of insulin on the IGF (insulin-like growth factor) receptors of the alveoli can have a carcinogenic action, especially when smoking that predisposes to cancer of the lungs coexists. The larger studies of treatment with inhaled insulin were careful to exclude smokers; therefore there are in sufficient data with regard to this matter. Evidence from small studies in experimental animals, however, is reassuring.

How is the action of inhaled insulin influenced by asthma and acute respiratory tract infections?

Individuals with asthma absorb less quantity of insulin from their lungs and thus need more units of inhaled insulin.

Acute respiratory tract infections do not appear to influence the absorption of inhaled insulin.

However, studies with regard to asthma and acute respiratory infections are still rare and it is expected that after the widespread use of treatment with inhaled insulin more explicit evidence will become available. Moreover, the use of different types of insulin and different inhalation appliances render any firm conclusions from the few publications and studies premature.

Has inhaled insulin been tried in all types of DM? What results were obtained?

Inhaled insulin has been tried in both Type 1 and Type 2 DM, compared to the subcutaneous administration of rapid-acting insulin, together with intermediate or slow-acting insulins. DM control in all cases was equally satisfactory. According to other studies, the treatment of Type 2 DM with inhaled insulin is superior to the combination of oral antidiabetic medicines.

TRANSPLANTATION OF KIDNEY AND PANCREAS

CASE STUDY 1

A 28 year old woman with Type 1 DM since the age of nine visits the outpatient Diabetes Clinic for follow-up. Her weight is 62 kg (136.7 lb) and height 1.55 m (5 ft 1 in). On physical examination she looks pale and oedematous. The thyroid gland is palpable. The heart sounds are normal, and an apical holosystolic murmur is heard (II/VI). The subcostal organs are not palpable. The Achilles and patellar reflexes were not produced and there was ankle oedema. There is no superficial or deep sensory neurologic disturbances. Fundoscopy reveals background diabetic retinopathy. The patient receives six units of intermediate-acting insulin every morning and 2–8 units of very-rapid-acting insulin analogue before meals, depending on the measurements of the blood glucose. She has nephrotic syndrome, diagnosed eight years ago, and receives treatment with felodipine, furosemide, perindopril, aluminum hydroxide (AluCap), calcium carbonate-glycine (Titralac) and erythropoietin 2,000 IU, three times per week.

Despite the not particularly high level of glycosylated haemoglobin (HbA$_{1c}$ 7.7 percent), the daily blood glucose levels range between severe hypoglycaemia and heavy hyperglycaemia, often expressed with ketoacidosis. Laboratory results are as follows: Hct 29.2 percent, Hb 9.5 g/dl, WBC 5,900/mm^3, PLT 373,000/mm^3, glucose 108 mg/dl (6.0 mmol/L), urea 210 mg/dl (34.9 mmol/L), creatinine 4.5 mg/dl (397.8 μmol/L), total cholesterol 253 mg/dl (6.08 mmol/L), LDL-cholesterol 141 mg/dl (3.65 mmol/L), HDL-cholesterol 69 mg/dl (1.78 mmol/L), triglycerides 124 mg/dl (1.4 mmol/L), uric acid 5.3 mg/dl (0.32 mmol/L), SGOT 16 U/L, SGPT 13 U/L: Urinalysis, protein 675 mg/dl, glucose > 1 g/dl.

From the recordings of her daily measurements, it is deduced that her DM is very unstable. All measurements range between 30 mg/dl (1.67 mmol/L) and 450 mg/dl (25.0 mmol/L) and no relation can be found between the units of consumed carbohydrates and the units of the insulin analogue injected before each meal. The patient reports that she was never able to control her blood sugar. Furthermore, she complains of severe gastroparesis symptoms and intense flatulence, which impede every effort to control her blood sugar, despite the use of prokinetic gastrointestinal medicines. A recent gastroscopy reveals bile-stained fluids in the stomach and food residuals, atrophy of the gastric and the duodenal mucosa and first degree oesophagitis in the distal part of the oesophagus. In the past she tried to manage the post-prandial hyperglycaemia by transferring the insulin injection after the meals, without success. A severe hypoglycaemic episode is manifested nearly once every two months.

At the first visit a statin was added and much time was spent trying to find some particular pattern in her blood glucose levels so useful advice could be offered. The effort was not successful, as seen during all the following visits.

Discussing the future, it was explained to the patient that the solution of choice, according to the international data, is a kidney and pancreas transplantation.

The patient did not wish to start renal replacement therapy straight away, despite the recommendations. Two years later, with levels of her serum creatinine ranging between 6.0–8.2 mg/dl (530.4–724.9 µmol/L), a simultaneous kidney and pancreas transplantation was performed.

After the successful transplantation of a cadaveric kidney and pancreas (drainage in the urinary bladder) the patient had normal pre-prandial and post-prandial blood sugar levels without the use of insulin, although a glucose tolerance test was abnormal. After another six months, the appearance of frequent complications (pancreatitis, urinary tract infections and acidosis) led to a new operation, during which the cadaveric pancreas was drained to an intestinal loop. After this operation, disturbances were cured. Four years after the transplantation, the patient has a normal glycosylated haemoglobin level, and there was no deterioration of her retinopathy or nephropathy.

Why is kidney and pancreas transplantation today considered to be the treatment of choice for patients with Type 1 DM with end stage renal disease? What are its advantages compared to the transplantation of the kidney alone?

The advantages of transplantation of the pancreas in combination with the kidney are better quality of life, stabilization of diabetic neuropathy and protection of the transplanted kidney from the consequences of hyperglycaemia. The allotransplantation of the kidney necessitates the administration of immunosuppressive therapy for life, which is accompanied by various undesirable effects. The transplantation of a pancreas together or after the transplantation of a kidney does not add any risks concerning the undesirable effects of the immunosuppressive medicines, which are taken anyway. According to one study, the survival of patients transplanted with a kidney and pancreas appears to be better than the survival of those transplanted with a kidney alone, although probably not statistically significant.

More analytically, the transplantation of the pancreas results in the secretion of insulin in a physiologic way after a glucose tolerance test. However, the insulin levels in the blood of transplanted individuals is double or triple that of normal persons, due to the bypass of the liver by the produced insulin (where its molecule is normally degraded to a great extent), and the intake of corticosteroids.

Generally, the recipients of a pancreas and kidney transplant have lower levels of triglycerides and LDL-cholesterol and higher levels of HDL-cholesterol than the recipients of a kidney transplant alone.

The secretion of counter-regulatory hormones, which is abnormal in patients with long-lasting DM, is improved or even restored after the transplantation of the pancreas. The ability to recognize hypoglycaemias is also corrected.

Moreover, the diabetic neuropathy of both the peripheral as well as the autonomous nervous system are stabilized or even improved. As regards diabetic retinopathy, the available data do not show any improvement.

The diabetic nephropathy of the transplanted kidney is prevented or minimized despite the nephrotoxic effects of cyclosporine. Even in pancreas transplantation alone, the damage of cyclosporine on the kidneys is less significant than the damage of the diabetic nephropathy in non-transplanted individuals.

There is also evidence that the microcirculation, but not the macro-angiopathy, is improved (less foot ulcers).

Finally, fertility of women with transplantation of kidney and pancreas is likely to be restored.

How is the transplantation of the kidney and pancreas done?

Usually the kidney is transplanted extraperitoneally in the left lower quadrant and the pancreas intraperitoneally with part of the duodenum in the right lower quadrant.

The pancreas is removed from the donor together with the liver, so that damage of the blood vessels that perfuse them is avoided, and then their separation follows. The pancreas can be maintained in a University of

Wisconsin solution (special buffer solution) for up to 30 hours. The arterial perfusion of the pancreas is ensured with a graft from the bifurcation of the donor's iliac artery, of a Y shape, while the internal iliac artery is anastomosed to the splenic artery and the common or external iliac artery is anastomosed to the superior mesenteric artery.

Afterwards, the Y-shaped arterial graft of the donor is anastomosed with the external iliac artery of the recipient. The portal vein of the graft is anastomosed with the iliac vein or with the portal vein of the recipient.

The exocrine part of the graft is drained either to the urinary bladder of the recipient or, more often, to an intestinal loop.

Why is intestinal drainage of the exocrine part of the transplanted pancreas preferred today compared to drainage in the urinary bladder of the recipient, which was preferred in the past?

Although the survival of both the graft and the recipient are similar in both techniques, intestinal drainage is nevertheless superior concerning the occurrence of metabolic complications (dehydration, acidosis due to bicarbonate loss, pancreatitis and urinary tract infections).

Which medicines are administered postoperatively, after a simultaneous kidney and pancreas transplantation?

The immunosuppressive therapy differs from hospital to hospital. A relatively common regimen is described below.

As an initial treatment, many transplant centres prefer a regimen of four medicines including:

- a polyclonal or monoclonal antibody against the T lymphocytes, such as the antilymphocyte globulin (ALG), or the antithymocyte globulin (ATG) or the OKT3;
- mycophenolate mofetil (MMF, Cellcept), which selectively inhibits the inosine monophosphate dehydrogenase (IMPDH) and hence inhibits purine synthesis on which the T and the B-lymphocyte proliferation depends (some clinicians use azathioprine, instead of the MMF);

- cyclosporine A, at a dose adjusted so that its levels in the blood are higher than 200 ng/ml or Tacrolimus Prograf (FK-506) 2 mg in the morning and in the evening, half an hour before meals (appearance of tremor and headache may constitute signs of overdosage);
- methylprednisolone (Medrol) or prednisone, received with the food and together with antacids.

The maintenance treatment usually includes cyclosporine, MMF or azathioprine and corticosteroids that are gradually decreased. Recently, Rapamycin (sirolimus) has been used as a maintenance treatment, or a medicine that inhibits the complete activation of T lymphocytes, or Daclizumab, an immunosuppressant humanized monoclonal antibody IgG1. This is selectively bound to the alpha-subunit (Tac subunit) of the interleukin-2 receptor, which is expressed on the surface of the activated lymphocytes.

Apart from the immunosuppressive medicines, the following are frequently prescribed on a chronic basis (indicative list):

- lansoprazole or omeparazole (proton pump inhibitors) and antacids for gastric protection;
- aspirin, for avoidance of thromboses;
- ganciclovir, for protection against megalocytovirus infections;
- co-trimoxazole, for the avoidance of infection from Pneumocystis carinii;
- florinef (fludrocortisone), for the avoidance of orthostatic hypotension;
- magnesium gluconate, for avoidance of serum magnesium decrease caused by the FK-506;
- potassium and perhaps sodium bicarbonate if their levels are low;
- clotrimazole (pills), for avoidance of mycoses from Candida;
- multivitamin preparations.

How is the transplanted patient monitored for episodes of rejection?

Usually, rejection concerns the cells of the exocrine part first, with the islets are rejected later. Therefore, monitoring of glycaemic control is not a reliable tool for the follow-up of the patient. The rejection of the pancreas only is less frequent than the rejection of both organs. In cases where the pancreas has been drained in the urinary bladder, the urinary amylase levels are monitored, which decrease when a rejection occurs; but in the case of intestinal drainage, this is not possible. The first clue is a rise of the serum creatinine. A transcutaneous biopsy of the organ and/or the duodenal graft, guided by ultrasound, or transurethral biopsy is performed and antirejection treatment is administered.

What are the pancreatic islets and how is their transplantation performed?

The pancreatic islets (or islets of Langerhans) are groups of cells that are scattered inside the pancreas and produce the pancreatic hormones – the α-cells produce glucagon, the β-cells insulin, the δ-cells somatostatin and the PP-cells the pancreatic polypeptide (Figure 29.1). The islets constitute 2–3 percent of the volume of the pancreas and number roughly one million in a pancreas. They can be isolated from the pancreas of a brain-dead donor and placed with a small intervention (usually through the portal vein, with local anaesthesia) inside the liver of the recipient. The

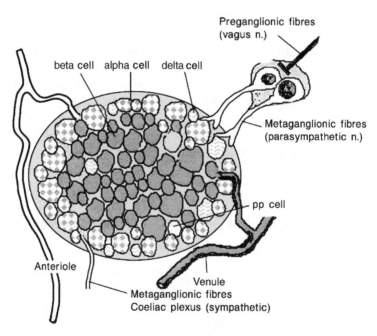

Figure 29.1. Schematic representation of the islet of Langerhans.

number of the transplanted islets determines the sufficient production of insulin. For a 70 kg (154.3 lb) individual, roughly 650,000 islets are needed.

What technical problems exist in the transplantation of the pancreatic islets?

Most research centres report that for every recipient, islets from two cadaveric pancreases are needed. Islet transplantation from only one donor has, however, been successful as well. The medicines that are usually given to a patient in an intensive care unit before he or she becomes an organ donor influence the quality of the islets. The process, from the moment of removal of the pancreas until the beginning of the islet isolation, should not exceed 18 hours, since the islets are destroyed quickly. Moreover, an islet transplantation centre has large expenses, since it employs very specialized personnel continuously on standby so that they can receive a cadaveric pancreas and process it to isolate the islets. During the isolation, around 30–50 percent of the cadaveric pancreatic islets are destroyed. It should be noted that every detail of the technique has not yet been determined, and it is not the same at all centres applying it. This entails different results and is one of the reasons why the number of islets received from a pancreas is not yet ideal.

The transplantation itself includes very few risks. The most common undesirable side effect is the thrombosis of a branch of the portal vein or bleeding, which however can be controlled. As is the case for the transplantation of the whole pancreas, immunosuppression is needed, with the same risks as involved in transplantation of the pancreas (risk of infections, small percentage of lymphomas).

What are the up to date results of the pancreatic islet transplantations?

From 1974 to the middle of 2004, the number of persons who were transplanted with islets and were published in medical journals was 750; from 1999 to 2003 this number was over 300. Before 2000 the rate of success was below 10 percent, and concerned individuals who had been transplanted with islets alone, or with islets and kidney simultaneously, or with islets after some time post-kidney transplantation. Today the best results from islet transplantations (in patients with Type 1 DM and good renal function), have been described with a combination of medicines that has been named 'the Edmonton Protocol', from the city in Canada where it was devised and reported in the year 2000. The particularity of this protocol is that it does not include any corticosteroids. It includes the medicines Daclizumab (a monoclonal antibody, inhibitor of the α-*subunit* of the interleukin-2 receptor) for induction, Sirolimus (a macrocyclic lactone) and Tacrolimus (an inhibitor of calsineurin) as maintenance therapy.

The success of the Edmonton protocol resulted in the attempt of other research centres in Europe and America to try and use it as well. The results of the 36 islet transplantation centres that exist internationally were very mixed: in some centres very successful, in some very poor. The successful transplantation of one recipient from only one donor has also been announced.

In Europe, a network of centres has been created by which cadaveric pancreases are dispatched to Germany (University of Giessen), Italy (Milan) or Switzerland (Geneva), where the islets are isolated and then sent back to the countries of origin, where they are transplanted, according to the Edmonton protocol. The results of this effort are pending. In the UK, there are islet transplantation centres in Leicester and London. There is also a centre in Finland, which does not follow the Edmonton protocol.

In January 2005 the transplantation of islets from a part of the pancreas of a living donor was also announced. The long-lasting results are pending.

In any case, until the methods of islet isolation are perfected and this protocol has been sufficiently carried out, islet transplantation should still be considered an experimental method of treatment, since the longevity of the transplanted islets is at present poor (up to five years).

What other research protocols for the treatment of DM with transplantation have been tried?

There have been experimental attempts to transplant porcine pancreatic islets to humans, since the insulin of the pig is almost identical to that of humans. The results are controversial and there is no unanimity for the methods and the real practical value of these experiments. The creation of experimental animals with human genes (transgenic animals), so that their organs are not rejected and an abundance of donors is created, will perhaps offer solutions in the future. The creation of β-cells in the laboratory from immature foetal cells (blastocytes or stem cells) and their transplantation is one more challenge for the researchers of the future.

Glucagon-like peptide 1 (GLP-1)

What is the Glucagon-like peptide 1 (GLP-1) and with what mechanisms does it act beneficially in Type 2 DM?

GLP-1 belongs to the peptides that are similar to glucagon, and is synthesized in the small intestine (L-cells of the jejunum). This, together with the gastric inhibitory polypeptide (or glucose-dependent insulino-tropic polypeptide, GIP), is 50 percent responsible for the secretion of insulin after a meal (entero-hepatic axis – incretin effect).

More specifically, GLP-1:

- stimulates the secretion of insulin;
- inhibits the secretion of glucagon;
- delays the stomach emptying;
- suppresses the appetite;
- stimulates the growth of β-cells.

Its action though is very short-lived because of its quick degradation by a ubiquitous enzyme, the dipeptidyl-peptidase IV (DPP-IV), and thus it has a half-life of only 1–2 minutes in the blood.

Are there data to show that GLP-1 improves the control of individuals with Type 2 DM?

There are studies of one week duration with the use of continuous intravenous infusion of GLP-1, in which the blood glucose level decreased under 125 mg/dl (6.9 mmol/L) in most diabetics, regardless of the previous antidiabetic treatment or their control. Also, studies with continuous subcutaneous infusion (using insulin pumps) of GLP-1 up to six weeks, showed improved glucose and insulin levels and decrease in HbA_{1c} of the patients treated with the infusion compared to placebo.

What is the big advantage of the use of GLP-1 in the treatment of Type 2 DM? What other advantages does it generally have?

The researchers hope that this substance will cause an increase in the β-cell mass and that in this way the deterioration of Type 2 DM will finally stop. Experimental animal data and indirect evidence from human studies corroborate this belief.

Another advantage is the avoidance of hypoglycaemias, since the GLP-1 induced secretion of insulin and suppression of glucagon depends on the presence of glucose. GLP-1 in high concentrations is not able on its own to stimulate the secretion of insulin, and it cannot impede the counter-regulation of hypoglycaemias.

One more advantage is the moderate weight loss associated with its use, most likely due to its gastric motility inhibitory actions.

What restrictions are there in the therapeutic use of GLP-1, and how were they overcome?

GLP-1 is destroyed by the enzymes of the gastrointestinal tract (since it is a protein) and by the enzyme dipeptidyl-peptidase IV (DPP-IV) in the blood in a few minutes. Consequently, it cannot be given by mouth. A continuous infusion (intravenous or subcutaneous) is not very practical.

For this reason, its molecule was subjected to chemical transformations, so that it can resist degradation by DPP-IV and act for a longer time. Such GLP-1 analogues are now in clinical trials (with very promising results), with the first agent of the class already having been approved.

The administration of DPP-IV inhibitors (small molecules that enhance the action of endogenous GLP-1 by inhibiting its degradation) has also been tried, so that its action can be prolonged.

What medicines of the GLP-1 type are in the pipeline?

One such medicine is exenatide, which is produced synthetically and is similar to the substance exendin-4. Exendin-4 is a natural protein found in the saliva of a large American lizard, the Heloderma suspectum or Gila monster. This substance is a full agonist of the GLP-1 receptor in humans, is resistant to DPP-IV and is cleared by the kidneys by glomerular filtration. Thus it can be used as a long-acting GLP-1 mimetic. Exenatide (produced by Amylin Pharmaceuticals and Eli Lilly and Co.) has already been tried in phase III clinical trials and was recently approved by the FDA (April 2005) for Type 2 diabetic patients who have not achieved adequate glycaemic control on metformin, sulfony-lureas or their combination. It is administered on a twice daily sub-cutaneous injection before meals, with the most frequent side effect being nausea and vomiting. A long-acting compound of Exenatide, which will be administered once weekly, is in clinical trials.

Liraglutide (produced by Novo Nordisk), another GLP-1 analogue, comprises a slightly modified GLP-1 sequence with a palmitoyl chain attached. This confers affinity for and binding to albumin, and thus protects the molecule both from DPP-IV and renal elimination. Its plasma half-life is 12 hours and thus it can be given in a once a day subcutan-eous injection. It is currently in phase III clinical studies.

CJC-1131 (ConjuChem Inc.) that can probably be administered once a week is a substance that is still in a very precocious stage of research.

DPP-IV inhibitors are the other class of compounds being tried as antihyperglycaemic agents of the incretin-mimetic effect, having the advantage of oral administration. The medicine LAF237 (Vildagliptin – Novartis) is the most advanced inhibitor of the class and has already been given to patients with good results. These compounds have the additional advantage that they do not cause as many gastrointestinal side effects as the GLP-1 analogues but on the other hand they do not cause any weight loss either. Other compounds of the class (sitagliptin, saxagliptin, etc.) are in early phases of development.

AMYLIN

What is amylin?

Amylin is a peptide with 37 amino-acids that is secreted by the pancreatic β-cells, together with insulin. The concentration of these two hormones in the plasma is parallel (low pre-prandial levels and high post-prandial increases). In individuals with Type 1 DM, the secretion of amylin is practically minimal as is that of insulin, whereas in individuals with Type 2 DM its secretion is decreased. Perhaps amylin contributes to the pathogenesis of Type 2 DM, since it has been found that it causes insulin resistance and/or inhibits its secretion from the pancreas.

Why isn't human amylin used in practice?

It is not used in practice because it is not adequately dissolved and tends to precipitate quickly in the various solvents. For this reason the equivalent amylin analogue, pramlintide, was created, that is administered with a subcutaneous injection and is cleared by the kidneys. When 30–60 µg of pramlintide are administered to individuals with Type 1 DM and 120 µg in individuals with Type 2 DM, the concentrations of pramlintide in the plasma amount to levels equivalent with the pre-prandial physiologic ones.

How does pramlintide act?

It decreases the post-prandial glucose levels, acting mainly during the first 30–60 minutes. The mechanisms that have been described concern the inhibition of glucagon secretion and the delay of gastric emptying. These effects are mediated through a central nervous pathway from the area postrema of the 4th ventricle, with centrifugal fibres to the adjacent nucleus of the vagus nerve. The area postrema contains a lot of binding sites for amylin (as well as for GLP-1) and is exposed to the changes of the plasma amylin and glucose, since it is located outside the blood-brain barrier. The presence of glucose is essential for the action of amylin and in the event of hypoglycaemia its actions are suppressed.

Are there studies showing that pramlintide is effective for the treatment of DM?

There are studies of patients with Type 1 and Type 2 DM in which pramlintide was added to the existing regimen of insulin therapy. The reduction in HbA_{1c} was 0.5 percent larger in the group who received pramlintide than the reduction that was produced by the placebo medicine, and more patients on the pramlintide group achieved HbA_{1c} levels <7 percent. Also they needed less units of insulin in order to get under control, did not suffer more hypoglycaemias (apart from the initial period) and did not manifest an increase of body weight.

The most common undesirable side effect is a moderate degree of nausea which is dose-dependent.

What is the current state of pramlintide in the market?

The substance (medicine Symlin, pramlintide acetate, produced by Amylin Works) has passed the phase III clinical studies and has been administered to a total of 4,800 individuals so far. In the year 2000, an application was submitted to the FDA to allow its promotion in the market but the FDA asked for more explanatory data in the following years. In March 2005 its circulation was approved in the USA as an adjunct treatment for Type 1 and 2 diabetics on insulin who have failed to achieve glycaemic control.

PPARαγ AGONISTS

This is a new class of compounds that is being tried in clinical studies for simultaneous treatment for hyperglycaemia and hypertriglyceridaemia. They act by stimulating the PPARγ nuclear receptors (similar action to the glitazones) and the PPARα nuclear receptors (similar action to the fibrates). Several compounds have reached phase III clinical trials (muraglitazar, tesaglitazar, MK0767, etc.) but none has yet been approved for clinical use. Concerns regarding their cardiovascular and renal safety, as well as regarding carcinogenicity issues in animals, have been raised.

ARTIFICIAL PANCREAS

This concerns appliances that measure the concentration of glucose and through special algorithms administer the proper dose of insulin to the patient, usually intravenously or/and subcutaneously. These appliances are currently used mainly for research reasons, and their perfection is anticipated. A serious technical problem derives from the fact that the electrode that measures the glucose concentration gets inactivated after some days. Significant contributions to this field have come from research efforts at the University of Ulm in Germany as well as in the USA.

For the time being, certain small-sized appliances that measure the glucose concentration continuously in the extracellular fluid are being evaluated with only relative success. A disadvantage is the lag time between any changes in the blood glucose concentration and its recording from the sensor of the appliance in the extracellular fluid. The ability of connecting this appliance with a continuous insulin infusion pump (intravenous or subcutaneous) and the automatic infusion of insulin at the proper rate (through a closed loop system) constitutes the ultimate ambition, with huge research efforts being expended chasing that dream. The future anyway is looking promising.

Further reading

American Diabetes Association (2004) ADA position statement: Continuous subcutaneous insulin infusion. *Diabetes Care*, **27** (Suppl 1), S110.

Ahren, B. and Pacini, G. (2005) Islet adaptation to insulin resistance: mechanisms and implications for intervention. *Diabetes, Obesity and Metabolism* 7:2–8.

Ahren, B., Simonsson, E., Larsson, H., Landin-Olsson, M., Torgeirsson, H., Jansson, P.A. (2002) Inhibition of dipeptidyl peptidase IV improves metabolic control over a 4-week study period in Type 2 diabetes. *Diabetes Care* **25**: 869–75.

Amiel, S. and Alberti, K.G.M.M. (2004) Inhaled insulin (editorial) *BMJ* **328**: 1215–6.

Bequette, B.W. **2005** A critical assessment of algorithms and challenges in the development of a closed-loop artificial pancreas. *Diabetes Technol Ther* **7**: 28–47.

Bode, B. (2004) Insulin pump therapy, in *Therapy for Diabetes Mellitus and Related Disorders*. 4th edn, American Diabetes Association. (ed. H. Lebovitz) Alexandria, *Virginia* pp. 224–31.

Buse, J., Weyer, C., Maggs, D.G. (2002) Amylin replacement with pramlintide in Type 1 and Type 2 diabetes: A physiological approach to overcome barriers with insulin therapy. *Clinical Diabetes* 3:137–44.

Diabetes Control and Complications Trial Research Group (DCCT) (1993) The effect of intensive treatment of diabetes on the development and progression of long-term complications in insulin-dependent diabetes mellitus. *N Engl J Med.,* **329**: 977–86.

El-Ouaghlidi, A., Nauck, M. (2004) Glucagon-like peptide 1: new therapies for Type 2 diabetes. *Diabetes Voice* **49**:24–6.

Heinemann, L., Heise, T. (2004) Current status of the development of inhaled insulin. *Br J Diabetes Vasc Dis* **4**: 295–301.

Holst, J.J. (2002) Therapy of Type 2 diabetes mellitus based on the actions of glucagon-like peptide-1. *Diabetes Metabolism Res Rev* **18**: 430–41.

Holst, J.J. (2006) Glucagon-like peptide-1. From extract to agent. The Claude Bernard Lecture, 2005. *Diabetologia* **49**: 253–60.

http://www.amylin.com/Pipeline/Symlin.cfm

Klonoff, D.C. (2005) Continuous glucose monitoring: Roadmap for 21st century diabetes therapy. *Diabetes Care* **28**:1231–9.

Kong, M-F., Stubbs, T.A., King, P., Macdonald, I.A., Blackshaw, P.E., Perkins, A.C., Tattersall, R.B. (1998) The effect of single doses of pramlintide on gastric emptying of two meals in men with IDDM. *Diabetologia* **41**: 577–83.

Mather, K.J., Paradisi, G., Leaming, R., Hook, G., Steinberg, H., Fineberg, N., Hamley, R., Baron, A. (2002) Role of amylin in insulin secretion and action in humans: antagonist studies across the spectrum of insulin sensitivity. *Diabet Metab Res Rev* **18**: 118–26.

Morel, P., Moudry-Munns, K., Najarian, J.S. *et al.* (1990) Influence of preservation time on outcome and metabolic function of bladder-drained pancreas transplants. *Transplantation* **49**:294.

Owens, D.R., Zinman, B., Bolli, G. (2003) Alternative routes of insulin delivery. *Diabet Med.* **20**: 886–98.

Pickup, J., Keen, H. (2002) Continuous subcutaneous insulin infusion at 25 years: Evidence base for the expanding use of insulin pump therapy in Type 1 diabetes. *Diabetes Care* **25**: 593–8.

Raptis, S., Mitrakou, A., Hadjidakis, D., Diamantopoulos, E., Anastasiou, C., Fountas, A., Muller, R. (1987) 24-h blood glucose pattern in type I and type II diabetics after oral treatment with pentoxyfilline as assessed with artificial endocrine pancreas. *Acta Diabetol Lat* **24**:181–92.

Robertson, R.P. (2004) Islet transplantation as a treatment for diabetes – a work in progress. *N Eng J Med* **350**: 694–705.

Rother, K.I., Harlan, D.M. (2004) Challenges facing islet transplantation for the treatment of Type 1 diabetes mellitus. *J Clin Invest* **114**: 877–83.

Royle, P., Waugh, N., McAuley, L., McIntyre, L., Thomas, S. (2003) Inhaled insulin in diabetes mellitus. *Cochrane Database Syst Rev* **3**: CD003890.

Schatz, H. (2004) Inhaled Insulin and the Dream of a Needle-Free Insulin Application. *Exp Clin Endocrinol Diabetes* **112**: 285–87.

Shapiro, A.M., Lakey, J.R., Ryan, E.A., Korbutt, G.S., Toth, E., Warnock, G.L., Kneteman, N.M., Rajotte, R.V. (2000) Islet transplantation in seven patients with Type 1 diabetes mellitus using a glucocorticoid-free immunosuppressive regimen. *N Eng J Med* **343**: 230–8.

Shapiro, A.M.J., Ricordi, C. (2004) Unraveling the secrets of single donor success in islet transplantation. *Am J Transpl* **4**: 295–8.

Shapiro, A.M.J., Ricordi, C., Hering, B. (2003) Edmonton's islet success has indeed been replicated elsewhere. *Lancet* **362**: 1242.

Weyer, C., Gottlieb, A., Kim, D.D., Lutz, K., Schwartz, S., Gutierrez, M., Wang, Y., Ruggles, J.A., Kolterman, O.G., Maggs, D.G. (2003) Pramlintide reduces post-prandial glucose excursions when added to regular insulin or insulin lispro in subjects with Type 1 diabetes. *Diabetes Care* **26**:3074–9.

30

Prevention of diabetes

Konstantinos Makrilakis

Why is there interest in the prevention of DM?

Diabetes mellitus is a chronic disease, the frequency of which has increased dramatically over the last decades. More specifically, the prevalence of Type 2 DM is reaching epidemic proportions worldwide, mainly because of the ageing of the population, the sedentary life-style and the increase of obesity. Around 5–8 percent of the population in various countries has been affected by the disease, and in certain countries and certain nationalities this percentage is even larger (e.g., in Pima Indians in America it approaches 50 percent). The undiagnosed DM in certain populations can be even more (roughly 2.5 times more). The future looks ominous since it is projected that an even more dramatic increase in the incidence of the disease will occur in the next few decades (the roughly 150 million diabetics in the year 2000 is expected to increase to about 300 million by 2025, more than 75 percent of which will be in developing countries, mainly because of the adoption of a 'Western' way of life). Furthermore, the frequency of Type 1 DM, for as yet unknown reasons, appears to be increasing as well, although not as dramatically as Type 2.

This common disease is associated with a variety of long-lasting and very serious complications, both microvascular (retinopathy, nephropathy, neuropathy) and macrovascular (coronary artery disease, strokes, peripheral arterial disease), and with increased mortality. This, added to the fact that therapeutic management of DM and its complications constitutes an enormous burden for society (medical and economical),

Diabetes in Clinical Practice: Questions and Answers from Case Studies. Nicholas Katsilambros *et al.*
© 2006 John Wiley & Sons, Ltd.

has caused the enormous interest in prevention of DM, with the final aim being the prevention of its complications and reduction of mortality. Also to be taken into account is that specifically for Type 2 DM (which constitutes 90 percent of diabetics) the risk of atherosclerotic complications probably begins even before the clinical appearance of the disease, at the stage of pre-diabetes (see Chapter 16), and that treatment of DM after its appearance is not satisfactory with regard to the reduction of complications (mainly from the cardiovascular system). Therefore, the ultimate aim of prevention of Type 2 DM is the likely reduction of the risk for cardiovascular diseases, before DM is clinically present.

Can DM be prevented?

Generally speaking, screening of asymptomatic populations for a particular disease should be performed when the following conditions are fulfilled:

1. The disease constitutes a serious health problem for the population.
2. The natural history of the disease is known and comprehensible.
3. There is a recognized pre-clinical (asymptomatic) stage during which the disease can be diagnosed.
4. The examinations for the diagnosis of the disease at this pre-clinical stage are reliable and acceptable.
5. The treatment after the precocious diagnosis of the disease is advantageous, more so than if diagnosis was delayed and treatment given later, at the clinical stage of the illness.
6. The cost for the precocious detection and treatment of the disease is reasonable, and there are resources available for this.
7. The screening can be repeated periodically and permanently and not only once.

For Type 1 DM, it appears that the above conditions are not fulfilled, since the natural history of the disease is not well understood (see Chapter 2, 'Pathophysiology of Type 1 Diabetes'), and it is unproven that any intervention during the pre-clinical stage of the disease is effective.

For Type 2 DM, conditions 1–4 are valid (see Chapter 3, 'Pathophysiology of Type 2 Diabetes'). The disease constitutes a very significant health problem for the population and its natural history is to a great extent comprehended, with the majority of Type 2 diabetics passing from the stage of normal glucose tolerance to the stage of impaired glucose tolerance (fasting or post-challenge), and afterwards to the stage of clinical diabetes. The examinations for the diagnosis of the disease in this pre-clinical stage of pre-diabetes (the examination of fasting plasma glucose for the diagnosis of Impaired Fasting Glucose [IFG] and the measurement of plasma glucose two hours after an oral glucose tolerance test with 75 g of glucose for the diagnosis of impaired glucose tolerance [IGT]) are simple, easy and reliable. Conditions 5–7, however, are not completely valid, since there are no randomized clinical studies yet that prove the effectiveness of screening in the reduction of morbidity and mortality of DM (although there are studies that provide powerful evidence for the reduction of the incidence of DM with various interventions, as will be discussed below). Also, there are disagreements with regard to the relation of cost-effectiveness of screening as well as whether these screening procedures can be permanently repeated and how often.

What are the risk factors for the development of DM?

Type 1 DM is due, in the majority of cases, to an autoimmune destruction of the insulin producing β-cells of the pancreatic islets (Type 1A DM) in contrast to the extremely infrequent non-autoimmune type (Type 1B DM). The process of autoimmune destruction presents in genetically predisposed individuals, is probably triggered by (presently unknown) environmental factors (viruses? antigens of diet?) and proceeds over a period of months to years. The genetic indices are present from birth and the immunologic ones (pancreatic auto-antibodies) present after the beginning of the autoimmune process. The metabolic indices can be detected with sensitive tests when enough destruction of the β-cell has occurred, but before the appearance of symptomatic hyperglycaemia (reduction of the first phase of insulin secretion during the intravenous glucose tolerance test). Thus, high-risk groups for the development of Type 1 DM are individuals with a certain genetic predisposition (certain combinations of genes of the Human Leukocytes Antigens [HLAs: DR3 and DR4]) and with existence of antibodies against certain pancreatic proteins (see also Chapter 2). The risk is increased in individuals with first degree relatives suffering from Type 1 DM, and is bigger when the sick relative is the father (diabetes risk 6 percent) or a sibling (risk 5 percent), rather than the mother (risk 2 percent), for unknown reasons (it is worth noting that the risk of Type 1 DM in the general population, when there are no first degree relatives who are Type 1 diabetics, is roughly 0.4 percent). The combination of family history of Type 1 DM with the presence of aggravating genes of the HLA system increases the risk much more (up to 25–50 percent).

For Type 2 DM, epidemiologic studies as well as data from its pathophysiology and natural history, have shown various factors that are related to an increased frequency of its appearance. These factors are age > 45 years, obesity (BMI $> 25\,\text{kg/m}^2$), family history of DM, a sedentary life-style, certain racial groups and nationalities (African Americans or Hispanics, Native Americans, Pacific Islanders, etc.), history of gestational DM or birth of a child $> 4\,\text{kg}$ (8.8 lb), history of hypertension or dyslipidaemia and the polycystic ovary syndrome. Also, a low birth weight and cigarette smoking have been associated epidemiologically with the risk of developing DM. However, the most powerful association has been found with the presence of Impaired Fasting Glucose (IFG) and/or Impaired Glucose Tolerance (IGT). IFG is defined as the presence of fasting plasma glucose levels between 110–125 mg/dl [6.1–6.9 mmol/L] for Europe 100–125 mg/dl [5.6–6.9 mmol/L] for America), and IGT is the presence of plasma glucose levels between 140–200 mg/dl (7.8–11.1 mmol/L) two hours after the intake of 75 g glucose by mouth during an oral glucose tolerance test. The individuals with IFG or IGT (conditions that only overlap in 20–25 percent of cases) have a probability of around 30 percent of developing clinically evident DM in the next five years. The presence of both of these conditions raises the risk to around 50 percent. Thus, these two conditions are rightly considered as a pre-clinical stage of DM and are called 'pre-diabetes'. The presence of IGT is usually also associated with other components of the metabolic syndrome (hypertension, dyslipidaemia, obesity) and with increased cardiovascular risk.

The studies of DM prevention have consequently been mainly focused on these high-risk groups.

What are the interventional methods for the prevention of DM?

In Type 1 DM, all interventions that have been tried so far for the prevention of the disease in high-risk individuals have unfortunately failed. Since the disease is in the majority of cases of autoimmune aetiology, immunomodulating factors were occasionally tried (azathioprine, cyclosporine, nicotinamide), as well as low doses of insulin, aiming at the possible delay of pancreatic function impairment, without success. The avoidance of cow-milk from the diet of the newborn and the additional administration of vitamin D, which were considered to be related with the pathogenesis of this type of DM, did not meet with any success either. As a consequence, research into the prevention of Type 1 DM is at the moment at a dead end, except for small continuing efforts directed towards special immunotherapeutic targeting of the onset of the autoimmune process in the pancreas.

For Type 2 DM, in which the main pathophysiologic characteristics are insulin resistance and impaired insulin secretion from the pancreas, its, prevention studies have been focused on the reduction of insulin resistance or the increase of the secretory capacity in high-risk persons. Thus, since changes in lifestyle (weight loss with diet and exercise) and, various medicines decrease insulin resistance, the interventional studies of DM prevention have been focused in this direction, mainly in obese and/or individuals with IGT. During the last five years, two well planned studies of lifestyle modification in Finland and USA proved that weight loss (5–7 percent of the initial weight) with diet and exercise (up to 150 min weekly) decreased the risk of DM development in obese persons with IGT by 58 percent. The use of various medicines to reduce insulin resistance also had beneficial effects as seen in various studies, but to a smaller degree than diet and exercise. Thus, metformin decreased the risk of DM development in individuals with IGT by 31 percent (mainly in young individuals [< 45 years old] with serious obesity [BMI > 35 kg/ m^2]), and acarbose by 25 percent. Troglitazone (a medicine of the thiazolidinedione category that has been now withdrawn from the market because of hepatotoxicity) decreased the risk by 56 percent in women with a previous history of gestational DM. Also orlistat, an anti-obesity medicine (it decreases the absorption of fat from the intestine) reduced the risk of DM development by 37 percent in obese individuals (21 percent of which had IGT) and by 45 percent when only those individuals with IGT were taken into consideration. Furthermore, two other medicines of the category of angiotensin converting enzyme (ACE) inhibitors (ramipril) and the category of angiotensin receptor blockers (ARBs) (losartan) were also found to decrease the risk of DM development mainly in studies of hypertensive individuals, with no completely satisfactory explanation for this. Presently, there are many ongoing studies of Type 2 DM prevention with pharmaceutical interventions (using medicines of the thiazolidinedione category, metformin, acarbose, meglitinides, ACE inhibitors, ARBs and insulin), the results of which are expected with great interest over the next few years.

What are the recommendations today for the prevention of DM?

For Type 1 DM, all interventional methods have up to now failed, and consequently trying to detect high-risk individuals (with genetic testing and testing for pancreatic auto-antibodies) is not even recommended, since no help can be offered to these people towards disease prevention. The knowledge of the risk for DM development will psychologically overload the individual and his or her family, without essential benefit as regards prevention of the disease in the future. The only advantage of knowing the risk would be useful information to the individual on the likely symptoms of the first appearance of DM (possible diabetic ketoacidosis), which can in a minority of cases be very harmful, or even lethal (in 1 per 200 children of the general population who present with Type 1 DM for the first time).

For Type 2 DM, the existing data show that it is possible to prevent or at least delay its development in high-risk individuals. Consequently, it is recommended to try and find individuals of high-risk and intervene to reduce this risk. As mentioned earlier, the best correlation of the risk for DM development has been found for individuals with glucose intolerance (IFG or IGT) and consequently it is recommended to find such individuals in the general population by measuring fasting plasma glucose and performing an oral glucose tolerance test. These tests should be focused on individuals with increased DM risk, such as those who are > 45 years of age, especially with obesity (BMI $> 25 \text{ kg/m}^2$) or even in younger individuals with BMI $> 25 \text{ kg/m}^2$ who have additional risk factors as follows: first degree relative with Type 2 DM; sedentary lifestyle; history of gestational DM or birth of a child with weight $> 4 \text{ kg}$ (8.8 lb); presence of hypertension or dyslipidaemia (HDL-cholesterol $< 35 \text{ mg/dl}$ [0.91 mmol/L] and/or triglycerides $> 250 \text{ mg/dl}$ [2.82 mmol/L]); polycystic ovary syndrome; history of angiopathy; or a previous examination that showed glucose intolerance (IFG or IGT). If the results are normal, it is recommended to repeat the screening tests every three years, because this time interval is considered insufficient for diabetic complications to develop in the event that DM does develop in the meantime. In the event of glucose intolerance, advice is recommended to change the lifestyle, aimed at the reduction of obesity and altering the sedentary life with diet and exercise. Screening for the possible development of DM is should be repeated every 1–2 years in these individuals (again with measurements of fasting plasma glucose or/and and oral glucose tolerance test). At the same time, screening and proper treatment of the other risk factors for athero-sclerosis are also recommended, such as hypertension, dyslipidaemia and smoking. Pharmaceutical treatment for the prevention of DM is not currently recommended for the individuals with IFG or IGT, since this is less effective than modification of the lifestyle (newer data from ongoing studies are expected).

An advantage of presymptomatic screening to detect the risk of developing DM by measuring a fasting plasma glucose level or by performing an oral glucose tolerance test is that screening will also detect a certain percentage of people who already have undiagnosed DM without knowing it. Furthermore, intervening and modifying the diet and exercise of pre-diabetic people also simultaneously helps to improve the other risk factors for heart disease (hypertension, dyslipidaemia, obesity). The big question is how much the high-risk individuals are able to change their lifestyle (losing weight with diet and exercise) and whether they can maintain these changes over a long period.

Can the prevention of DM decrease the morbidity and mortality associated with it?

This has not yet been proven in prevention studies. The only study that showed some evidence for such a reduction is the STOP-NIDDM study of acarbose use for the prevention of DM in individuals with IGT (Chiasson *et al.*, 2002), where the acarbose group had a reduction of the cardiovascular events by 49 percent compared to the placebo group. This matter, however, has not been completely clarified and ongoing studies with other medicines (e.g., thiazolidinediones, ACE inhibitors) are also examining it.

CASE STUDY 1

A mother of two children, one nine years old who has had Type 1 DM for three years and the other six years old with no health problems up to now, comes to

the Diabetes Clinic asking about the risk of her second child developing DM and what she can do to prevent it.

The existence of a first child with Type 1 DM, means that the second child has a higher risk than children of the general population of developing DM (around 5 percent compared to 0.4 percent for the general population). If this child also has aggravating genes (HLA DR3/DR4), the risk increases even more (50 percent) and if pancreatic auto-antibodies are already present, the probability of developing DM in the next five years increases even further (75 percent). What should be explained to the mother is that even if her child were found to have such a high risk, nothing can be done for the time being to reduce this risk. Consequently, it should be discussed with the mother (and perhaps with the child) how much they could bear the psychological weight of learning about the possible risk of the appearance of a disease that cannot currently be prevented (in the event that the results of screening turn out negative, of course, the agony would be reduced). Moreover, knowledge that the appearance of the disease is probably imminent (if the results indicate this), does present the opportunity for the family and the child to prepare for its management when DM occurs for the first time (a small percentage of newly developing cases of Type 1 DM with ketoacidosis may even have a fatal result, which could be avoided). In consequence, the answer to the question is that every case should be individualized, after discussion with, and informing the affected individuals.

CASE STUDY 2

A 45 year old man, obese (BMI 31 kg/m², with a history of hypertension and dyslipidaemia for six years, and family history of Type 2 DM on both his parents' side, presents to the Diabetes Clinic because at a routine blood examination a fasting blood glucose level of 118 mg/dl (6.6 mmol/L) was found (the lab technician told him to 'take a look at it'). He denies any symptoms of polyuria, polydipsia or polyphagia and his body weight has been stable for several months. His question is, how much risk is he at now, or in the future, of having a problem with blood sugar, and if the risk is high, what can he do about it?

The blood glucose level of this person is increased and is within the limits defined as impaired fasting glucose (IFG: 110–126 mg/dl [6.1–7.0 mmol/L] for Europe, 100–126 mg/dl [5.6–7.0 mmol/L] for America), but not yet in the diabetic range. It is always recommended to repeat the measurement on a second day for confirmation. The presence of a family history of DM, and of obesity, hypertension and dyslipidaemia, constitute risk factors for the development of Type 2 DM on their own, but the presence of IFG constitutes the most powerful risk factor (this patient has a probability around 30 percent of developing clinically evident DM in the next five years). If at the same time our patient also has IGT (the two conditions IFG and IGT do not usually effect the same individuals, and overlap only in 20–25 percent of cases) the risk for DM development is even higher (50 percent in five years). Thus, even though the therapeutic approach will not change (recommendation for change of lifestyle, with weight loss through diet and exercise), it would be useful for this patient to perform a 2-hour oral glucose tolerance test with 75 grams of glucose (oGTT), in order to clarify the existence (or not) of IGT. It should also be mentioned here that it is not impossible for the glucose tolerance test to prove that the patient is already a diabetic (that is, have a blood sugar level two hours after the glucose challenge > 200 mg/dl [11.1 mmol/L]). In its initial stages, DM can have fasting blood glucose levels < 126 mg/dl [7.0 mmol/L) and be diagnosed only with the post-challenge blood glucose levels at the OGTT. In this case the therapeutic and diagnostic approach will probably need to change (that is, examinations for HbA_{1c}, examinations of the eyes, kidneys etc., and probably initiation of anti-diabetic medicines).

For this patient, the oral glucose tolerance test (oGTT) showed fasting blood glucose levels of 105 mg/dl (5.8 mmol/L) and two hours after the glucose challenge 168 mg/dl (9.3 mmol/L). The patient came back even more alarmed.

The existence of both IFG and IGT is confirmed with the oGTT, but no evidence of DM. The risk, however, of future development of DM is very significant. This enormous risk should be explained to the patient, as well as the fact that he is already at risk of developing cardiovascular complications even before the clinical manifestation of DM, and that he should take drastic measures for their prevention. He should try to lose weight (by 5–10 percent) with diet and exercise (at least 150 min every week) and optimize the therapeutic management of hypertension and dyslipidaemia. Collaboration with a dietitian will be very useful. He should also be informed about the first symptoms of DM manifestation and of cardiovascular events (myocardial or cerebral ischaemia), so that he visits his doctor in time if these events occur. Repeat of blood tests (for fasting blood glucose and oGTT) should be performed every 1–2 years, provided that he remains asymptomatic. The use of medicines to prevent

DM is not yet recommended. However, if the patient is unable to change his lifestyle and achieve and maintain a weight loss with diet and exercise (and pending the results of more studies in this area), the use can be considered of pharmaceutical substances (metformin, acarbose) which have data showing they help in the prevention of DM (studies with the thiazolidinediones rosiglitazone and pioglitazone are still under development).

Further reading

American Diabetes Association (2004) Clinical Practice Recommendations. Prevention or delay of Type 2 diabetes. *Diabetes Care* **27** (Suppl 1): S47–S54.

Buchanan, T.A., Xiang, A.H., Peters, R.K., *et al.* (2002) Prevention of pancreatic beta-cell function and prevention of Type 2 diabetes by pharmacological treatment of insulin resistance in high risk Hispanic women. *Diabetes* **51**, 2796–803.

Chiasson, J-L., Josse, R.G., Gomis, R., *et al.* (2002) Acarbose for prevention of Type 2 diabetes mellitus: the STOP-NIDDM randomized trial. *Lancet* **359**, 2072–7.

Knowler, W.C., Barrett-Connor, E., Fowler, S., *et al.* (2002) (for the Diabetes Prevention Program Research Group) Reduction in the incidence of Type 2 diabetes with lifestyle intervention or metformin. *N Engl J Med* **346**, 393–403.

Seissler, J., Hatziagelaki, E., Scherbaum, W.A. (2001) Modern concepts for the prediction of Type 1 diabetes. *Exp Clin Endocrinol diabetes* **109** (Suppl 2): S304–S316.

Torgerson, J.S., Hauptman, J., Boldrin, M.N., Sjöström, L. (2004) XENical in the Prevention of Diabetes in Obese Subjects (XENDOS) Study: A randomized study of orlistat as an adjunct to lifestyle changes for the prevention of Type 2 diabetes in obese patients. *Diabetes Care* **27**, 155–61.

Tuomilehto, J., Lindstrom, J., Ericsson, J.G., Valle, T.T., Hamalainen, H., Ilanne-Parikka, P., Keinanen-Kiukaanniemi, S., Laasko, M., Louheranta, A., Rastas, M., Salminen, V., Uusitupa, M. (2001) (for the Finnish Diabetes Prevention Study Group) Prevention of Type 2 diabetes mellitus by changes in lifestyle among subjects with impaired glucose tolerance. *N Engl J Med* **344**, 1343–50.

Yusuf, S., Sleight, P., Pogue, J., Bosch, J., Davies, R., Dagenais, G. (2000) Effects of an angiotensin-onverting-enzyme inhibiter, ramipril, on cardiovascular events on high risk patients. The Heart Outcomes Prevention Evaluation Study Investigators. *N Engl J Med* **342**, 145–53.

Index

Diabetes in Clinical Practice: Questions and Answers from Case Studies.   Nicholas Katsilambros *et al.*
© 2006 John Wiley & Sons, Ltd.